a Lange medical book

Current Procedures: Pediatrics

Denise M. Goodman, MD, MSc

Associate Professor of Pediatrics
Northwestern University Feinberg School of Medicine
Division of Critical Care Medicine
Children's Memorial Hospital
Chicago, Illinois

Thomas P. Green, MD

Professor and Chairman
Department of Pediatrics
Northwestern University Feinberg School of Medicine
Division of Pulmonary Medicine
Children's Memorial Hospital
Chicago, Illinois

Sharon M. Unti, MD

Assistant Professor of Pediatrics
Northwestern University Feinberg School of Medicine
Pediatric Residency Program Director
Children's Memorial Hospital
Chicago, Illinois

Elizabeth C. Powell, MD, MPH

Associate Professor of Pediatrics
Northwestern University Feinberg School of Medicine
Division of Pediatric Emergency Medicine
Children's Memorial Hospital
Chicago, Illinois

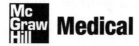 **Medical**

New York   Chicago   San Francisco   Lisbon   London   Madrid
Mexico City   Milan   New Delhi   San Juan   Seoul   Singapore   Sydney   Toronto

Current Procedures: Pediatrics

1 2 3 4 5 6 7 8 9 0 QPD/QPD 0 9 8 7

ISBN 13: 978-0-07-145908-2
ISBN 10: 0-07-145908-1
ISSN: 1933-7884

Notice

Medicine is an ever-changing science. As new research and clinical experience broaden our knowledge, changes in treatment and drug therapy are required. The authors and the publisher of this work have checked with sources believed to be reliable in their efforts to provide information that is complete and generally in accord with the standards accepted at the time of publication. However, in view of the possibility of human error or changes in medical sciences, neither the authors nor the publisher nor any other party who has been involved in the preparation or publication of this work warrants that the information contained herein is in every respect accurate or complete, and they disclaim all responsibility for any errors or omissions or for the results obtained from use of the information contained in this work. Readers are encouraged to confirm the information contained herein with other sources. For example and in particular, readers are advised to check the product information sheet included in the package of each drug they plan to administer to be certain that the information contained in this work is accurate and that changes have not been made in the recommended dose or in the contraindications for administration. This recommendation is of particular importance in connection with new or infrequently used drugs.

This book was set in Minion by Silverchair Science + Communications, Inc.
The editors were Anne Sydor, Harriet Lebowitz, and Penny Linskey.
The production supervisor was Catherine H. Saggese.
The design and illustration manager was Charissa Baker.
Project management was provided by Silverchair Science + Communications, Inc.
The designer was Alan Barnett Design.
The illustrator was Susan Gilbert, CMI.
The cover designer was Mary McKeon.
Cover photo: © Janine Wiedel Photolibrary/Alamy.
The index was prepared by Patricia Perrier.
The printer was Quebecor World Dubuque.

This book is printed on acid-free paper.

[CONTENTS]

SECTION 5: Genitourinary System

SECTION 6: Nervous System

SECTION 7: Skin

SECTION 8: Ears, Nose, Throat, and Eyes

SECTION 9: Musculoskeletal System

PART III SUBSPECIALTY PROCEDURES

[AUTHORS]

Lina AbuJamra, MD
Assistant Professor, Department of Pediatrics, Northwestern University Feinberg School of Medicine; Division of Pediatric Emergency Medicine, Children's Memorial Hospital, Chicago, Illinois

Mark Adler, MD
Assistant Professor, Department of Pediatrics, Northwestern University Feinberg School of Medicine; Division of Pediatric Emergency Medicine, Children's Memorial Hospital, Chicago, Illinois

Frederique Bailliard, MD
Fellow, Division of Cardiology, Children's Memorial Hospital; Department of Pediatrics, Northwestern University Feinberg School of Medicine, Chicago, Illinois

Marybeth Browne, MD
Chief Surgery Resident, Department of Surgery, Northwestern University Feinberg School of Medicine; Department of Surgery, Northwestern Memorial Hospital, Chicago, Illinois

Sarah Chamlin, MD
Assistant Professor, Department of Pediatrics and Department of Dermatology, Northwestern University Feinberg School of Medicine; Division of Dermatology, Children's Memorial Hospital, Chicago, Illinois

Anthony Chin, MD
Pediatric Surgery Fellow, Department of Surgery, Northwestern University Feinberg School of Medicine; Division of Pediatric Surgery, Children's Memorial Hospital, Chicago, Illinois

Stephen Crotty, MD
Pediatric Emergency Medicine Fellow, Department of Pediatrics, Northwestern University Feinberg School of Medicine; Division of Pediatric Emergency Medicine, Children's Memorial Hospital, Chicago, Illinois

Barbara J. Deal, MD
M. E. Wodika Professor of Pediatrics, Northwestern University Feinberg School of Medicine; Director of Electrophysiology Services, Division of Cardiology, Children's Memorial Hospital, Chicago, Illinois

Renee Dietz, RN
Ambulatory Patient Care Services, Post Anesthesia Care Unit, Children's Memorial Hospital, Chicago, Illinois

Kimberley Dilley, MD, MPH
Assistant Professor, Department of Pediatrics, Northwestern University Feinberg School of Medicine; Division of Hematology/Oncology/Transplant, Children's Memorial Hospital, Chicago, Illinois

Bradley Dunlap, MD
Resident, Department of Orthopedic Surgery, Northwestern University Feinberg School of Medicine; Division of Orthopedic Surgery, Children's Memorial Hospital, Chicago, Illinois

Wayne H. Franklin, MD, MPH
Associate Professor, Department of Pediatrics, Northwestern University Feinberg School of Medicine; Division of Cardiology, Children's Memorial Hospital, Chicago, Illinois

Joshua Goldstein, MD
Assistant Professor, Department of Pediatrics, Northwestern University Feinberg School of Medicine; Division of Neurology, Children's Memorial Hospital, Chicago, Illinois

Ty Hasselman, MD
Cardiology Fellow, Department of Pediatrics, Northwestern University Feinberg School of Medicine; Division of Cardiology, Children's Memorial Hospital, Chicago, Illinois

Lauren Holinger, MD
Professor, Department of Otolaryngology and Neck Surgery, Northwestern University Feinberg School of Medicine; Paul H. Holinger, MD Professor, Head, Division of Otolaryngology, Children's Memorial Hospital, Chicago, Illinois

Russ Horowitz, MD
Instructor, Department of Pediatrics, Northwestern University Feinberg School of Medicine; Division of Pediatric Emergency Medicine, Children's Memorial Hospital, Chicago, Illinois

Yiannis L. Katsogridakis, MD, MPH
Instructor, Department of Pediatrics, Northwestern University Feinberg School of Medicine; Division of Pediatric Emergency Medicine, Children's Memorial Hospital, Chicago, Illinois

Rae-Ellen W. Kavey, MD
Professor, Department of Pediatrics, Northwestern University Feinberg School of Medicine; Division of Cardiology, Children's Memorial Hospital, Chicago, Illinois

Janine Y. Khan, MD
Assistant Professor, Department of Pediatrics, Northwestern University Feinberg School of Medicine; Division of Neonatology, Children's Memorial Hospital, Chicago, Illinois

Sue Kim, MD
Otolaryngology Fellow, Department of Surgery, Northwestern University Feinberg School of Medicine; Division of Otolaryngology, Children's Memorial Hospital, Chicago, Illinois

Jerome C. Lane, MD
Assistant Professor, Department of Pediatrics, Northwestern University Feinberg School of Medicine; Division of Kidney Diseases; Children's Memorial Hospital, Chicago, Illinois

B U.K. Li, MD
Adjunct Professor, Department of Pediatrics, Northwestern University Feinberg School of Medicine, Chicago, Illinois; Program Director, Functional Gastroenterology Disorders, Children's Hospital of Wisconsin, Milwaukee, Wisconsin

Robert I. Liem, MD
Assistant Professor, Department of Pediatrics, Northwestern University Feinberg School of Medicine; Division of Hematology, Oncology and Stem Cell Transplant, Children's Memorial Hospital, Chicago, Illinois

Kelly Michelson, MD
Assistant Professor, Department of Pediatrics, Northwestern University Feinberg School of Medicine; Division of Critical Care Medicine, Children's Memorial Hospital, Chicago, Illinois

Zehava Noah, MD
Associate Professor, Department of Pediatrics, Northwestern University Feinberg School of Medicine; Attending Physician, Division of Critical Care Medicine, Children's Memorial Hospital, Chicago, Illinois

Stephen Pophal, MD
Assistant Professor of Pediatrics, Northwestern University Feinberg School of Medicine; Division of Cardiology, Children's Memorial Hospital, Chicago, Illinois

Adrienne Prestridge, MD
Instructor, Department of Pediatrics, Northwestern University Feinberg School of Medicine; Division of Pulmonary Medicine, Children's Memorial Hospital, Chicago, Illinois

Marleta Reynolds, MD
Professor, Department of Surgery, Northwestern University Feinberg School of Medicine; Division of Pediatric Surgery, Children's Memorial Hospital, Chicago, Illinois

Ranna A. Rozenfeld, MD
Associate Professor, Department of Pediatrics, Northwestern University Feinberg School of Medicine; Division of Critical Care Medicine, Children's Memorial Hospital, Chicago, Illinois

Alexandra Ryan, MD
General Academic Pediatric Fellow, Department of Pediatrics, Northwestern University Feinberg School of Medicine; Division of General Academic Pediatrics, Children's Memorial Hospital, Chicago, Illinois

Sandra M. Sanguino, MD, MPH
Assistant Professor, Department of Pediatrics, Northwestern University Feinberg School of Medicine; Division of General Academic Pediatrics, Children's Memorial Hospital, Chicago, Illinois

John F. Sarwark, MD
Professor, Department of Orthopedic Surgery, Northwestern University Feinberg School of Medicine; Division of Orthopedic Surgery, Children's Memorial Hospital, Chicago, Illinois

Robin H. Steinhorn, MD
Professor, Department of Pediatrics, Northwestern University Feinberg School of Medicine; Division of Neonatology, Children's Memorial Hospital, Chicago, Illinois

Boris Sudel, MD
Fellow, Department of Pediatrics, Northwestern University Feinberg School of Medicine, Division of Gastroenterology, Hepatology and Nutrition, Children's Memorial Hospital, Chicago, Illinois

Jennifer Trainor, MD
Assistant Professor, Department of Pediatrics, Northwestern University Feinberg School of Medicine; Division of Pediatric Emergency Medicine, Children's Memorial Hospital, Chicago, Illinois

Sabrina Tsao, MD
Program Director, Functional Gastroenterology Disorders, Children's Hospital of Wisconsin, Milwaukee, Wisconsin

Sharon M. Unti, MD
Assistant Professor of Pediatrics, Northwestern University Feinberg School of Medicine; Pediatric Residency Program Director, Children's Memorial Hospital, Chicago, Illinois

Thomas J. Valvano, MD
Assistant Professor, Department of Pediatrics, Medical College of Wisconsin; Attending Physician, Children's Hospital of Wisconsin, Milwaukee, Wisconsin

Kendra M. Ward, MD
Assistant Professor, Department of Pediatrics, Northwestern University Feinberg School of Medicine; Division of Cardiology, Children's Memorial Hospital, Chicago, Illinois

David Wax, MD
Instructor, Department of Pediatrics, Northwestern University Feinberg School of Medicine; Division of Cardiology, Children's Memorial Hospital, Chicago, Illinois

Luciana T. Young, MD
Associate Professor, Department of Pediatrics, Northwestern University Feinberg School of Medicine; Division of Cardiology, Children's Memorial Hospital, Chicago, Illinois

PREFACE

The scope of practice for a pediatrician is broad, and continues to expand. The clinician must understand physiology, disease processes, and interventions in patients ranging in age from neonates to young adults. Moreover, as a result of medical progress, children with chronic and complicated illnesses are seen in general pediatrics settings for their regular childhood care. The evolving knowledge base is matched by a growing repertoire of technical procedures for delivering healthcare. General pediatricians must be proficient in many of these and conversant in many others to properly counsel the families for whom they provide care.

The intent of *Current Procedures: Pediatrics* is to provide a comprehensive review of technical medical procedures applicable to pediatric patients. The content of the book particularly targets the general pediatrician but is also appropriate for other practitioners taking care of children, as well as medical students and residents. The material focuses exclusively on procedures and is not meant to be a comprehensive textbook of pediatric medicine. Rather, the aim is to provide a clinically useful, accessible guide with step-by-step instructions in an easy-to-use format.

The text is divided into three parts; the first covers the ABCs: **a**irway stabilization, assisted **b**reathing, and **c**irculatory support and vascular access. The second part contains the rest of the alphabet—procedures organized by organ system. It encompasses those most likely to be used by general pediatricians. Each chapter focuses on a specific procedure, accompanied by instructive illustrations and presented in a standard format featuring:

- Indications
- Contraindications
- Equipment needed
- Risks
- Pearls and tips
- Patient preparation and positioning
- Review of anatomy
- Step-by-step procedure instructions
- Monitoring
- Complications
- Caveats
- Follow-up

The innovative third part addresses a need unmet in other similar texts. In recognition of the fact that generalists will often be the clinicians suggesting subspecialty evaluation and providing initial counseling to families, this text offers an overview of a number of subspecialty procedures. The generalist, while not actually performing the procedure, may need information (a general overview, reasons for referral, indications, risks, and benefits) to demystify the patient's and family's encounter with the subspecialist. This part is organized by organ system and comprises a wide range of procedures, such as echocardiography, endoscopy, and electroencephalography. Finally, the appendix lists recommended equipment for a general pediatrics office.

The chapter authors are recognized authorities in their field and have drawn on their experience, as well as the published literature, to offer complete, lucid discussions of each procedure. We hope this text will become a well-thumbed reference kept in the most easily reached section of the bookshelf. We welcome the comments of our readers in improving and revising future editions.

Denise M. Goodman, MD, MSc
Thomas P. Green, MD
Sharon M. Unti, MD
Elizabeth C. Powell, MD, MPH

[PART I]

THE ABCs: AIRWAY, BREATHING, CIRCULATORY SUPPORT

CHAPTER 1

Bag-Mask Ventilation

Ranna A. Rozenfeld, MD

INDICATIONS

- To ventilate and oxygenate a patient.
- A ventilation face mask may be used with an oropharyngeal or nasopharyngeal airway during spontaneous, assisted, or controlled ventilation.

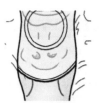
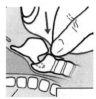

CONTRAINDICATIONS

Relative

- In patients with full stomach, cricoid pressure must be maintained to avoid vomiting and aspiration.

EQUIPMENT

- Ventilation bags (manual resuscitator) come in 2 types: self-inflating bag and flow-inflating ("anesthesia") bag.
- Ventilation bags used for resuscitation should be self-inflating.
- Ventilation bags come in different sizes: infant, child, and adult.
- Face masks come in many sizes.
- A ventilation mask consists of a rubber or plastic body, a standard connecting port, and a rim or face seal.
- Supplemental oxygen can be attached to ventilation bags to provide oxygen to the patient.

RISKS

- Vomiting and aspiration.

PEARLS AND TIPS

- Bag-mask ventilation gives the clinician time to prepare for more definitive airway management.
- Good technique involves preserving good mask-face seal, inflating the chest with minimal required pressure, and maintaining the optimal patency of the upper airway through manipulation of the mandible and cervical spine.

- The clinician should only use the force and tidal volume necessary to cause the chest to rise visibly.
- The mask should extend from the bridge of the nose to the cleft of the chin, enveloping the nose and mouth but avoiding compression of the eyes.
- The mask should provide an airtight seal.
- The goal of ventilation with a bag and mask should be to approximate normal ventilation.

PATIENT PREPARATION

- Sedation may be required before beginning.

PATIENT POSITIONING

- A neutral "sniffing" position without hyperextension of the neck is usually appropriate for infants and toddlers.
- Avoid extreme hyperextension in infants because it may produce airway obstruction.
- In patients with head or neck injuries, the neck must be maintained in a neutral position.

ANATOMY REVIEW

- The upper airway consists of the oropharynx, the nasopharynx, and supraglottic structures.
- The cricoid cartilage is the first tracheal ring, located by palpating the prominent horizontal band inferior to the thyroid cartilage and cricothyroid membrane.
- Cricoid pressure occludes the proximal esophagus by displacing the cricoid cartilage posteriorly. The esophagus is compressed between the rigid cricoid ring and the cervical spine.

PROCEDURE

Sequence
- Open the airway via chin lift/jaw thrust maneuver.
- Seal the mask to the face.
- Deliver a tidal volume that makes the chest rise.

E-C Clamp Technique
- Tilt the head back and place a towel beneath the head.
- If head or neck injury is suspected, open the airway with the jaw thrust technique without tilting the head.
  - If a second person is present, have that person immobilize the spine.
- Apply the mask to the face.
  - Lift the jaw using the third, fourth, and fifth fingers from the left hand under the angle of the mandible; this forms the "E" (Figure 1–1).

- The thumb and forefinger form a "C" shape to tightly seal the mask onto the face while the remaining fingers of the same hand form an "E" shape to lift the jaw, pulling the face toward the mask.

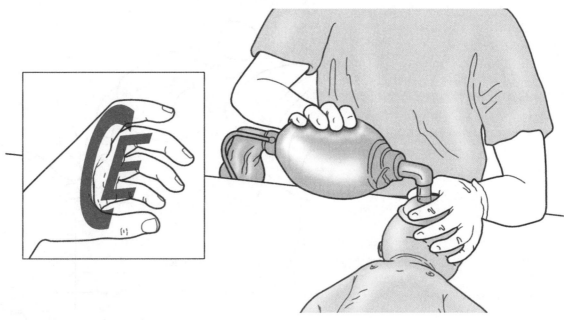

Figure 1–1. *E-C clamp technique.*

- When lifting the jaw, the tongue is also lifted away from the posterior pharynx.
  - Do not put pressure on the soft tissues under the jaw because this may compress the airway.
- Place the thumb and forefinger of the left hand in a "C" shape over the mask and exert downward pressure (see Figure 1–1).
  - Create a tight seal between the mask and the patient's face using the left hand and lifting the jaw.
  - Compress the ventilation bag with the right hand.
  - Be sure the chest rises visibly with each breath.
- If 2 people are present, then 1 person can hold the mask to the face while the other person ventilates with the bag.
  - One person uses both hands to open the airway and maintain a tight mask-to-face seal (Figure 1–2).
  - The second person compresses the ventilation bag.
- If 2 or 3 people are present, someone can apply pressure to the cricoid cartilage (termed "Sellick maneuver") to limit gastric distention in unconscious patients (Figure 1–3).
  - The Sellick maneuver may also prevent regurgitation and aspiration of gastric contents.
  - Avoid excessive cricoid pressure because it may produce tracheal compression and obstruction or distortion of the upper airway anatomy.
- To relieve gastric distention, a nasogastric tube can be placed (if not contraindicated).

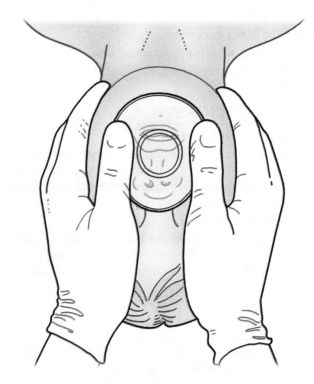

Figure 1–2. *Two-handed mask technique.*

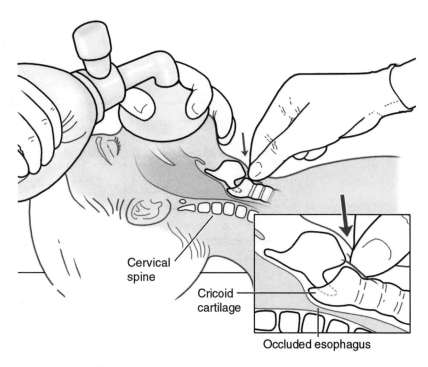

Figure 1–3. *Sellick maneuver.*

MONITORING

- Use pulse oximetry to measure oxygen saturation levels continuously.
- Measure heart rate continuously.
- Check blood pressure using a noninvasive device.
- Ensure the chest rises visibly.

COMPLICATIONS

- Reduction in cardiac output.
  - Excessive ventilation volume and airway pressure may lower cardiac output by raising intrathoracic pressure and distending alveoli, increasing afterload of the right heart, and decreasing venous return.
- Vomiting and aspiration.
- Air trapping, barotrauma, air leak, and reduced cardiac output can be caused by excessive tidal volume and rate in patients with small airway obstruction (eg, asthma and bronchiolitis).

CAVEATS

- It is important to coordinate bag-mask ventilation with the patient's spontaneous breaths in a patient who is spontaneously breathing. Dyssynchrony can predispose patients to barotrauma and air leak.
- While performing bag-mask ventilation, it is important for someone with more advanced airway skills to be preparing for intubation, or for someone to be arranging for the patient's transport to a facility where definitive airway management can be performed.
- No muscle relaxant should be given unless a person trained in advanced airway skills is present.

REFERENCES

Hazinski MF et al, eds. *PALS Provider Manual.* Dallas, Texas: American Heart Association; 2002:53–55, 92–98.

Holinger LD, Lusk RP, Green CG, eds. *Pediatric Laryngology and Bronchoesophagology.* Philadelphia: Lippincott-Raven Publishers; 1997:19–25, 117–133.

Mondolfi AA, Grenier BM, Thompson JE, Bachur RG. Comparison of self-inflating bags with anesthesia bags for bag-mask ventilation in the pediatric emergency department. *Pediatr Emerg Care.* 1997;13:312–316.

Sullivan KJ, Kissoon N. Securing the child's airway in the emergency department. *Pediatr Emerg Care.* 2002;18:108–121.

CHAPTER 2

Placement of Oropharyngeal Airway

Ranna A. Rozenfeld, MD

INDICATIONS

- Oropharyngeal airways provide a conduit for airflow through the mouth to the pharynx.
- Oropharyngeal airways prevent mandibular tissue from obstructing the posterior pharynx.
- Oropharyngeal airways may be used in the unconscious infant or child if procedures (ie, head tilt-chin lift or jaw thrust) to open the airway fail to provide and maintain a clear, unobstructed airway.

CONTRAINDICATIONS

Absolute

- Avoid inserting an oropharyngeal airway in conscious or semiconscious patients because it may stimulate gagging and vomiting.

EQUIPMENT

- Oropharyngeal airways come in various sizes ranging from 4 cm to 10 cm.
- Oropharyngeal airways consist of a flange, a short bite-block segment, and a curved body usually made of plastic and shaped to provide an air channel and suction conduit through the mouth.

PEARLS AND TIPS

- Oropharyngeal airways do not prevent aspiration.

PATIENT PREPARATION

- Measure the distance from the central incisors to the angle of the mandible to approximate the correct size oral airway.

PATIENT POSITIONING

- Head and airway must be positioned properly to maintain a patent airway even after insertion of an oropharyngeal airway.

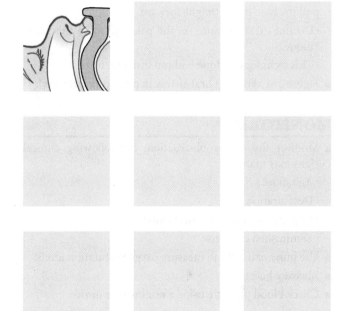

ANATOMY REVIEW

■ The upper airway consists of the oropharynx, the nasopharynx, and supraglottic structures.

PROCEDURE

■ The airway can be placed with a tongue blade holding the tongue on the floor of the mouth.

■ Depress the tongue and gently glide the airway with the concave side downward, following the curvature of the tongue.

■ The airway can also be introduced upside down and gently rotated to the proper position, using rotation to pull the base of the tongue forward.

  • Do not exert pressure on the palate if using this technique.

  • This technique is done without instrumentation.

■ Figure 2–1 shows an oral airway in place (sagittal view).

MONITORING

■ Monitor for airway obstruction; the following clinical signs may manifest:

  • Agitation.

  • Desaturation.

  • Impaired air exchange when auscultated.

  • Diminished chest rise.

■ Use pulse oximetry to measure oxygen saturation levels.

■ Measure heart rate.

■ Check blood pressure using a noninvasive device.

COMPLICATIONS

■ If the oropharyngeal airway is too large, it may obstruct the larynx, make a tight mask fit difficult, and traumatize laryngeal structures.

■ If the oropharyngeal airway is too small or is inserted improperly, it pushes the tongue posteriorly, obstructing the airway.

■ If the oral airway is placed in the awake patient, it may induce vomiting, aspiration, and laryngospasm.

■ If the airway is too long, it may induce vomiting and aspiration.

CAVEAT

■ The oropharyngeal airway may not be sufficient to relieve upper airway obstruction, and the patient may subsequently require intubation.

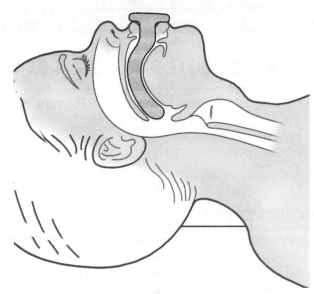

Figure 2–1. *Sagittal view of oral airway in place.*

REFERENCES

Hazinski MF et al, eds. *PALS Provider Manual.* Dallas, Texas: American Heart Association; 2002:90–91.

Holinger LD, Lusk RP, Green CG, eds. *Pediatric Laryngology and Bronchoesophagology.* Philadelphia: Lippincott-Raven Publishers; 1997:117–133.

Kharasch M, Graff J. Emergency management of the airway. *Crit Care Clin.* 1995;11:53–66.

Tong JL, Smith JE. Cardiovascular changes following insertion of oropharyngeal and nasopharyngeal airways. *Br J Anaesth.* 2004;93:339–342.

CHAPTER 3

Placement of Nasopharyngeal Airway

Ranna A. Rozenfeld, MD

INDICATIONS

- Nasopharyngeal airways provide a conduit for airflow between the nares and the pharynx.
- Nasopharyngeal airways prevent mandibular tissue from obstructing the posterior pharynx.
- Nasopharyngeal airways may be used in conscious patients (unlike oropharyngeal airways).
- Nasopharyngeal airways may be used in children with impaired consciousness or in neurologically impaired patients with poor pharyngeal tone leading to upper airway obstruction.
- Nasopharyngeal airways can be used to suction secretions.

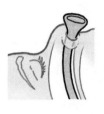

CONTRAINDICATIONS

Absolute

- Nasal airway occlusions.
- Nasal fractures.
- Coagulopathy (because of the risk of epistaxis).
- Cerebrospinal fluid leak.
- Basilar skull fracture.
- Adenoidal hypertrophy.

EQUIPMENT

- A nasopharyngeal airway is a soft rubber or plastic tube.
- Nasopharyngeal airways come in various sizes ranging from 12F to 36F.
- A shortened tracheal tube may be used as a nasopharyngeal airway.
- Lubrication jelly.

RISKS

- Nasal bleeding.

■ When using a shortened tracheal tube instead of a soft nasopharyngeal airway, injury to the soft tissues of the nasal passages may occur because of the rigid stiff plastic.

PEARLS AND TIPS

■ Nasopharyngeal airways do not prevent aspiration.

PATIENT PREPARATION

■ Measure the distance from the nares to the tragus of the ear to approximate the appropriate size and length of tube.

PATIENT POSITIONING

■ Head and airway must be positioned properly to maintain a patent airway even after insertion of a nasopharyngeal airway.

ANATOMY REVIEW

■ The upper airway consists of the oropharynx, the nasopharynx, and supraglottic structures.

PROCEDURE

■ The tube is lubricated and inserted into the nostril and positioned into the posterior pharynx.
■ Advance the tube gently, following the natural curvature of the nasal passage to direct the tube in a posterior inferior position.
■ After measuring as above, use the largest diameter tube that can fit into the nose without causing blanching of the nares.
■ If passage does not occur easily, attempt the other nostril because patients may have different size nasal passages.
■ Figure 3–1 shows a nasopharyngeal airway in place (sagittal view).

MONITORING

■ Because the nasopharyngeal airway has a small internal diameter, it can be obstructed with mucus, blood, vomit, or the soft tissues of the pharynx.
■ When necessary, suction the airway frequently to ensure patency.
■ Use pulse oximetry to measure oxygen saturation levels.
■ Measure heart rate.
■ Check blood pressure using a noninvasive device.

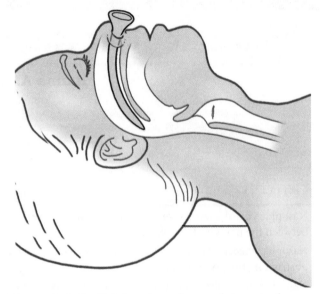

Figure 3–1. *Sagittal view of nasopharyngeal airway in place.*

COMPLICATIONS

- If the nasopharyngeal airway is too long, it may cause bradycardia through vagal stimulation or it may injure the epiglottis or vocal cords.
- Physical irritation of the larynx or lower pharynx may stimulate coughing, vomiting, or laryngospasm (if the tube is too long).
- Nasopharyngeal airways can cause a pressor response with increased blood pressure.
- Failure of insertion.
- Epistaxis (due to mucosal tears or avulsion of turbinates).
- Submucosal tunneling and pressure sores.
- Perforation of cartilage into the sinuses.
- Stimulation of nasal secretions with obstruction of the tube.
- Prolonged placement of a tight fitting tube may lead to nasal necrosis.

CAVEAT

- The nasopharyngeal airway may not be sufficient to relieve upper airway obstruction, and the patient may subsequently require intubation.

REFERENCES

Hazinski MF et al, eds. *PALS Provider Manual.* Dallas, Texas: American Heart Association; 2002:91–92.

Holinger LD, Lusk RP, Green CG, eds. *Pediatric Laryngology and Bronchoesophagology.* Philadelphia: Lippincott-Raven Publishers; 1997:117–133.

Kharasch M, Graff J. Emergency management of the airway. *Crit Care Clin.* 1995;11:53–66.

Tong JL, Smith JE. Cardiovascular changes following insertion of oropharyngeal and nasopharyngeal airways. *Br J Anaesth.* 2004;93:339–342.

CHAPTER 4

Placement of Endotracheal Tube

Ranna A. Rozenfeld, MD

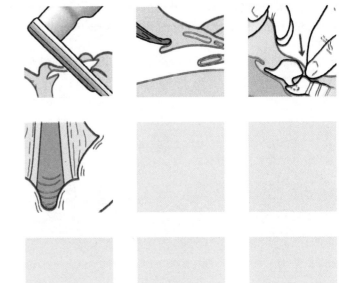

INDICATIONS

Respiratory

- Apnea.
- Acute respiratory failure (PaO_2 < 50 mm Hg in patient with fraction of inspired oxygen [FIO_2] > 0.5 and $PaCO_2$ > 55 mm Hg).
- Need to control oxygen delivery (eg, institution of positive end-expiratory pressure [PEEP], accurate delivery of FIO_2 > 0.5).
- Need to control ventilation (eg, to decrease work of breathing, to control $PaCO_2$, to provide muscle relaxation).

Neurologic

- Inadequate chest wall function (eg, in patient with Guillain-Barré syndrome, poliomyelitis).
- Absence of protective airway reflexes (eg, cough, gag).
- Glasgow Coma Score ≤ 8.

Airway

- Upper airway obstruction.
- Infectious processes (eg, epiglottis, croup).
- Trauma to the airway.
- Burns (concern for airway edema).

CONTRAINDICATIONS

Absolute

- Nasotracheal intubation is contraindicated in patients with nasal fractures or basilar skull fractures.

EQUIPMENT

- Suction.
  - Should have a tonsil-tipped suction device or a large-bore suction catheter as well as a suction catheter of appropriate size that fits into the endotracheal tube.

- Oxygen.
- Resuscitation bags.
- Masks (appropriate sizes for ventilation).
- Laryngoscope (blade, handle, bulb, battery).
- Endotracheal tubes (appropriate sizes, cuffed, uncuffed).
- Forceps.
- Oropharyngeal airway.
- Tongue blade.
- Bite block.
- Tape (to secure tube).
- Stylet (appropriate sizes).
- CO_2 detector device.
- Syringe to inflate the endotracheal tube balloon on cuffed tubes.

RISKS

- Desaturation.
- Bradycardia.
- Inability to intubate.
- Tracheal tear or rupture.

PEARLS AND TIPS

- Table 4–1 lists the suggested sizes for endotracheal tubes.
- Uncuffed tubes are generally recommended in children younger than 8 years, except in cases of severe lung disease.
- Laryngoscopes.
  - Handle with battery and blade with light source. Adult and pediatric handles fit all blades, and differ only in handle diameter.
  - A straight blade provides greater displacement of the tongue into the floor of the mouth and visualization of a cephalad and anterior larynx (Figure 4–1A).
  - A curved blade may be used in the older child; the broader base and flange allow easier displacement of the tongue (Figure 4–1B).
- Table 4–2 lists the suggested sizes of blades.
- If a difficult intubation is anticipated due to altered supraglottic anatomy, absolutely no irreversible anesthetics or muscle relaxants should be administered.
  - Such patients should generally be intubated awake or in the operating room with halothane.
  - For difficult intubations, other techniques, such as fiberoptic intubation, may be used.

PATIENT PREPARATION

- Preoxygenate with 100% F_{IO_2}.
- In an older child, explain each step as it is done.

Table 4–1. Suggested endotracheal tube size.[a]

Age	Internal Diameter (mm)
Premature infant	2.5–3.0
Newborn	3.0
Newborn–6 months	3.5
6 months–12 months	3.5–4.0
12 months–2 years	4.0–4.5
3–4 years	4.5–5.0
5–6 years	5.0–5.5
7–8 years	5.5–6.0
9–10 years	6.0–6.5
11–12 years	6.5–7.0
13–14 years	7.0–7.5

[a]Useful formula: $\dfrac{16 + \text{age}}{4}$

PATIENT POSITIONING

- A neutral "sniffing" position without hyperextension of the neck is usually appropriate for infants and toddlers.
  - Avoid extreme hyperextension in infants because it may produce airway obstruction.
- It is sometimes helpful to place a towel under the patient's shoulders.
- In patients with head or neck injuries, the neck must be maintained in a neutral position.

ANATOMY REVIEW

- Following are the distinguishing features of the infant and child airway compared with adults:
  - The larynx is more cephalad.
  - The epiglottis is omega shaped.
  - In children younger than 8 years, the cricoid is the narrowest part of the airway.
  - The infant larynx is one-third the size of the adult larynx.
  - The vocal cords are short and concave.
  - Aligning the mouth, pharynx, and glottis to create a visual field is difficult.
  - The endotracheal tube size relates to the cricoid ring.
  - In children, the lower airways are smaller, have less supporting cartilage, and may easily obstruct.
  - A small reduction in diameter results in a large reduction in the cross-sectional area and therefore increased airway resistance.

PROCEDURE

Prior to Intubation

- Check the intubation equipment before beginning.
- Attach the blade to the handle and be sure that the bulb illuminates.
- Attach suction to a suction machine and be sure that suction is turned on.
- If using a stylet, insert stylet into endotracheal tube.
  - The tip of the stylet should be 1–2 cm proximal to the distal end of the endotracheal tube, ensuring that the stylet does not go through the Murphy eye.
- Prepare to monitor the patient's heart rate, oxygen saturation levels, and blood pressure.

Sequence

- Preoxygenate with 100% oxygen.
- Administer 0.01–0.02 mg/kg IV of atropine (minimum dose, 0.1 mg). Atropine may not be indicated in cases of significant tachycardia.

A

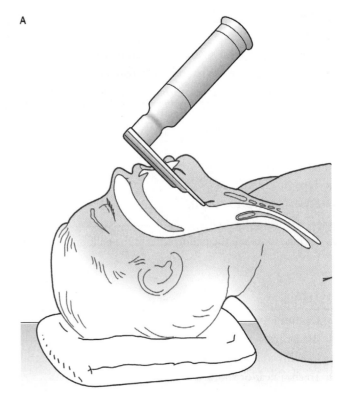

B

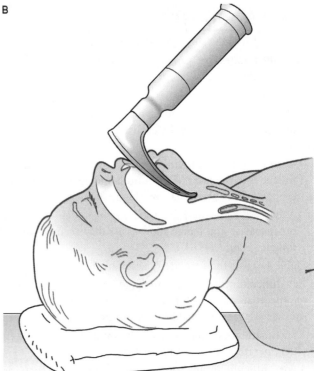

Figure 4–1. *Sagittal view of laryngoscopes.* **A:** *Straight blade.* **B:** *Curved blade.*

- Administer IV sedation (eg, fentanyl, morphine, midazolam, etomidate, thiopental, ketamine). (Dosages, indications, and contraindications are listed below.)
- Apply cricoid pressure (Figure 4–2).
- Perform bag-mask ventilation with 100% oxygen.
- Give an IV muscle relaxant.
- Open the mouth and insert the laryngoscope (Figure 4–3).
- Avoid positioning the blade against the teeth, gums, or lips.
- Visualize the glottic opening.
- Suction any secretions that may obscure visualization.
- Insert endotracheal tube; observe the tube to pass through the glottic opening.
- Remove the stylet while holding the tube securely in place, and ventilate the patient.
- Secure the tube to the face.

Confirm Correct Position of Tube

- Auscultation for symmetric breath sounds.
- Good chest excursion.
- Effective oxygenation.
- Disposable colorimetric capnometer (color should change from purple to yellow if patient has a perfusing rhythm) or capnograph.
- Obtain chest radiograph.
- Absence of breath sounds over the upper abdomen.
- If unilateral breath sounds are heard on the right, pull back the tube slowly while ventilating and listen for breath sounds on the left (probable intubation of right main bronchus).

Table 4–2. Suggested blade size.

Age	Laryngoscope Blade Size
Newborn–6 months	Miller 0-1, Wis Hipple 1
1 year	Miller 1, Wis Hipple 1.5
Child	Miller 2
8–12 years	Miller 2, Macintosh 2
Adolescent	Miller 3, Macintosh 3

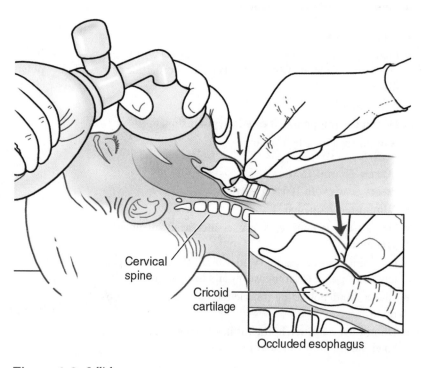

Cervical spine

Cricoid cartilage

Occluded esophagus

Figure 4–2. *Sellick maneuver.*

Special Circumstances

A. "FULL STOMACH"

■ When patients are at risk for aspiration, they should be intubated either awake (the patient may protect his or her own airway) or using a **rapid sequence induction.**

■ Rapid sequence induction involves the following steps:

· Preoxygenate with 100% oxygen.

· Administer 0.01–0.02 mg/kg IV of atropine (minimum dose, 0.1 mg). Atropine may not be indicated in cases of significant tachycardia.

· Apply cricoid pressure to prevent regurgitation.

· Apply oxygen without active mask ventilation ("apneic preoxygenation").

· Give a rapid-acting anesthetic (eg, thiopental, ketamine, midazolam). (Dosages, indications, and contraindications are listed below.)

· Administer a rapid-acting muscle relaxant (eg, succinylcholine, rocuronium). (Dosages, indications, and contraindications are listed below.)

B. ELEVATED INTRACRANIAL PRESSURE

■ Preoxygenate with 100% oxygen.

■ Thiopental provides relatively deep anesthesia associated with a rapid decline in cerebral metabolic oxygen requirement.

■ **Do not use ketamine; it causes increased intracranial pressure.**

■ Lidocaine, 1.0–1.5 mg/kg IV, effectively blocks the systemic and intracranial hypertensive response as well as the cough reflex.

■ Administer a muscle relaxant.

C. HYPOVOLEMIA

■ Preoxygenate with 100% oxygen; this is especially important in hypovolemia when patients have a borderline cardiac output.

■ Administer ketamine.

■ **Do not use thiopental; it causes hypotension.**

■ Administer a muscle relaxant.

D. OPEN GLOBE INJURY

■ Preoxygenate with 100% oxygen.

■ Administer thiopental.

■ **Do not use ketamine; it causes increased intraocular pressure.**

■ Lidocaine, 1.0–1.5 mg/kg IV, may blunt the ocular hypertensive response to laryngoscopy and intubation.

■ Give a nondepolarizing muscle relaxant, such as rocuronium.

■ **Do not use succinylcholine; it has been associated with an elevation of intraocular pressure.**

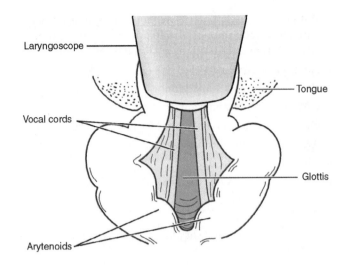

Figure 4–3. *Head-on view of airway as seen with laryngoscope.*

■ There is a risk of aspiration in patients who have eaten less than 4–8 hours before intubation, have undergone a traumatic event, have gastroesophageal reflux, have abdominal distention (eg, ileus, ascites, pregnancy), or are obese.

■ Intubation is a likely stimulus for further and potentially lethal intracranial hypertension.

■ Correction of hypovolemia should be begun immediately, along with establishing a secure airway.

■ If intraocular pressure increases, vitreous humor may leak from the open globe.

Medications

- Sedation and analgesia medications should be given before the neuromuscular blocking agents. Examples include benzodiazepines, opioids, ketamine, etomidate, and barbiturates.

A. BENZODIAZEPINES

- Most commonly used medications.
- Provide amnesia, not analgesia.
- Examples include midazolam and lorazepam.
- Consider starting at the lower end of the dosage range and repeating as necessary.
- Flumazenil reverses the effects of benzodiazepines.
  - Dose: 0.01 mg/kg/dose IV up to 0.2 mg/dose; may repeat every 1 minute to maximum dose of 1 mg.
  - Flumazenil is contraindicated in patients with seizure disorder, tricyclic antidepressant ingestion, or long-term benzodiazepine use.

1. Midazolam—

- Dose: 0.1–0.25 mg/kg IV.
- Onset of action: Within 1–5 minutes.
- Maximal depression may not be achieved for 5–7 minutes.
- Duration of effect: Approximately 20–30 minutes.
- May cause apnea in some patients.

2. Lorazepam—

- Dose: 0.05–0.1 mg/kg IV.
- Onset of action: 15–30 minutes.
- Duration of effect: 8–12 hours.
- Metabolized in the liver to inactive compounds, excreted in the urine.
- May not be optimal for intubation because of prolonged onset.

B. OPIOIDS

- Second most commonly used medications.
- Provide analgesia, not amnesia.
- Differences among drugs include chemical structure, half-life, potency, cardiovascular effects, and metabolic products.
- Naloxone is reversal agent.
  - Dose: 0.01–0.1 mg/kg/dose IV, up to 2 mg/dose; may repeat every 3–5 minutes.

1. Morphine—

- Dose: 0.05–0.1 mg/kg IV.
- Onset of action: Peak 20 minutes.
- Duration of effect: 3–5 hours.

- Metabolized in the liver to inactive and active compounds.
- Excreted in urine.
- Cardiovascular effects: Peripheral vasodilation.
- Respiratory depression may occur.

2. Fentanyl—

- Dose: 1–2 mcg/kg IV
- Peak onset of respiratory depression is approximately 15 minutes.
- Onset of action: Almost immediate.
- Duration of effect: 30–60 minutes.
- Respiratory depression may last longer than analgesia.
- May provide adequate anesthesia (and analgesia), especially in combination with other drugs and in patients with serious cardiovascular limitations.
- Unlike morphine, fentanyl rarely decreases blood pressure, even in patients with poor left ventricular function (no histamine release).
- Incidence of chest wall rigidity ranges from 0% to 100%.
  - Rigidity usually begins as patient is losing consciousness.
  - Succinylcholine reliably and rapidly terminates rigidity.
  - Rigidity is related to both dose and rate of infusion.

C. KETAMINE

- Dose: 0.5–2 mg/kg IV.
- Onset of action: Within 30 seconds.
- Duration of effect: 5–10 minutes.
- Recovery: 1–2 hours.
- Provides amnesia and analgesia.
- A "dissociative anesthetic," may cause hallucinations in older children and adults; should pretreat with a benzodiazepine.
- Increases blood pressure and heart rate.
- Ventilation is maintained.
- Bronchial smooth muscle tone is relaxed.
- Preferred in patients with heart disease and may be the drug of choice in patients with asthma.
- Disadvantages include increased secretions (should always give vagolytic agent, such as atropine); dysphoria; and increased skeletal muscle tone, often requiring muscle relaxation.
- Contraindications include elevated intracranial pressure, hypertension, and increased intraocular pressure.

D. ETOMIDATE

- Dose: 0.3 mg/kg IV.
- Onset of action: 30–60 seconds.
- Duration of effect: 4–10 minutes.

- Nonbarbiturate, anesthetic agent.
- Decreases cerebral metabolic rate and intracranial pressure.
- Maintains cerebral perfusion pressure.
- Minimal changes in mean arterial pressure, cardiac output, or systemic vascular resistance.
- Disadvantages include pain on injection, myoclonus, nausea and vomiting, and adrenal suppression.

E. BARBITURATES: THIOPENTAL

- Dose: Children < 12 years, 5–6 mg/kg; children > 12 years, 3–5 mg/kg IV.
- Onset of action: 30–60 seconds.
- Duration of effect: 5–30 minutes.
- Provides sedation and amnesia, not analgesia.
- Decreases cerebral metabolic rate and intracranial pressure.
- Decreases cardiac output.
- Often causes severe hypotension.
- Often results in apnea.
- Contraindicated in patients with hemodynamic instability.

F. NEUROMUSCULAR BLOCKING AGENTS

- No analgesic or amnestic properties.
- **Must be able to manage the airway.**

1. Succinylcholine—

- Dose: 1–2 mg/kg IV; can be given IM 2.5–4.0 mg/kg.
- Onset of action: 30–60 seconds.
- Duration of effect: 4–6 minutes.
- Major disadvantage is vagal stimulation, which can result in bradycardia and cardiac arrest, especially after second dose.
- Should always be preceded by atropine.
- Metabolized by plasma pseudocholinesterase.
- Contraindications include the following:
  - Traumatic and burn injuries (increased receptor density 24 hours to 6 months after injury; **note:** not contraindicated at time of injury).
  - Hyperkalemia.
  - Neuromuscular disease (including muscular dystrophy but not cerebral palsy).
  - Renal failure.
  - Severe intra-abdominal infection.
  - Raised intraocular pressure.
  - Personal or family history of malignant hyperthermia.

- Succinylcholine is a **depolarizing** neuromuscular blocking agent.

2. Rocuronium—

- Dose: 0.6–1.2 mg/kg IV.
- Dose for rapid sequence intubation: 1.2 mg/kg IV.

- Rocuronium is a **nondepolarizing** neuromuscular blocking agent.

- Onset of action: 30–60 seconds.
- Duration of effect: 30–40 minutes.
- Excretion: Primarily biliary, with some renal.

MONITORING

- Use pulse oximetry to measure oxygen saturation levels continuously.
- Measure heart rate continuously.
- Check blood pressure frequently using a noninvasive device.

COMPLICATIONS

- Esophageal intubation.
- Perforation of trachea.
- Intubation of right main bronchus.
- Aspiration.
- Dental damage.
- Laceration of lips or gums.

FOLLOW-UP

- The importance of follow-up is to make sure that the endotracheal tube remains in the correct position and is not obstructed.
- Monitor end tidal CO_2 using capnography.
- Monitor oxygen saturation levels.
- Check heart rate.

REFERENCES

Bledsoe GH, Schexnayder SM. Pediatric rapid sequence intubation. *Pediatr Emerg Care.* 2004;20:339–344.

Hazinski MF et al, eds. *PALS Provider Manual.* Dallas, Texas: American Heart Association; 2002:99–109.

Holinger LD, Lusk RP, Green CG, eds. *Pediatric Laryngology and Bronchoesophagology.* Philadelphia: Lippincott-Raven Publishers; 1997:19–25.

Sullivan KJ, Kissoon N. Securing the child's airway in the emergency department. *Pediatr Emerg Care.* 2002;18:108–121.

Taketomo CK, Hodding JH, Kraus DM. *Lexi-Comp's Pediatric Dosage Handbook.* 11th edition. Hudson, Ohio: Lexi-Comp; 2004.

CHAPTER 5

Cricothyrotomy

Kelly Michelson, MD

INDICATIONS

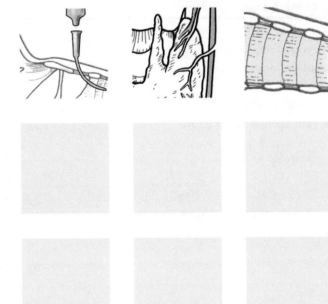

- Patients who cannot be adequately oxygenated or venti-
lated using bag-mask ventilation.
- Patients in whom it is impossible to establish an airway
via oral or nasal endotracheal intubation due to any of the
following:
  - Bleeding from upper airway structures.
  - Massive emesis.
  - Masseter spasm.
  - Spasm of the larynx or pharynx.
  - Laryngeal stenosis.
  - Structural deformities of the upper airway.
- To avoid delay in airway control in patients with upper airway
obstruction, thus preventing or shortening periods of anoxia.
- Patients with maxillofacial trauma, laryngeal trauma
(except for tracheal transection), and unstable cervical
spine fractures to minimize movement of the neck.
- An elective situation when a patient is undergoing surgery
of the head, face, or neck.

CONTRAINDICATIONS

Absolute

- Cricothyrotomy should not be performed in any patient who
can quickly and easily be intubated using nonsurgical means.
- Patients with a fractured or significantly damaged larynx.
- Patients with tracheal transection.
  - The cervical fascia may be tenuously holding the airway
  together.
  - The incision required to perform a cricothyrotomy may
  transect the fascia causing the distal airway to retract into
  the mediastinum.
  - In such cases, tracheostomy is the preferred method for
  controlling the airway.

Relative

- Coagulopathy.

- Preexisting infection.
- Significant neck distortion.
- Massive neck edema.
- In children younger than 5 years, needle cricothyrotomy with transtracheal jet ventilation is recommended due to the difficulty of performing a surgical cricothyrotomy. (Some clinicians recommend transtracheal jet ventilation for children younger than 12 years.)
- Establishing an airway should supersede any relative contraindication in a patient in extremis.

EQUIPMENT

Surgical Cricothyrotomy

- Scalpel.
- Tracheal dilator (Trousseau dilator) or spreader or hemostat.
- Appropriate size tracheostomy or endotracheal tube.
- 25-gauge needle and syringe with 1% lidocaine (for local anesthesia).
- Preparation solution (either 2% chlorhexidine-based preparation in patients older than 2 months of age or 10% povidone-iodine).
- Sterile gauze pads.
- Ties for tracheostomy tube.
- Oxygen source and suction.
- Bag-valve device.

Needle Cricothyrotomy

- 12- or 14-gauge needle or over-the-needle catheter.
- 5- or 10-mL syringe.
- High-pressure tubing.
- Stopcock.
- High-pressure oxygen source at 50 psi.
  - If a high-pressure oxygen source is not available, use a bag-valve device with the proximal connector of an 8.0 endotracheal tube and 3-mL syringe or the proximal connector of a 3.0 endotracheal tube.

PEARLS AND TIPS

- Remember, the thyroid gland lies inferior to the larynx. Therefore, if the thyroid gland is visualized, the incision should be extended cranially, toward the larynx.
- After making an incision through the cricoid membrane, it may be necessary to lift and hold the larynx anteriorly with a tracheal hook in order to avoid posterior displacement of the larynx.
- If needle cricothyrotomy is performed and there is no pressurized oxygen source available, the patient can be ventilated using a bag-valve apparatus connected to the catheter (Figure 5–1).

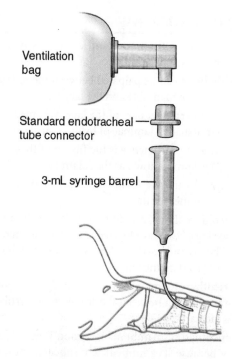

Ventilation bag

Standard endotracheal tube connector

3-mL syringe barrel

Figure 5–1. *Setup for translaryngeal ventilation.*

• Attach a 3-mL syringe to the needle/catheter and then the proximal end of an 8.0 endotracheal tube connector into the back of the 3-mL syringe.

• Alternatively, attach the proximal end of a 3.0 endotracheal tube connector to the needle/catheter, and then, connect a bag-valve apparatus to the distal side of the endotracheal tube connector.

PATIENT PREPARATION

■ Time permitting, sterilize the patient's neck with either 2% chlorhexidine-based preparation in patients older than 2 months or 10% povidone-iodine. Then, administer local anesthesia using a 25-gauge needle and syringe with 1% lidocaine.

■ Sedation can be used sparingly in patients whose agitation may hinder the procedure; however, sedation may cause respiratory depression in patients with an already compromised airway.

■ In emergent situations, there may not be time to administer local anesthesia or sedation.

PATIENT POSITIONING

■ Place the patient supine with the head midline.

■ If possible, hyperextend the patient's neck to expose the anatomic landmarks.

■ Hyperextension is contraindicated in patients with known or suspected cervical spine injury.

ANATOMY REVIEW

■ Figure 5–2 shows the important landmarks with which practitioners must be familiar.

■ The **hyoid bone** can be palpated between the mental protuberance of the mandible and the larynx.

■ The **thyroid cartilage,** part of the larynx, is made up of 2 quadrilateral-shaped laminae of hyaline cartilage.

• The laryngeal prominence is the fusion of these 2 pieces of cartilage and is known as the Adam's apple.

• The thyroid cartilage forms the superior border of the cricothyroid membrane.

■ The **cricoid cartilage,** also part of the larynx, is a circumferential ring of cartilage located caudal to the thyroid cartilage. The cricoid cartilage forms the inferior border of the cricothyroid membrane.

■ The **cricothyroid membrane** is the dense fibroelastic membrane located between the cricothyroid cartilage and the thyroid cartilage.

• The cricothyroid membrane is a good way to access the airway because it is immediately subcutaneous, it does

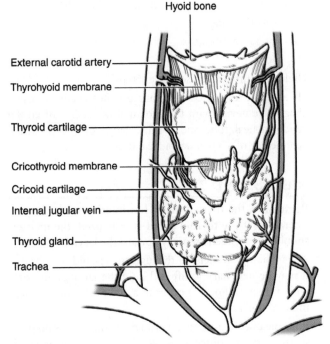

Figure 5–2. *Anatomic landmarks.*

Hyoid bone

External carotid artery

Thyrohyoid membrane

Thyroid cartilage

Cricothyroid membrane

Cricoid cartilage

Internal jugular vein

Thyroid gland

Trachea

Table 5–1. Tracheostomy tube sizes.

Age	Internal Diameter of Tracheostomy Tube (mm)	Holinger or Magill Tube Size	Internal Diameter of Endotracheal Tube (mm)
Premature (< 1.8 kg; < 4 lb)	—	000	2.5
Premature (≥ 1.8 kg; ≥ 4 lb)	—	00	2.5
Newborn	2.5	00 or 0	3.0
0–6 mo	3.5	0	3.5
6–12 mo	4.0–4.5	1	4.0
1 yr	4.5–5.0	1 or 2	4.5
2 yr	5.0	2	5.0
4 yr	5.5	3	5.5
6 yr	6.0	4	6.0
8 yr	6.5	4	6.5
10 yr	7.0	4	7.0
12 yr	7.5	5	7.5
14 yr	8.0	5	7.5
Adult female	8.0–8.5	5	7.5–8.5
Adult male	8.5–9.5	6	8.0–9.0

not calcify with age, and there are no major overlying blood vessels or nerves.
- The **tracheal rings** are located caudal to the cricothyroid cartilage.
  - Of note, the thyroid gland overlies the second and third tracheal rings.

PROCEDURE

Basic Steps
- Palpate the larynx and identify the cricothyroid membrane.
- Make a midline vertical skin incision approximately 2–4 cm long.
- While stabilizing the larynx between the nondominant thumb and middle finger, make a short horizontal incision in the cricothyroid membrane close to the cricothyroid cartilage.
- Insert a curved Mayo scissors, Trousseau dilator, tracheal hook, hemostat, or blade handle into the opening.
- Insert an appropriately sized tracheostomy tube into the airway.
  - Typically, a number 5 or 6 Shiley is appropriate for an adult or adolescent female or male, respectively (Table 5–1).

• An endotracheal tube can also be used if a tracheostomy tube is not available.

■ Secure the tracheostomy tube with tracheostomy ties around the neck or suture the tube in place.

The Four-Step Technique

■ Palpate the cricoid membrane.

■ Make a horizontal incision through the cricoid membrane.

■ Use a tracheal hook to create caudal traction on the cricoid ring.

■ Pass a tracheostomy or endotracheal tube through the opening created.

Percutaneous Transtracheal Ventilation—Needle Cricothyrotomy

■ Identify the cricothyroid membrane via palpation.

■ Insert a 12- to 14-gauge needle or catheter-over-needle caudally at a 30–45% angle through the cricothyroid membrane into the airway while aspirating as the needle is inserted (Figure 5–3). When air is aspirated, the needle tip is in the trachea.

■ Attach the needle/catheter to a pressurized oxygen source that can deliver approximately 50 psi for adults and 30 psi for children using oxygen tubing.

■ To achieve intermittent ventilation, either cut a small hole in the oxygen tubing or attach a stopcock to the catheter before attaching the oxygen tubing.

• Provide inflations at a rate of 12–20 bursts per minute by covering the hole in the oxygen tubing or closing the stopcock.

• Allow for expiration by uncovering the hole in the oxygen tubing or opening the stopcock for approximately 2–9 seconds.

MONITORING

■ Throughout the procedure, the patient should be observed using a cardiopulmonary monitor, continuous pulse oximetry, and frequent assessment of vitals signs.

■ While a patient can be adequately oxygenated and ventilated after a surgical cricothyrotomy with a tracheostomy tube in place, the same is not true for patients after a needle cricothyrotomy.

■ Needle cricothyrotomy is a temporary procedure.

• Typically, patients can only be oxygenated for approximately 30 minutes and lack of adequate ventilation causes rapid hypercapnia.

• These patients require urgent placement of a more stable airway.

■ This technique is an alternative approach to the Basic Steps in the preceding description; however, studies have shown that this technique is associated with a higher incidence of complications.

■ For children younger than 5 years, needle cricothyrotomy is recommended.

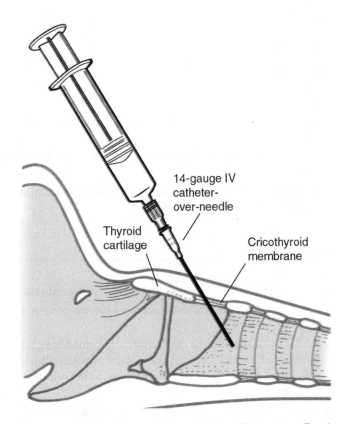

14-gauge IV
catheter-
over-needle

Thyroid
cartilage

Cricothyroid
membrane

Figure 5–3. *Percutaneous transtracheal ventilation or needle cricothyrotomy.*

COMPLICATIONS

Early

- Bleeding or hematoma formation.
- Inability to place the tube correctly.
- Hypoxia.
- Inadequate ventilation.
- Subcutaneous or mediastinal emphysema.
- Pneumothorax.
- Pneumomediastinum.
- Esophageal laceration.
- Vocal cord injury.
- Thyroid perforation.
- Posterior tracheal wall perforation.
- Aspiration.

Late

- Infection.
- Dysphonia.
- Subglottic or glottic stenosis.
- Persistent stoma.
- Tracheoesophageal fistula.
- Tracheomalacia.

FOLLOW-UP

- Given the potential long-term complications, patients who have undergone a cricothyrotomy should be monitored by a pediatric ear, nose, and throat surgeon.

REFERENCES

Advanced Trauma Life Support Program for Doctors. 7th ed. Chicago, IL: American College of Surgeons; 2004.

Blanda M, Gallo UE. Emergency airway management. *Emerg Med Clin North Am.* 2003;21:1–26.

Butler KH, Clyne B. Management of the difficult airway: alternative airway techniques and adjuncts. *Emerg Med Clin North Am.* 2003;21:259–289.

Chan TC, Vilke GM, Bramwell KJ, Davis DP, Hamilton RS, Rosen P. Comparison of wire-guided cricothyrotomy versus standard surgical cricothyrotomy technique. *J Emerg Med.* 1999;17:957–962.

Davis DP, Bramwell KJ, Vilke GM, Cardall TY, Yoshida E, Rosen P. Cricothyrotomy technique: standard versus the Rapid Four-Step Technique. *J Emerg Med.* 1999;17:17–21.

Gunn VL, Nechyba C, Johns Hopkins Hospital. Children's Medical and Surgical Center. *The Harriet Lane Handbook: A Manual for Pediatric House Officers.* 16th ed. Philadelphia: Mosby; 2002.

Hazinski MF et al, eds. *PALS Provider Manual.* Dallas, Texas: American Heart Association; 2002:155–172.

Mace SE, Hedges JR. Cricothyrotomy and translaryngeal jet ventilation. In: Roberts JR, Hedges JR, eds. *Clinical Procedures in Emergency Medicine.* 4th ed. Philadelphia: WB Saunders; 2004:115–132.

Marr JK, Yamamoto LG. Gas flow rates through transtracheal ventilation catheters. *Am J Emerg Med.* 2004;22:264–266.

American Society of Anesthesiologists Task Force on Management of the Difficult Airway. Practice guidelines for management of the difficult airway: an updated report by the American Society of Anesthesiologists Task Force on Management of the Difficult Airway. *Anesthesiology.* 2003;98: 1269–1277.

Roberts JR, Hedges JR, Chanmugam AS. *Clinical Procedures in Emergency Medicine.* 4th ed. Philadelphia: WB Saunders; 2004.

Rosen P. *Emergency Medicine Concepts and Clinical Practice.* 5th ed. St. Louis, MO: MD Consult LLC; 2002.

CHAPTER 6

Chest Compression

Ty Hasselman, MD and Wayne H. Franklin, MD, MPH

INDICATIONS

- Chest compressions are started once signs of circulatory arrest are identified.
  - For the layperson, these include absence of breathing, coughing, and movement.
  - In addition, for the healthcare worker, lack of an identifiable pulse is a sign of circulatory arrest.
- Chest compressions are started in infants and children if their heart rate is less than 60 beats per minute with signs of poor perfusion; the main mechanism for increasing cardiac output is by increasing heart rate.
- The combination of bradycardia and poor perfusion is a sign of imminent cardiac arrest.

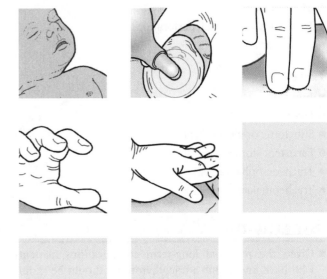

CONTRAINDICATIONS

Absolute

- None. However, compressions should be started with caution if the patient has a known period of prolonged asystole.
- Do-not-resuscitate orders are respected in patients with prior orders.

EQUIPMENT

- No equipment is necessary when patient is on a firm, flat surface.
- A resuscitation board is used when hospitalized patients are in a soft bed.
  - It is placed underneath the patient for effective compressions.
  - The board extends from the shoulders to the waist and across the width of the bed.

RISKS

- Multiple studies have shown significant complications during resuscitation of adults.

- However, cardiopulmonary resuscitation of children results in significant injuries only about 3% of the time.

PEARLS AND TIPS

- Cardiac arrest in pediatric patients is most commonly due to respiratory failure. The rescuer attempts to correct any obvious respiratory compromise.
- Infants with no signs of head or neck trauma may be carried on the rescuer's forearm during resuscitation, which allows the lone rescuer to continue resuscitation while seeking help.
- Compressions are coordinated with ventilation in an unintubated patient.
  - Once the patient has been intubated, it is no longer necessary to coordinate compressions and ventilations.
  - However, coordinating compressions and ventilations is suggested in newborns because it may facilitate adequate ventilation.

PATIENT POSITIONING

- The patient is placed supine on a firm flat surface.
- If the patient is in bed, then a resuscitation board is placed underneath him or her.
- Any bulky clothing that will interfere with compressions or assessment is removed or opened up.
- The head and neck are placed in a neutral position.

ANATOMY REVIEW

- The heart lies centrally in the chest between the lower part of the sternum and the thoracic spine.
- Effective compressions squeeze the heart between the sternum and spine to eject blood; for this reason, hand placement is over the lower portion of the sternum.
- The central pulse is located by palpating the brachial, femoral, or carotid arteries (Figure 6–1).
  - The preferred location for checking the pulse depends on the patient's age as well as the number and skill of the rescuers.
  - In infants, the brachial pulse is preferred but the femoral pulse can be used alternatively.
  - In older children and adults, the carotid pulse is preferred but a second or third rescuer may be better able to use the femoral pulse to monitor compressions.
  - The brachial artery is palpated just above the elbow, medial to the biceps (see Figure 6–1A).
  - The femoral artery is palpated just below the inguinal ligament half-way between the anterior superior iliac spine and the pubic tubercle (see Figure 6–1B).

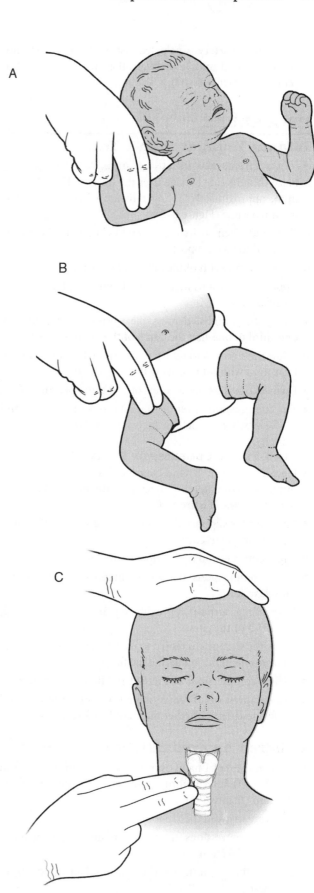

Figure 6–1. *Locating the central pulse.*

• The carotid artery is palpated just medial to the sterno-cleidomastoid muscle (between the muscle and the trachea) (see Figure 6–1C).

PROCEDURE

Infants Younger than 1 Year

A. Two Thumb-Encircling Hands Technique

■ Place thumbs side by side over the lower half of the sternum, approximately 1 finger breadth below the intermammary line (Figure 6–2).

■ The hands then encircle the infant's chest with the fingertips used to give support to the back.

■ Avoid compression of the xiphoid process.

■ Apply compressions in a smooth manner with equal time for relaxation.

■ Using the thumbs, depress the sternum approximately one-third to one-half the depth of the infant's chest.

■ Allow the sternum to return to its original position during relaxation without removing the fingers.

■ Deliver compressions at a rate of 100 times per minute.

■ The compression to ventilation ratio is 5:1 for infants and 3:1 for newborns whether there are 1 or 2 rescuers.

B. Two-Finger Compression Technique

■ Place 2 fingers of 1 hand over the lower half of the sternum, approximately 1 finger breadth below the intermammary line (Figure 6–3).

■ The infant is supported on a firm surface or on the other forearm of the rescuer.

■ Avoid compression of the xiphoid process.

■ Apply compressions in a smooth manner with equal time for relaxation.

■ Depress the sternum approximately one-third to one-half the depth of the chest.

■ Allow the sternum to return to its original position during relaxation without removing the fingers.

■ Deliver compressions at a rate of 100 times per minute.

■ The compression to ventilation ratio is 5:1 for infants and 3:1 for newborns whether there are 1 or 2 rescuers.

Children Approximately 1 to 8 Years

■ Place the heel of 1 hand over the lower half of the sternum between the intermammary line and the bottom of the sternum (Figure 6–4).

■ Take care to avoid the xiphoid process.

■ Deliver compressions in a smooth manner allowing equal time for relaxation.

■ Depress the sternum one-third to one-half the depth of the chest.

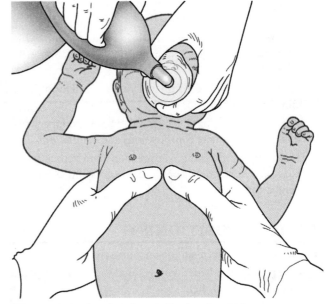

Figure 6–2. *Two thumb-encircling hands technique.*

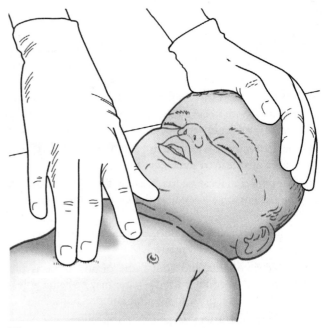

Figure 6–3. *Two-finger compression technique.*

- Allow the sternum to return to its original position during relaxation without removing the hand.
- Deliver compressions at a rate of 100 times per minute.
- Chest compressions and ventilations are always performed at a ratio of 5:1 whether 1 or 2 rescuers are present.

Patients Over 8 Years of Age

- Place the heel of 1 hand on the lower half of the sternum at the level of the intermammary line.
- Place the heel of the other hand on top of the first, being careful not to put pressure on the xiphoid process.
- Interlock the fingers of both hands and lift the fingers off the chest to avoid pressure on the ribs (Figure 6–5).
- Position yourself vertically above the patient with arms straight.
- Depress the sternum 1.5 to 2 inches. (**Note:** This is a defined value, not a proportion of the depth of the chest.)
- Deliver compressions in a smooth manner allowing equal time for relaxation.
- Allow the sternum to return to its original position during relaxation without removing the hands.
- Deliver compressions at a rate of 100 times per minute.
- In the unintubated patient, pause compressions after every 15 to give 2 ventilations whether there are 1 or 2 people present.
- If the patient is intubated, then the compression to ventilation ratio is 5:1.

MONITORING

- Once chest compressions are begun, they are continued for approximately 1 minute or 20 cycles and then paused to reassess the patient.
- After the initial reassessment, compressions are paused every few minutes for reassessment.
- If multiple rescuers are present, then the adequacy of chest compressions can be monitored by palpating the pulse.
- When the compressions are being performed effectively, a pulse is felt with every compression.

COMPLICATIONS

- Complications are rare in the pediatric population.
- The most common injuries are chest contusions and abrasions.
- Significant complications occur in 3% of cases and include the following:
  - Rib fracture.
  - Retinal hemorrhages.
  - Retroperitoneal hematoma.

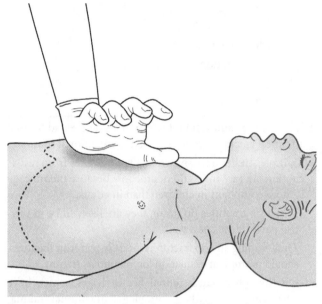

Figure 6–4. *One-hand technique for children aged 1–8 years.*

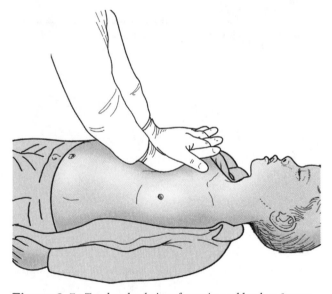

Figure 6–5. *Two-hand technique for patients older than 8 years.*

• Pneumothorax.
• Pulmonary hemorrhage.
• Epicardial hematoma.
• Gastric perforation.

CAVEATS

■ Rib fractures and retinal hemorrhages deserve additional attention as they have been linked to intentional trauma.

■ Multiple studies have shown that rib fractures from resuscitation are rare in children, probably because the rib cage is more compliant in children than in adults.

• When rib fractures do occur, they are likely to be in ventral parts of the chest wall.

• Thus, finding any rib fracture, especially posterior fractures, should prompt an evaluation for intentional trauma.

• On the other hand, retinal hemorrhages, which have been considered pathognomonic for intentional trauma, have been attributed to resuscitation.

FOLLOW-UP

■ No specific follow-up is recommended.

■ However, patients who have undergone resuscitation are evaluated for transient or permanent end-organ damage.

■ When traumatic injury from chest compressions is suspected, serial examinations and imaging studies are performed.

REFERENCES

Stapleton EF, Aufderheide TP, Hazinski MF, Cummins RO, eds. *BLS for Healthcare Providers*. Dallas, Texas: American Heart Association; 2001.

Bush CM, Jones JS, Cohle SD, Johnson H. Pediatric injuries from cardiopulmonary resuscitation. *Ann Emerg Med*. 1996; 28:40–44.

Feldman KW, Brewer DK. Child abuse, cardiopulmonary resuscitation, and rib fractures. *Pediatrics*. 1984;73:339–342.

Hazinski MF et al, eds. *PALS Provider Manual*. Dallas, Texas: American Heart Association; 2002.

Kramer K, Goldstein B. Retinal hemorrhages following cardiopulmonary resuscitation. *Clin Pediatr*. 1993;32:366–368.

Spevak MR, Kleinman PK, Belanger PL, Primack C, Richmond JM. Cardiopulmonary resuscitation and rib fractures in infants: a postmortem radiologic-pathologic study. *JAMA*. 1994;272:617–618.

CHAPTER 7

Cardioversion and Defibrillation

Sabrina Tsao, MD and Barbara J. Deal, MD

INDICATIONS

- Rapid termination of tachycardia that is either unresponsive to medications or pacing interventions or is hemodynamically compromising, necessitating more urgent intervention.

Cardioversion

- Tachycardia, either supraventricular or ventricular, with regular ventricular response with mild to moderate hypotension.
- Mechanisms of supraventricular tachycardia include the following:
  - Atrial reentry tachycardia.
  - Reciprocating tachycardia utilizing an accessory connection.
  - Atrial flutter.
  - Atrioventricular nodal reentry tachycardia.

Defibrillation

- The most effective treatment for ventricular fibrillation and pulseless ventricular tachycardia (Table 7–1).
- Its effectiveness diminishes rapidly over time; therefore, early defibrillation is recommended in patients who have suffered cardiac arrest.
- Atrial fibrillation.
- Supraventricular tachycardia with rapid conduction via an accessory connection.
- Ventricular fibrillation.
- Torsades de pointes.

CONTRAINDICATIONS

Absolute

- A patient directive regarding resuscitation.

Relative

- Cardioversion of a rhythm known to be automatic in origin is not indicated.

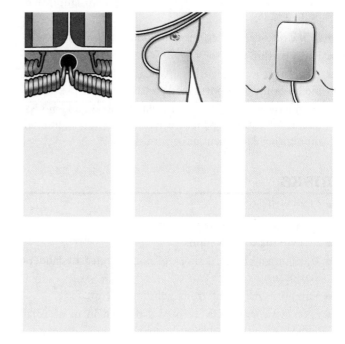

[■■■]

- Cardioversion: Can be performed using medications, electrical pacing, or electrical direct current shock synchronized to QRS complex to correct an abnormal rapid cardiac rhythm.
- Defibrillation: Uses electrical energy delivered transthoracically, nonsynchronously, and in a random fashion during the cardiac cycle to correct a very rapid rhythm.
- Benefits of cardioversion are restoration of a sinus or slower rhythm, improving cardiac output and function, and decreasing the risk of thromboembolism, cardiac dysfunction, and sudden death associated with the tachycardia.

■ Digoxin toxicity-induced arrhythmia.

• With digoxin toxicity, there is a high incidence of post-cardioversion ventricular tachycardia and fibrillation.

■ Elective cardioversion of a hemodynamically stable patient with a known atrial thrombus; however, the likelihood of impending cardiovascular compromise can outweigh the risk of thromboembolism.

■ Repeated cardioversion of a rhythm where the predisposing cause is not eliminated.

EQUIPMENT

■ External defibrillator, either manual or semi-automated (Figure 7–1).

■ Skin electrode patches, wires to connect to defibrillator.

■ Heart rhythm monitor.

■ Equipment to protect the airway as well as resuscitation medications to support blood pressure.

■ Do not delay cardioversion or defibrillation in a hemodynamically unstable patient while waiting for additional monitoring equipment or personnel.

RISKS

■ Chest wall lesions.

■ Neurologic complications.

■ Arrhythmia complications.

■ Transmitted electrical shock of nonprotected bystanders may occur.

■ Skin burns may result from high-dose energy.

■ Excessive energy delivery may also result in myocardial damage and irreversible cardiomyopathy.

■ Stroke may result from thromboembolism of atrial or ventricular thrombus with energy delivery.

■ Anticoagulation and assessment of risk of thrombus with transesophageal echocardiogram may minimize but not eliminate risk of stroke, which occurs in 1–3% of cardioversions.

■ In very ill patients or patients with longstanding arrhythmia or underlying sinus or junctional node disease, cardioversion may result in asystole or profound bradycardia, which may not respond to medications or temporary pacing.

■ Cardioversion may convert a stable arrhythmia into an unstable tachycardia, particularly with asynchronous cardioversion of a regular tachycardia producing ventricular fibrillation.

■ Immediate defibrillation is necessary in such cases.

PEARLS AND TIPS

■ Most failures of cardioversion relate to any of the following:

• Improper lead positioning.

• Energy selection.

Table 7–1. Treating tachycardia.

Tachycardia	Specific rhythm	Treatment
Narrow QRS complex	Sinus tachycardia	Treat underlying cause
Narrow QRS complex	Supraventricular tachycardia	Medications
		Vagal maneuvers
		Pacing
		Cardioversion
Wide QRS complex	Ventricular tachycardia	Medications
	SVT with aberrant conduction	Cardioversion
	SVT with antegrade conduction over an accessory connection	
Pulseless rhythm	Very rapid atrial or ventricular tachycardia	Defibrillation
	Atrial or ventricular fibrillation	
	Torsades de pointes	

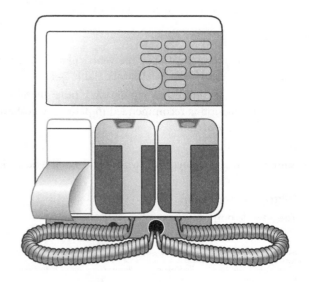

Figure 7–1. *Cardioverter/defibrillator.*

- Synchronization.
  - Use of cardioversion for an automatic rhythm not responsive to cardioversion (sinus tachycardia, automatic atrial tachycardia).
- Lead positioning should direct the current of energy across the chamber to be cardioverted.
- Cardioversion of ventricular tachycardia should direct energy across the ventricle: Position 1 electrode near the cardiac apex.
- Atrial tachycardia requires the current of energy to be directed across the atria; an anterior-posterior pad configuration may be preferable.
- Patients with repaired congenital heart disease resulting in dilated atria and atrial tachycardia are candidates for anterior-posterior pad configuration.
- In dextrocardia, the pads need to positioned across the right chest.
- Energy selection.
  - Regular rhythms (atrial flutter, supraventricular tachycardia, ventricular tachycardia) require low-dose energy, up to 1 J/kg.
  - Irregular tachycardias (atrial fibrillation, ventricular fibrillation) require high-dose energy, at least 2 J/kg.
- **Regular** rhythms should receive energy **synchronized** to the QRS.
  - Check the rhythm monitor to verify that the QRS, not the T wave, is being sensed.
  - **Asynchronous** energy delivered into a **regular** rhythm may fire on the T wave and produce ventricular fibrillation.
  - In such cases, immediate **asynchronous** defibrillation is required.
- **Irregular** rhythms require **asynchronous** cardioversion because the QRS timing cannot be predicted.
- Remember that the default setting on a defibrillator is **asynchronous** and must be reset to **synchronous** if so desired after every discharge.
- When an arrhythmia is due to a reentrant circuit, a **synchronized** shock depolarizes all excitable tissue within the circuit, making tissue refractory; therefore, the electrical circuit is no longer able to propagate and terminates.
- Rhythms due to abnormal accelerated automaticity are not reliant upon a reentrant circuit and do not respond to cardioversion or defibrillation.
  - Examples of such rhythms are automatic (ectopic) atrial tachycardia or arrhythmias due to drug toxicity or profound metabolic derangement.

PATIENT PREPARATION

- For elective cardioversion, patient should follow protocol for sedation and have a functional peripheral IV.

- Consent for the procedure and sedation is obtained.
- With hands-off electrode pads, if anterior-posterior position is preferred, pads should be placed before the patient is sedated.
- If the patient has a pacemaker/implantable cardioverter defibrillator (ICD) in place, the electrode pads or paddles should not be placed directly over the device.
- The device should be interrogated before and after the procedure to ensure proper lead and device functions.
- In the presence of excessive thoracic hair, the chest should be shaved.
- For emergent cardioversion associated with significant hypotension, sedation is optimal depending on the clinical scenario, and fasting is clearly not an option.

PATIENT POSITIONING

- Supine, with adequate airway protection and support.

ANATOMY REVIEW

- Dextrocardia: Place anterior pad in the left upper sternum and the lateral pad in the right-sided apex.
- The *anteroposterior* pad configuration has a higher rate of success in converting atrial fibrillation in adults, and atrial reentry tachycardia/atrial flutter/atrial fibrillation in patients with congenital heart disease.
- Congenital heart disease diagnoses typically associated with the development of atrial tachycardia include the following:
  - Repaired atrial septal defects.
  - Ebstein anomaly of the tricuspid valve.
  - Transposition of the great arteries.
  - Fontan-type repairs of single ventricle anatomy.
  - Chronic mitral valve disease, such as secondary to rheumatic fever.
- Lesions at higher risk for developing ventricular tachycardia include the following:
  - Tetralogy of Fallot.
  - Double outlet right ventricle.
  - Ventricular conduit-type repairs.
  - Transposition of the great arteries.
- Torsades de pointes, a nonperfusing ventricular tachycardia associated with prolongation of the QT interval, is due to any of the following:
  - A congenital cardiac ion channelopathy.
  - Drug administration (eg, adenosine, ibutilide, procainamide, sotalol, and amiodarone).
  - Electrolyte or metabolic derangement (such as low potassium or magnesium).

- Special considerations in children are related to structural congenital heart disease and arrhythmias that are more common in childhood.

- Congenital long QT syndrome often presents in infancy or childhood and may be misdiagnosed as seizures or vasovagal syncope.

PROCEDURE

- Adequate sedation is essential and is generally given by an anesthesiologist or an intensivist.
- Emergent airway management equipment should be available.
- The patient should be preoxygenated before elective cardioversion.
- There are 2 conventional electrode configurations: anterior-lateral and anterior-posterior.
  - Anterior-lateral: Pads are positioned at right upper sternal border and cardiac apex.
  - Anterior-posterior: Pads are positioned over upper midsternal border and between scapulae.
- Electrode size is an important determining factor of the transthoracic current flow and success of cardioversion.
  - Pad size should be adjusted for patient body surface area.
  - Pediatric pads are necessary in infants and small children to avoid delivery of excessive energy.
- A larger paddle surface is associated with decreased resistance and increase in current delivery.
- Self-adhesive pads can be used in the standard anterior-lateral or anterior-posterior paddle positions in place of paddles (Figures 7–2 and 7–3).

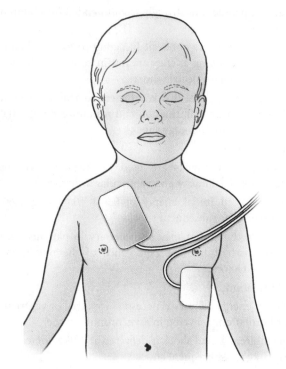

Figure 7–2. *Anterior-lateral pad and paddle positioning.*

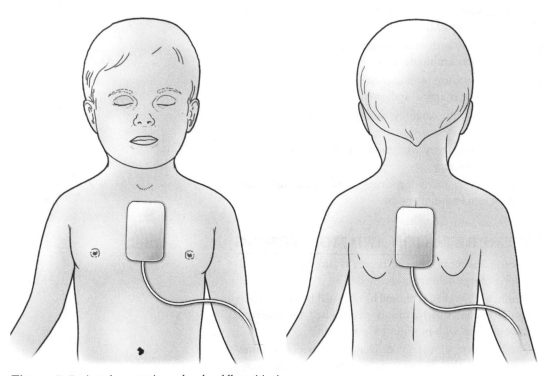

Figure 7–3. *Anterior-posterior pad and paddle positioning.*

- Pediatric paddles are strongly recommended for children below 10 kg.
- If pediatric pads are not available, adult paddles and pads can be used as long as they are not in contact with each other (to avoid an electric short).
- Select an energy level that is sufficient to achieve prompt cardioversion or defibrillation and minimize myocardial damage from high-energy shocks.
- Cardioversion.
  • Lower energy shocks are used for regular rhythms, including atrial flutter and ventricular tachycardia.
  • Synchronized initial energy of 0.5–1 J/kg is selected, increasing for subsequent shocks.
- Repeat cardioversion may be necessary in patients with chronic arrhythmias, or persistence of the underlying causative factors.
- Defibrillation.
  • Higher energy delivery is necessary for atrial or ventricular fibrillation, delivered in asynchronous mode.
  • In children, initial shock is delivered at 2 J/kg, increasing to 4 J/kg for subsequent shocks.
  • In adults, initial shock is delivered at 200 J, second shock at 200–300 J, third and subsequent shocks 360 J.
- Charge the defibrillator to the desired energy.
- Ensure all medical personnel, including the one responsible for holding oxygen for the patient, are cleared from contact with the patient and bed before discharge.
  • The phrase "I'm clear, you're clear, oxygen clear" is used.
  • Oxygen should either be removed or pointed away from the electrode paddles.
- Deliver energy with shock command or by depressing the shock buttons simultaneously.
- Interpret response to energy delivery, assess efficacy, and deliver repeat energy as indicated.
- Monitor rhythm carefully during and following energy delivery.
- Cardiopulmonary resuscitation may be necessary following energy delivery.
- Appropriate resuscitation drugs should be readily available for rapid administration.

INTERPRETATION AND MONITORING

- Continuous monitoring of heart rhythm during and following energy delivery is required.
- Ideally, a 12-lead ECG should be obtained before and after cardioversion; clearly, this is not advised for emergent interventions with profound hypotension.
- The response to energy delivery is immediately interpreted, and the decision about whether repeat energy

Special Considerations for the Use of Automated Defibrillators

- The use of semi-automatic external defibrillators (AED) requires less operator manipulation.
- The AED is turned on, and either voice or visual prompts guide the operator.
- Operator applies self-adhesive pads on the patient's chest, and the AED analyzes the rhythm.
- The machine advises the operator if "shock advised, deliver energy."
- The operator presses the "shock button" to deliver the recommended energy to the unconscious patient.
- An AED will not allow energy delivery to a rhythm it does not interpret as requiring cardioversion or defibrillation.
- Caution is necessary in the setting of a pacemaker because the AED may interpret pacer spikes as a stable rhythm and not allow energy delivery.
- A manual defibrillator will then be required for energy delivery.

delivery is needed is made while adequate anesthesia is still present.

■ For subsequent shocks, increased energy or asynchronous mode (or both) may be necessary.

■ Suspect an automatic rhythm when repeated energy delivery that is done correctly does not affect the rhythm.
  •Mechanism of tachycardia should be reassessed.
  •Pharmacologic rate control may be advised.

CAVEATS

■ Patients with repaired congenital heart disease are at increased risk for life-threatening arrhythmias.

■ Due to their underlying anatomy, they may not tolerate persistent tachycardia for prolonged periods, even hours.

■ Patients with single ventricle physiology are at particularly high risk for hemodynamic compromise, stroke, or sudden death if tachycardia persists.

■ In patients with congenital heart disease who have an internal implanted pacemaker, antitachycardia pacemaker, or defibrillator in place, avoid energy delivery over the implanted device.

■ Be aware of pitfalls with automated defibrillators and pacing spikes.

FOLLOW-UP

■ Patients undergoing cardioversion should undergo continuous rhythm monitoring for at least 4 hours after the procedure.

■ Post-sedation monitoring is required.

■ Children undergoing cardioversion tend to have recurrent tachyarrhythmias, unless the arrhythmia occurred in the setting of a reversible initiating event, such as acute electrolyte derangement.

■ Long-term antiarrhythmic therapy or pacing therapy may be necessary to decrease the risk of recurrent tachycardia.

■ Outpatient monitoring with Holter monitors or event recorders may help document the frequency and duration of arrhythmia recurrences or predisposing premature beats or bradycardia.

■ Anticoagulation is frequently advised for at least 4 weeks following cardioversion.

■ Long-term anticoagulation may be necessary in patients who are not aware of the onset of arrhythmia and are at risk for recurrent tachycardia.

■ The incidence of intracranial hemorrhage is relatively low in pediatric patients.

■ Patients with recurrent arrhythmias and sinus node dysfunction may benefit from placement of an antitachycardia pacemaker or defibrillator.

■ Certain patients with recurrent atrial fibrillation may benefit from atrial dynamic overdrive pacing.

REFERENCES

AFFIRM Investigators. A comparison of rate control and rhythm control in patients with atrial fibrillation. *N Engl J Med.* 2002;347:1825–1833.

Bjerkelund CJ, Orning OM. The efficacy of anticoagulant therapy in preventing embolism related to DC electrical conversion of atrial fibrillation. *Am J Cardiol.* 1969;23:208–216.

Botto GL, Politi A, Bonini W, Broffoni T, Bonatti R. External cardioversion of atrial fibrillation: role of paddle position on technical efficacy and energy requirements. *Heart.* 1999;82: 726–730.

Carlson MD, Ip J, Messenger J et al. A new pacemaker algorithm for the treatment of atrial fibrillation: results of the Atrial Dynamic Overdrive Pacing Trial (ADOPT). *J Am Coll Cardiol.* 2003;42:627–633.

Dalzell GW, Cunningham SR, Anderson J, Adgey AA. Electrode pad size, transthoracic impedance and success of external ventricular defibrillation. *Am J Cardiol.* 1989;64:741–744.

Hohnloser SH, Kuck KH, Lilienthal J. Rhythm or rate control in atrial fibrillation: Pharmacological Intervention in Atrial Fibrillation (PIAF); a randomised trial. *Lancet.* 2000;356: 1789–1794.

Kerber RE, Jensen SR, Grayzel J, Kennedy J, Hoyt R. Elective cardioversion: influence of paddle-electrode location and size on success rates and energy requirements. *N Engl J Med.* 1981;305:658–662.

Kirchhof P, Eckardt L, Loh P et al. Anterior–posterior versus anterior–lateral electrode positions for external cardioversion of atrial fibrillation: a randomized trial. *Lancet.* 2002;360: 1275–1279.

Minczak BM, Krimm JR. Assessment of Implanted Pacemaker/ AICD Devices. In: Roberts JR, Hedges JR, eds. *Clinical Procedures in Emergency Medicine*, 4th ed. Philadelphia: WB Saunders; 2004.

Ornato JP. Public Access Defibrillation (PAD) Trial. American Heart Journal 2004 Apr; 147(4) AHJ at the meetings Session Late-breaking trials.

Rashba EJ, Gold MR, Crawford FA, Leman RB, Peters RW, Shorofsky SR. Efficacy of transthoracic cardioversion of atrial fibrillation using a biphasic, truncated exponential shock waveform at variable initial shock energy. *Am J Cardiol.* 2004;94:1572–1574.

Snow V, Weiss KB, LeFevre M et al; AAFP Panel on Atrial Fibrillation; ACP Panel on Atrial Fibrillation. Management of newly detected atrial fibrillation: a clinical practice guideline from the American Academy of Family Physicians and the American College of Physicians. *Ann Intern Med.* 2003;139: 1009–1016.

Valenzuela TD, Roe DJ, Cretin S, Spaite DW, Larsen MP. Estimating effectiveness of cardiac arrest interventions: a logistic regression survival model. *Circulation.* 1997;96:3308–3313.

Van Gelder IC, Hagens VE, Bosker HA et al; Rate Control versus Electrical Cardioversion for Persistent Atrial Fibrillation Study Group. A comparison of rate control and rhythm control in patients with recurrent persistent atrial fibrillation. *N Engl J Med.* 2002;347:1834–1840.

CHAPTER 8

Peripheral IV Insertion

Zehava Noah, MD

INDICATIONS

- Vascular access in nonemergent situations or temporary access in emergent situations.
- Administration of fluids and electrolytes.
- Administration of intravenous medications.
- Administration of blood and blood products.
- Blood sampling.

CONTRAINDICATIONS

Absolute

- Do not insert through an infected site.
- Do not insert through a burn.
- Do not insert in an injured site.

Relative

- Avoid a paralyzed extremity.
- Do not insert in a massively edematous extremity.
- Do not insert an IV distal to injured organs (eg, do not use lower extremities when treating abdominal injuries).
- Avoid joint area.

EQUIPMENT

- Gloves.
- Tourniquet or rubber band.
- Tape and occlusive transparent dressing.
- Alcohol wipes.
- Povidone or chlorhexidine.
- Syringe filled with injectable saline.
- Gauze pads.
- IV device: catheter or butterfly of appropriate size to fit the patient and the task.
- Topical anesthetic cream.
- Ultrasound guiding equipment (if available and if trained in its use).

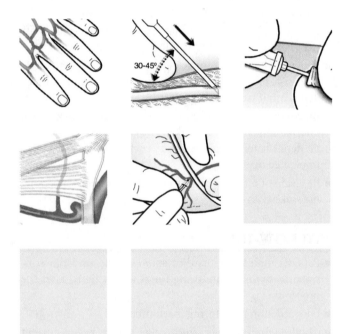

- **Caution: All equipment must be latex free.**

RISKS

- Infection.
- Hematoma.
- Extravasation.
- Compartment syndrome.
- Severe vasoconstriction if vasoactive medications are infused through a peripheral IV and extravasate.
- Venous thrombosis.
- Embolization of air or catheter fragment.

PEARLS AND TIPS

- Plan the procedure.
- Limit the procedure time.
- Have a backup plan.
- Examine all possible sites carefully before choosing one.
- Apply gentle circumferential pressure with 1 hand on the extremity to fill up the veins, which helps identify the most appropriate site.
- In choosing the equipment and the site for the line, consider the patient's needs.
  - A trauma patient will require a large bore line, preferably a short one in order to avoid high resistance with high flows.

PATIENT PREPARATION

- Introduce yourself to the parents and to the patient.
- Explain to the parents and the child, if appropriate, the procedure and its purpose.
- Choose 1 or more possible sites, and apply topical anesthetic cream.
- Answer all of the parents' and patient's questions.

PATIENT POSITIONING

- Position the patient with the chosen site closest to you.
- Have a helper gently restrain and distract the child.
- Have the patient at a comfortable working height.
- For external jugular line placement, have the patient's head lower than the trunk (Trendelenburg).

ANATOMY REVIEW

- Accessible peripheral veins that are usually available include the following (Figure 8–1):
  - On the dorsum of the hands.
  - On the radial side of the hand.
  - In the antecubital fossa.
  - The saphenous vein at the medial aspect of the ankle.

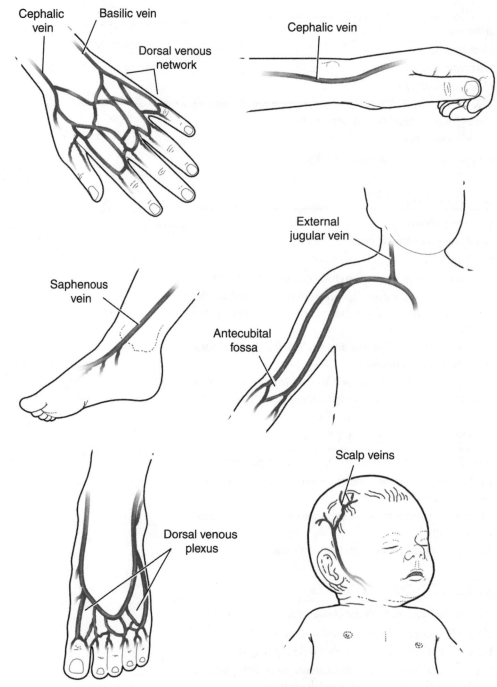

Figure 8–1. *Common sites for insertion.*

- The dorsum of the feet.
- External jugular vein.
- In infants, additional sites include scalp veins.

PROCEDURE

- Wash your hands thoroughly.
- Assemble the equipment at the bedside.

- Observe universal precautions.
- Follow the patient's specific isolation instructions.

Upper and Lower Extremities

- Apply tourniquet.
- Identify the blood vessel by palpation, visualization, transillumination, or ultrasound.
- Release the tourniquet, cleanse the site.
- Inspect the integrity of the catheter/stylet assembly.
- Flush the catheter and the connecting tube with saline (omit this step if you intend to draw blood through this catheter).
- Reapply the tourniquet.
- Use your nondominant hand to apply traction on the skin linearly or circumferentially in order to stabilize the vein.
- Enter the skin at a 30- to 45-degree angle proximal to or alongside the vein (Figure 8–2).
- Reduce the angle as you advance the catheter and enter the vein.
- Watch for blood flashback in the hub of the catheter.
- Stabilize the catheter with the thumb and middle finger of your dominant hand and advance the catheter over the stylet using the tip of your index finger (Figure 8–3).
- Remove the stylet.
- Do not reinsert the stylet once it has been removed; it may damage the catheter.
- Release the tourniquet.
- Connect the extension tubing and saline-filled syringe to the catheter.
- Gently flush the catheter; observe for swelling, mottling, or color changes in the extremity.
- Secure the IV with occlusive transparent dressing and tape.
- Make a small loop in the IV tubing and tape it across. Attach the line to an IV infusion assembly and turn the pump on.
- Dispose of all sharp instruments in the proper secure container.

External Jugular Vein

- Bundle infant or child.
- Have an assistant position the patient in the Trendelenburg position with the head toward you.
- Turn the patient's head away from the jugular vein you intend to use.
- Elevate the patient's shoulders and neck.
- Apply traction with your nondominant hand to the skin over the jugular vein.
- Nick the skin with a large bore needle at a shallow angle below or alongside the vein in order to facilitate the catheter's entry.

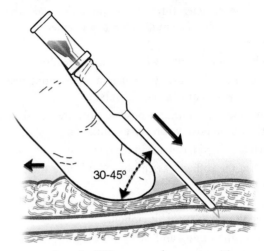

Figure 8–2. *Inserting IV in upper or lower extremities.*

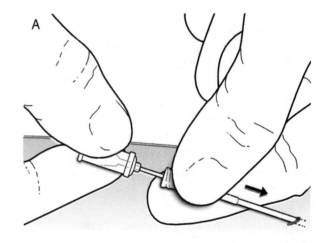

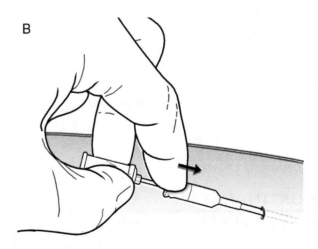

Figure 8–3. *Advancing the catheter over the stylet.*

- Insert the catheter through the puncture and advance subcutaneously a few millimeters before entering the vein (Figure 8–4).
- Synchronize your entry with the child's breathing.
  - Enter the vein during exhalation in a spontaneously breathing patient to avoid air embolus.
  - Enter the vein during a positive pressure breath if the patient is on positive pressure ventilation.
- Watch for blood flashback in the hub.
- Stabilize the catheter assembly and advance the catheter over the stylet.
- Withdraw the stylet and occlude the catheter with your gloved thumb to avoid air embolus.
- Connect the tubing and saline-filled syringe, draw back, and flush.
- Secure the line with occlusive transparent dressing and tape.
- Reposition the child and retest the line.
  - The jugular vein has a number of valves that can obstruct the catheter when the neck position is altered.
  - Traction may be needed or the catheter may need to be withdrawn slightly to ensure proper function.

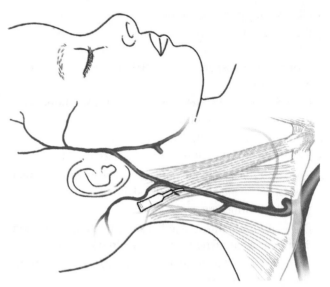

Figure 8–4. *Inserting IV into external jugular vein.*

Scalp IV

- Inspect the scalp for appropriate veins.
- A rubber band may be used to help fill the scalp veins.
- The area of the scalp over the vein may need to be shaved.
- Palpate for pulse in order to avoid inadvertent arterial cannulation.
- Cleanse the skin.
- Apply traction with your nondominant hand.
- Insert the catheter proximal to the site of the vein, advance slightly subcutaneously, then enter the vein (Figure 8–5).
- Watch for blood flashback.
  - If the vein is very small, there may be none.
  - If there is no flashback, rely on the change in resistance as you enter the vein.
- Advance the catheter over the stylet.
- Remove the rubber band (if used).
- Flush the assembly gently; watch for blanching, swelling, or mottling.
- Secure the IV with transparent occlusive dressing and tape.
- Attach to an infusion assembly.

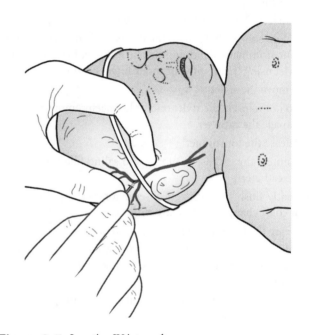

Figure 8–5. *Inserting IV into scalp.*

MONITORING

Peripheral IV in Extremity

- Compare extremity's color and temperature; watch for congestion and swelling.
- Watch for signs of occlusion.

- Palpate pulses.
- Ensure skin integrity.
- Check tightness of dressing.
- Inspect IV tubing for blood or precipitation.
- Monitor IV pump for increased resistance that may indicate clotting.
- Watch for pump malfunction.

Jugular Vein

- Monitor for swelling.
- Assess for signs of occlusion.

Scalp IV

- Monitor for swelling and blanching.
- Watch for signs of occlusion.
- Assess skin integrity.

Complications

- Infection.
- Hematoma.

- Skin ulceration.
- Air or particle embolism.
- Blood clot.
- Local ischemia.
- Phlebitis.

REFERENCES

Couzigou C, Lamory J, Salmon-Ceron D, Figard J, Vidal-Trecan GM. Short peripheral venous catheters: effect of evidence-based guidelines on insertion, maintenance and outcomes in a university hospital. *J Hosp Infect.* 2005;59:197–204.

Kahn JM, Kress JP, Hall JB. Skin necrosis after extravasation of low-dose vasopressin administered for septic shock. *Crit Care Med.* 2002;30:1899–1901.

Hazinksi MF et al, eds. *PALS Provider Manual.* Dallas, Texas: American Heart Association; 2002:159–160, 165–166.

Sandhu NP, Sidhu DS. Mid-arm approach to basilic and cephalic vein cannulation using ultrasound guidance. *Br J Anaesth.* 2004;93:292–294.

Straussberg R, Harel L, Bar-Sever Z, Amir J. Radial osteomyelitis as a complication of venous cannulation. *Arch Dis Child.* 2001;85:408–410.

CHAPTER 9

Intraosseous Line Insertion

Zehava Noah, MD

INDICATIONS

- Emergent temporary vascular access during cardiopulmonary resuscitation or during the treatment of uncompensated shock when unable to insert an intravenous line.
- Volume resuscitation.
- Administration of blood and blood products.
- Administration of fluids and electrolytes.
- Administration of medications.
- Infusion of inotropes and pressors.
- Sampling of blood and bone marrow.

CONTRAINDICATIONS

Absolute

- Do not insert in a recently fractured bone.
- Do not insert through an infected site.
- Osteogenesis imperfecta.
- Osteopetrosis.

Relative

- Osteoporosis or osteopenia.
- Cystic bones.

EQUIPMENT

- Intraosseous needle (18 or 20 gauge) or bone marrow aspiration needle.
- Povidone, chlorhexidine, and alcohol wipes.
- Gauze.
- Tape.
- Extension tubing.
- T-connector.
- Syringe.
- Gloves.

RISKS

- Infection.

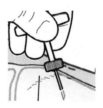

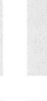

- **Caution: All equipment must be latex free.**

- Each of the risks listed is < 1%.

- Injury to growth plate.
- Bone fracture.
- Hematoma.
- Extravasation.
- Compartment syndrome.
- Severe vasoconstriction if vasoactive substances extravasate.

PEARLS AND TIPS

- Do not place hands under the site of insertion.
- Avoid administration of bone marrow–suppressing drugs.
- Avoid prolonged use. Replace with an intravenous line after the patient is stabilized.
- A properly placed unsupported needle will remain upright.
- Fluid should flow freely through the needle, and the line should flush without resistance.

PATIENT PREPARATION

- Introduce yourself to the parents and the patient.
- Explain the procedure.
- Choose the most appropriate site.
- Inject local anesthetic if the patient is conscious.

PATIENT POSITIONING

- Support the site of insertion over a firm surface.
- Hold the extremity above and below the insertion site.
- Position the patient with the selected site closest to where you are standing.

ANATOMY REVIEW

Recommended Sites of Intraosseous Insertion

A. INFANT
- Medial flat surface of the anterior tibia 1–2 cm below the tibial tuberosity.
- Direct the needle caudally to avoid the growth plate.
- Alternate site is the distal femur.

B. CHILD
- Medial flat surface of the anterior tibia 1–2 cm below the tibial tuberosity.
- Alternate site is the distal tibia.

C. ADOLESCENT
- Medial flat surface of the anterior tibia.
- Alternate sites include the following:
  - Distal tibia proximal to the medial malleolus.
  - Distal femur.

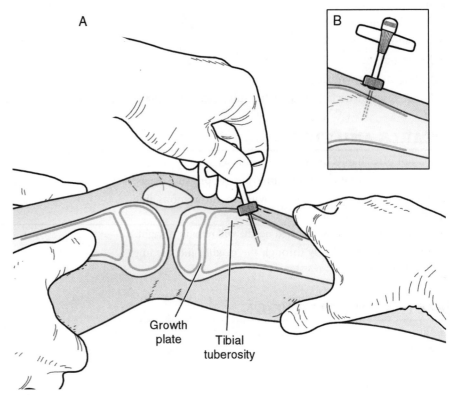

Figure 9–1. *Insertion site of intraosseous line.*

• Anterior superior iliac spine.

• Posterior superior iliac spine.

• Iliac crest.

PROCEDURE

■ Sanitize or wash your hands thoroughly and don gloves.

■ Use universal precautions or isolation precautions as appropriate.

■ Cleanse the site with antiseptic solution.

■ Support the leg on a firm surface and have an assistant support the leg above and below the insertion site.

■ Ensure no hand is under the site.

■ Administer local anesthetic if the patient is conscious.

■ Align needle bevel and stylet.

■ Insert needle assembly through the skin and advance to bone cortex.

■ Hold the needle perpendicular to the bone, and direct it away from the nearest joint (Figure 9–1).

■ Use a twisting motion when advancing the needle.

■ Stop advancing the needle when you feel a sudden decrease in resistance.

■ Unscrew the cap, remove the stylet, and attempt to aspirate bone marrow.

- The unsupported needle should remain upright if properly placed (see Figure 9–1).
- Flush the line with normal saline.
- Watch for increased resistance to the flush or swelling of the extremity.
- If no marrow is aspirated but you think you are in the bone marrow, attempt to flush.
- If you encounter resistance, advance needle assembly and reattempt aspiration.
- Fluid should flow freely through the needle and the line should flush without resistance.
- Use tape and gauze to secure the line.

MONITORING

- Watch for signs of compartment syndrome (pain, pallor, loss of pulses, and paresthesia or paralysis).
- Look for swelling, redness, blanching, and leakage.
- Assess for vasoconstriction.

COMPLICATIONS

- Extravasation.
- Compartment syndrome.
- Infection.
- Fracture.
- Injury to growth plate.

REFERENCES

Boon JM, Gorry DLA, Meiring JH. Finding an ideal site for intraosseous infusion of the tibia: an anatomical study. *Clin Anat.* 2002;16:15–18.

Bowley DM, Loveland J, Pitcher GJ. Tibial fracture as a complication of intraosseous infusion during pediatric resuscitation. *J Trauma.* 2003;55:786–787.

Claudet I, Baunin C, Laporte-Turpin E, Marcoux MO, Grouteau E, Cahuzac JP. Long-term effects on tibial growth after intraosseous infusion: a prospective radiographic analysis. *Pediatr Emerg Care.* 2003;19:397–401.

Hazinski MF et al. *PALS Provider Manual.* Dallas, Texas: American Heart Association; 2002:155–158.

Stoll E, Golej J, Burda G, Hermon M, Boigner H, Trittenwein G. Osteomyelitis at the injection site of adrenalin through an intraosseous needle in a 3-month-old infant. *Resuscitation.* 2002;53:315–318.

CHAPTER 10

Femoral Venous Catheterization

Kelly Michelson, MD

INDICATIONS

- Any situation that requires central venous access or venous access that cannot be obtained peripherally.
- An emergency resuscitation requiring administration of large amounts of fluids.
- The need for central venous pressure monitoring.
- Placement of a pulmonary artery catheter.
- The need for frequent blood draws.
- Infusion of hyperalimentation, concentrated solutions (ie, KCl, dextrose concentrations greater than 12.5%, chemotherapeutic agents, hyperosmolar saline).
- Infusion of vasoactive substances (ie, dopamine and norepinephrine) that can extravasate and cause soft-tissue necrosis.
- The need for hemodialysis.

Advantages of Catheter Placement at Femoral Site

- It does not interfere with procedures or monitoring involving the head, neck, or chest (such as cardiopulmonary resuscitation).
- Pressure can be applied easily in the event of femoral artery puncture or catheterization.
- It leaves the patient's neck free of devices.

Disadvantages of Catheter Placement at Femoral Site

- It is a relatively "dirty" area (though this can be managed with good sterile technique and dressing changes).
- Placement of a long line is required for central venous pressure monitoring.
- It can be challenging to place a pulmonary artery catheter through a femoral venous catheter.

CONTRAINDICATIONS

Absolute

- Severe abdominal trauma (provided that adequate venous access can be obtained elsewhere).

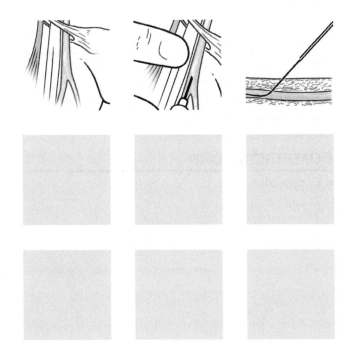

Relative

- A patient with distorted anatomy or landmarks.
- Risk factors for excessive bleeding, such as thrombocytopenia, coagulopathy, and anticoagulant or thrombolytic therapy.
- Skin lesions (such as cellulitis, burns, abrasions, or dermatitis).
- Conditions that predispose the patient to sclerosis or thrombosis (such as vasculitis).
- Known thrombus of the femoral vein.

EQUIPMENT

- The catheter.
- An appropriate size guidewire (at least 2 times the length of the catheter).
- An appropriate size introducer needle.
- A tissue dilator if the catheter is larger than 3F.
- Two or three 3- to 5-mL syringes.
- 1% lidocaine and a 26-gauge needle to inject the lidocaine.
- Skin preparation solution (either 2% chlorhexidine-based preparation for patients older than 2 months or 10% povidone-iodine).
- Sterile drapes.
- Scalpel blade.
- Suture (ie, 3.0 silk).
- Sterile gauze pads.

RISKS

- Bleeding (can usually be managed by applying pressure to the site).
- Infection (can be minimized with the use of good sterile technique during placement and regular catheter care).
- Embolization of the guidewire if the operator does not use proper technique.
- Vessel perforation.
- Embolization of a preexisting thrombus.

PEARLS AND TIPS

- Attach the insertion needle so that the numbers on the syringe are facing up when the bevel is in the upward position. This way, you will always know how to hold the syringe so that the bevel is facing upward.
- After the skin is punctured with the insertion needle, inject a small amount of saline (approximately 0.2 mL) into the subcutaneous tissue.
  - This will clear the needle of any skin plugs.
  - Alternatively, make a small knick in the skin with a 12- or 14-gauge needle at the puncture site prior to the procedure.

■ After the guidewire is passed through the catheter, attach a Kelly clamp to the wire. This will ensure that the wire does not get lost or hidden in the catheter and frees both hands to pass the catheter over the wire and into the vessel.

■ The distal end of the guidewire must be visible at all times.

PATIENT PREPARATION

■ The patient must be able to lie comfortably in the supine position and remain still throughout the procedure.

■ In the case of a child whose respiratory status is compromised in the supine position, it may be necessary to obtain definitive airway control (ie, intubate the patient) prior to the procedure.

■ Children who can comfortably lie supine may require conscious sedation so that they remain still throughout the procedure.

■ To avoid aspiration during intubation or conscious sedation, the procedure should be delayed 6 hours after the ingestion of solid food and 4 hours after the ingestion of clear liquids, unless central access is needed emergently.

PATIENT POSITIONING

■ Place the patient in the supine position.

■ Raise the hips slightly to flatten the inguinal area.

■ Position the patient with his or her legs extended or with the hips and knees slightly flexed in the "frog" position.

ANATOMY REVIEW

■ The important anatomic landmarks in femoral artery catheter placement include the femoral artery and the femoral vein (Figure 10–1).

■ The femoral artery and vein run in parallel with the artery lateral to the vein.

■ The inguinal ligament runs from the anterior superior iliac spine to the pubic tubercle.

■ Remember the mnemonic "NAVEL" (*n*erve, *a*rtery, *v*ein, *e*mpty space, *l*ymph), which describes the structures' anatomic location from lateral to medial.

PROCEDURE

■ The operator should wear a cap and mask, be scrubbed, and use a sterile gown and gloves for this procedure.

■ Prepare the area using either 2% chlorhexidine-based preparation for patients older than 2 months of age or 10% povidone-iodine.

■ Using the nondominant hand, palpate the femoral artery in 2 to 3 places to get a sense for the path of the artery (Figure 10–2).

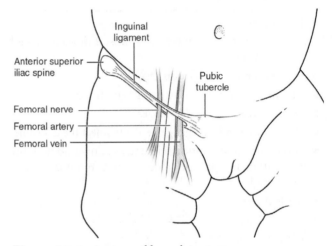

Figure 10–1. *Anatomy of femoral structures.*

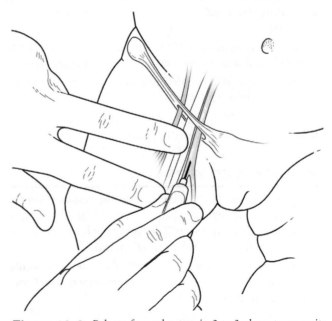

Figure 10–2. *Palpate femoral artery in 2 to 3 places to assess its path.*

- The femoral vein lies just medial to the artery and typically follows in parallel.
- Inject a local anesthetic (1% lidocaine) in the area of the venipuncture site and the tissues deep to the venipuncture site. Always withdraw the plunger slightly before injecting lidocaine to avoid injecting intravascularly.
- Flush all ports of the catheter with normal saline or heparinized saline prior to the procedure.
- The technique for placing the catheter is called the **Seldinger technique** (Figure 10–3).
- Attach the insertion needle to a syringe partially filled with saline.
- With the bevel of the insertion needle facing up (toward the ceiling) hold the needle and syringe at a 30- to 45-degree angle directing the needle toward the patient's umbilicus.
- Puncture the skin approximately 1–2 cm distal to the inguinal ligament in the location of the femoral vein (just medial to the palpated femoral artery).
- As the needle is slowly advanced, gently draw back on the syringe.
- When a free flow of blood appears remove the syringe.
- Insert the guidewire into the needle.
- The guidewire should pass easily through the needle into the vessel.
- Leave the distal end of the guidewire exposed.
- If resistance is met, redirect the needle or remove the guidewire and needle, apply pressure until the bleeding stops and begin the process over.
- **Do not force the guidewire into place.**
- Using the scalpel, make a small (approximately 2 mm) incision at the venipuncture site.
- Apply gentle pressure to the venipuncture site and remove the needle, leaving the guidewire in place.
- If the catheter is larger than 3F, thread the tissue dilator over the wire and advance it into the venipuncture site.
- It may be necessary to use a twisting action to advance the tissue dilator.
- Remove the tissue dilator.
- The guidewire should be exposed and visible continuously.
- Hold the guidewire with the nondominant hand and thread the catheter over the guidewire until the guidewire protrudes from the distal end of the catheter.
- It may be necessary to hold a little pressure at the insertion site if there is a significant amount of bleeding.
- Take the end of the guidewire with the nondominant hand and pass the catheter over the wire and into the vessel.
- Remove the guidewire.
- There should be good blood flow from all ports.
- Flush each port with attention to removing any air bubbles before flushing.

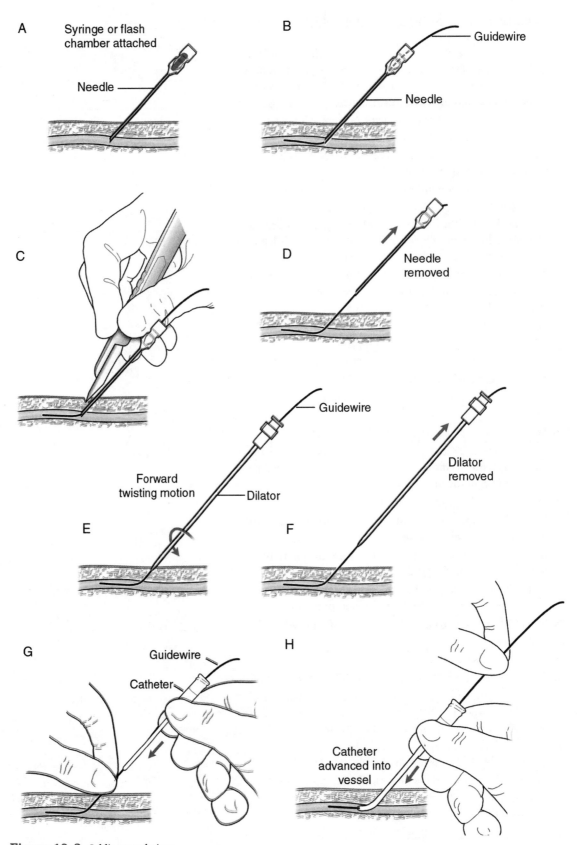

Figure 10–3. *Seldinger technique.*

- Suture the catheter in place.
- Cap off the catheter or attach it to IV tubing.

MONITORING

- If the catheter is correctly placed in the femoral vein, blood flow from the catheter should be steady, but not pulsatile.
- Verify correct placement by obtaining a venous gas and documenting an appropriate venous saturation.
- However, remember that placement confirmation using a blood gas can be unreliable in patients who have significant cardiopulmonary disease whose arterial oxygen saturation may be abnormally low or in hyperoxygenated patients whose venous oxygen saturation may be abnormally elevated.
- A more reliable method for verifying catheter placement is to transduce the catheter and confirm a venous waveform and pressure.

COMPLICATIONS

During Catheter Placement

- Bleeding, the main complication, often results from inadvertent artery puncture.
- Local hematomas.
- Bowel or bladder perforation.
- Air embolus.
- Catheter embolus.
- Creation of an arteriovenous fistula.

With Catheter in Place

- Infection.
- Current recommendations for limiting infectious complications include the following:
  - Strict adherence to sterile technique during catheter placement.
  - Use of 2% chlorhexidine-based preparation in patients older than 2 months of age.
  - Use of a catheter with the fewest number of lumens that is essential for treatment.
- Swelling of the lower extremity, resulting from impaired venous return.
  - The swelling can often be managed by elevating the leg.
  - Care should be taken to confirm palpable distal pulses in such cases.
- Deep venous thrombosis or inferior vena cava thrombosis.
- Catheter knotting.
- Catheter malposition (ie, insertion into the lumbar venous plexus, a potentially lethal complication).

FOLLOW-UP

- The catheter should be removed as soon as it is not needed.
- When catheter is no longer needed, remove the sutures and pull the catheter slowly and carefully.
- Apply pressure to the insertion site until the bleeding stops.

REFERENCES

Advanced Trauma Life Support Program for Doctors. 6th ed. Chicago, IL: American College of Surgeons; 1997.

Domino KB, Bowdle TA, Posner KL, Spitellie PH, Lee LA, Cheney FW. Injuries and liability related to central vascular catheters: a closed claims analysis. *Anesthesiology.* 2004;100: 1411–1418.

Gunn VL, Nechyba C, Johns Hopkins Hospital, Children's Medical and Surgical Center. *The Harriet Lane Handbook: A Manual for Pediatric House Officers.* 16th ed. Philadelphia: Mosby; 2002.

Gutierrez JA, Bagatell R, Samson MP, Theodorou AA, Berg RA. Femoral central venous catheter-associated deep venous thrombosis in children with diabetic ketoacidosis. *Crit Care Med.* 2003;31:80–83.

Hazinski MF et al, eds. *PALS Provider Manual.* Dallas, Texas: American Heart Association; 2002.

Journeycake JM, Buchanan GR. Thrombotic complications of central venous catheters in children. *Curr Opin Hematol.* 2003;10:369–374.

Lavandosky G, Gomez R, Montes J. Potentially lethal misplacement of femoral central venous catheters. *Crit Care Med.* 1996;24:893–896.

Merrer J, De Jonghe B, Golliot F et al; French Catheter Study Group in Intensive Care. Complications of femoral and subclavian venous catheterization in critically ill patients: a randomized controlled trial. *JAMA.* 2001;286:700–707.

Mickiewicz M, Dronen SC, Younger JG. Central Venous Catheterization and Central Venous Pressure Monitoring. In: Roberts JR, Hedges JR, eds. *Clinical Procedures in Emergency Medicine.* 4th ed. Philadelphia: WB Saunders; 2004.

O'Grady NP, Alexander M, Dellinger EP et al. Guidelines for the prevention of intravascular catheter-related infections. The Hospital Infection Control Practices Advisory Committee, Center for Disease Control and Prevention, u.s. *Pediatrics.* 2002;110(5):e51.

Roberts JR, Hedges JR, Chanmugam AS. *Clinical Procedures in Emergency Medicine.* 4th ed. Philadelphia: WB Saunders; 2004.

Rosen P. *Emergency Medicine Concepts and Clinical Practice.* 5th ed. St. Louis, MO: MD Consult LLC; 2002.

Shefler A, Gillis J, Lam A, O'Connell AJ, Schell D, Lammi A. Inferior vena cava thrombosis as a complication of femoral vein catheterisation. *Arch Dis Child.* 1995;72:343–345.

Talbott GA, Winters WD, Bratton SL, O'Rourke PP. A prospective study of femoral catheter-related thrombosis in children. *Arch Pediatr Adolesc Med.* 1995;149:288–291.

CHAPTER 11

Arterial Puncture

Zehava Noah, MD

INDICATIONS

- Collection of arterial blood for blood gas analysis to manage cardiopulmonary disorders and maintain acid-base balance.
- Collection of arterial blood when unable to sample venous blood to help manage fluid and electrolyte imbalance.

CONTRAINDICATIONS

Absolute

- Allen test indicates that collateral circulation is compromised.
- Circulatory defects.
- Sampling area is infected.

Relative

- Coagulation abnormalities, such as hypercoagulability or hypocoagulability.
- Patient has disease associated with hypercoagulability or hypocoagulability.
- Hematoma at site.
- Anatomic abnormalities in limb.

EQUIPMENT

- Gloves.
- 23-gauge or smaller butterfly needle.
- 1-mL heparinized syringe for blood gas sampling.
- Syringes for blood sampling.
- Disinfectant (povidone-iodine, chlorhexidine, and alcohol) swabs.
- Sterile gauze pads.
- Topical anesthetic.

RISKS

- Ischemia.
- Hematoma.

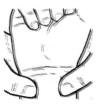
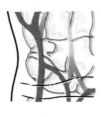
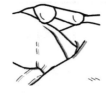

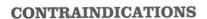

- Caution: All equipment must be latex free.

PEARLS AND TIPS

■ Use smallest gauge needle to minimize arterial trauma.

■ Hold pressure over puncture to prevent hematoma formation and bleeding.

■ The radial artery and the femoral artery are the preferred sites for arterial puncture.

■ If the pulse is hard to palpate, use Doppler and mark the location.

■ In small infants, the radial artery may be located by transillumination.

■ The Allen test involves the following:

  • Localizing and assessing the radial pulse.

  • Encircling the patient's wrist with your hand and elevating the hand.

  • Applying occlusive pressure on the radial and the ulnar arteries.

  • Releasing the ulnar artery and continuing to apply occlusive pressure on the radial artery.

  • Monitoring palmar blush.

PATIENT PREPARATION

■ Introduce yourself to the patient and parents.

■ Explain the procedure to the patient (if appropriate) and the parents.

■ Choose site of puncture.

■ Apply topical anesthetic to the site.

PATIENT POSITIONING

■ Position the patient with the puncture site within easy reach.

■ Have an assistant gently immobilize the extremity.

■ If using the femoral artery, open the femoral joint by elevating it over a rolled up towel.

ANATOMY REVIEW

Radial Artery

■ The palmar arch is composed of the radial and ulnar arteries and connecting palmar arteries (Figure 11–1).

■ The radial artery is located at the wrist proximal to the head of the radius.

■ In most patients, collateral circulation is dependent on an intact ulnar artery.

Femoral Artery

■ The femoral artery is located below the inguinal ligament over the femoral gutter halfway between the pubic symphysis and the anterior superior iliac spine (Figure 11–2).

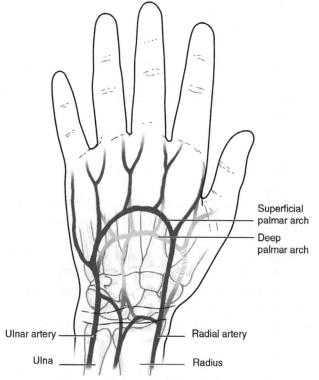

Figure 11–1. *Anatomy of radial artery.*

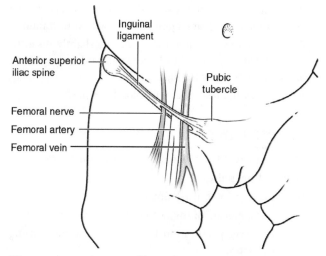

Figure 11–2. *Anatomy of femoral structures.*

- The femoral artery lies in the gutter lateral to the femoral vein.

PROCEDURE

- Assemble equipment.
- Review collection syringes and test tubes.
- Don gloves.
- Remove butterfly needle from packaging.

Radial Artery

- Have assistant gently hold the forearm.
- Palpate the radial pulse.
- Perform Allen test; proceed only if test demonstrates collateral circulation (Figure 11–3).
- With your nondominant hand, hold the patient's hand palm up in a neutral position.
- Hold all the patient's fingers in the palm of your nondominant hand.
- Palpate radial artery with your dominant hand.
- Disinfect site.
- Break the skin with the butterfly needle at a 30- to 45-degree angle proximal to the crease between the hand and the wrist (Figure 11–4).
- Flatten the angle and advance the butterfly needle proximally until blood flashback is seen in the tubing.
- If the needle perforates the artery, gently withdraw it until flashback is seen in the tubing.
- Fill syringe and test tubes with arterial blood sample.

Femoral Artery

- Palpate the pulse with your nondominant hand.
- Don gloves.
- Disinfect puncture site.
- Palpate the artery with the second and third fingers of your nondominant hand, and apply traction with your thumb.
- Break the skin with the butterfly needle slightly distal to the palpated pulse at an 80-degree angle and advance until blood appears in the tubing.
- Fill syringes and test tubes with blood samples.

MONITORING

- Monitor extremity for hematoma formation.
- Palpate distal pulses.
- If unable to palpate, use Doppler.
- Assess temperature of the extremity.
- Measure oxygen saturation levels of the extremity using pulse oximetry.

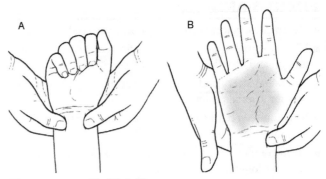

A   B

Figure 11–3. *Modified Allen test.*

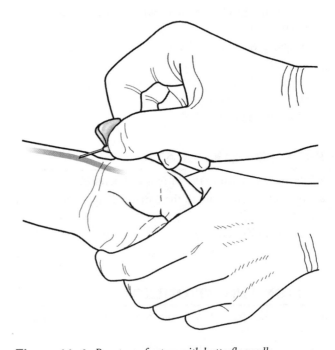

Figure 11–4. *Puncture of artery with butterfly needle.*

COMPLICATIONS

- Hematoma.
- Infected hematoma.
- Ischemia.
- Thrombus.

REFERENCES

Barbeau GR, Arsenault F, Dugas L, Simard S, Lariviere MM. Evaluation of the ulnopalmar arterial arches with pulse oximetry and plethysmography: comparison with the Allen's test in 1010 patients. *Am Heart J.* 2004;147:489–493.

Davison BD, Polak JF. Arterial injuries: a sonographic approach. *Radiol Clin North Am.* 2004;42:383–396.

Hazinski MF et al, eds. *PALS Provider Manual.* Dallas, Texas: American Heart Association; 2002.

CHAPTER 12

Umbilical Artery Cannulation

Janine Y. Khan, MD and Robin H. Steinhorn, MD

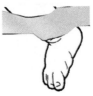

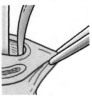

INDICATIONS

- Frequent or continuous measurement of blood gases.
- Continuous monitoring of arterial blood pressure.
- Infusion of maintenance glucose-electrolyte solutions.
- Exchange transfusion.

CONTRAINDICATIONS

Absolute

- Local vascular compromise in lower extremities or buttock area.
- Omphalitis.
- Abdominal wall defects (eg, omphalocele, gastroschisis).
- Necrotizing enterocolitis.

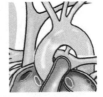

Relative

- Peritonitis.

EQUIPMENT

- Sterile catheter
  - Use 3.5F catheter for patients weighing < 1500 g.
  - Use 5F catheter for patients weighing > 1500 g.
- Sterile umbilical catheter tray includes the following:
  - Sterile drapes.
  - Povidone-iodine and alcohol swabs.
  - Umbilical tie.
  - Toothed iris forceps.
  - 2 curved non-toothed hemostats.
  - Suture scissors.
  - Small needle holder.
  - 3-0 silk suture on small curved needle.
  - 3-way stopcock with Luer-Lok.
  - 3-mL and 1-mL syringes with needles.
  - 2 × 2 gauze.

• 4 × 4 gauze.

• Saline solution with heparin 1 unit/mL.

RISKS

■ Although serious complications have been reported from arterial catheterization, very few are seen in practice if adequate precautions are observed.

■ Bacterial colonization of umbilical arterial catheters has been reported to be as high as 60%; however, bacteremia occurs in less than 5% of infants.

  • The risk of infection is minimized by placing the catheter under sterile conditions and using a sterile technique for blood sampling from the catheter.

  • Infection risks are low because most infants who require an umbilical arterial catheter are receiving antibiotic therapy for other reasons.

■ Hemorrhage may occur if the catheter inadvertently becomes disconnected or dislodged; however, this is avoided by maintaining exposure of the umbilical site at all times in an isolette or radiant warmer, together with constant nursing supervision.

■ Approximately 5% of catheters decrease circulation to 1 or both legs, especially in infants weighing < 1000 grams.

  • If this occurs, the catheter should be removed.

  • Circulation usually returns to the extremity within an hour.

■ Embolization and thrombosis can occur.

PEARLS AND TIPS

■ Always observe the infant's face, chest, and lower extremities during catheter placement.

■ Carefully dilate the lumen of the artery before attempting to introduce the catheter.

■ Do not attempt to force the catheter past an obstruction; this may result in vessel perforation requiring surgical intervention and blood volume replacement.

■ Once secured, never advance nonsterile portions of the catheter into the vessel. If the catheter needs to be advanced, it should be replaced.

■ Insertion of an umbilical arterial catheter to a "high" position is associated with fewer complications and is generally preferred.

■ Always confirm catheter position on radiograph before use.

PATIENT PREPARATION

■ Place the infant on a radiant warmer.

■ Place chest leads for continuous cardiorespiratory monitoring and a sensor for pulse oximetry monitoring throughout the procedure.

■ Measure the distance from the tip of the shoulder to the umbilicus, and calculate the length of catheter insertion needed (Figure 12–1).
- High line: shoulder to umbilical distance + 2 cm; **or** 3 × birth weight (kg) + 9 cm
- Low line: birth weight (kg) + 7 cm

PATIENT POSITIONING

■ Place the infant in the supine position, and secure the upper and lower extremities (see Figure 12–1).

ANATOMY REVIEW

■ Umbilical artery traverses downward and then upward into the internal iliac artery.

■ The umbilical arteries are the direct continuation of the internal iliac arteries and bypass branches to the superior and inferior gluteal arteries.

■ Umbilical artery continues from internal iliac artery to common iliac artery and subsequently into the aorta.

PROCEDURE

■ Assistant should grasp cord with forceps and pull cord vertically out of the sterile field.

■ Clean cord and surrounding skin with povidone-iodine and alcohol solutions.

■ Place umbilical tie loosely at the base of the umbilicus to control bleeding.

■ Drape the infant with sterile drapes with head and feet visible.

■ Cut the cord horizontally with a scalpel, approximately 1–2 cm from the skin.

■ Identify vessels—usually 2 arteries and 1 vein (Figure 12–2).
- The arteries are white thick structures with pinpoint opening sometimes protruding slightly from the Wharton's jelly.
- The vein is a large, thin-walled gaping vessel lying superiorly.

■ Apply 2 curved, non-toothed hemostats to the Wharton's jelly on opposite sides of the cord and apply traction to stabilize the cord for cannulation (Figure 12–3).

■ Gently introduce 1 point of the fine curved iris forceps into the lumen to a depth of 0.5 cm.

■ Withdraw forceps from the lumen, insert the closed tip of the iris forceps gently into the lumen to a depth of 1 cm.
- Allow the tips of the forceps to spread apart.
- Maintain forceps in this position for approximately 1 minute to overcome arterial spasm (see Figure 12–3).

■ Grasp the heparinized saline–filled catheter between the points of a second iris forceps, and introduce the catheter

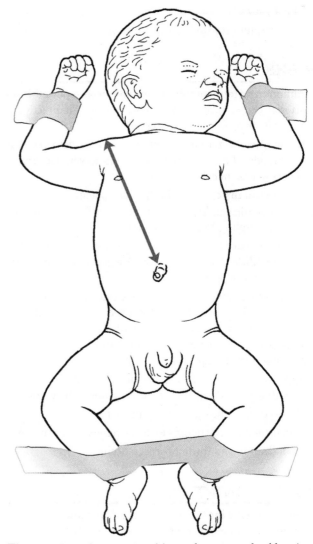

Figure 12–1. *Secure extremities and measure shoulder tip to umbilicus.*

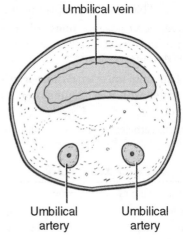

Figure 12–2. *Cross sectional view of umbilical arteries and vein.*

between the separated points of curved forceps in the vessel lumen to approximately 1–2 cm.

- Remove the initial curved forceps and apply traction to the cord, pulling the stump toward the infant's head to straighten the artery as it makes the angle between the umbilicus and the anterior abdominal wall.
- **At this stage, false passages into the vessel wall can be created, resulting in failed cannulation.**
- Continue to gently advance the catheter to approximately 5 cm, and aspirate for blood return to confirm intraluminal placement.
- **Never force the catheter through an obstruction.**
- Once the anterior abdominal wall angle is passed, there is a second sharp turn in the vessel as it angles around the bladder toward the internal iliac artery (Figure 12–4).
- Once this second angle is passed, the catheter may be advanced to the estimated distance required.
- Check lower extremities for discoloration.
- Secure catheter in position with a purse-string suture to the base of the cord with several loops around the catheter.
- Once hemostasis is achieved, remove the umbilical tie at the base of the umbilicus.
- Obtain a chest and abdominal film to check catheter tip position and adjust position to safe level between T6–T10 (or below L3–L4 if a low position is desired).

MONITORING

- High line placement is above the diaphragm at T8–T10 (above the origin of the celiac axis).
- Low line placement is at L3–L4 (just above the aortic bifurcation and below the origin of the inferior mesenteric artery).
- Avoid placing the catheter tip below the diaphragm or above L3.

COMPLICATIONS

- Because complications are usually related to the catheter tip, avoid positioning the tip at the level of the inferior mesenteric artery (L3–L4), renal artery (L1–L2), superior mesenteric artery (L1–L2), or celiac axis (T12–L1).

Complications Resulting from Impaired Circulation

- Pale, mottled legs, thighs, or buttocks.
- Discolored toes.
- Hematuria.
- Abdominal distention.
- Blood in stool.

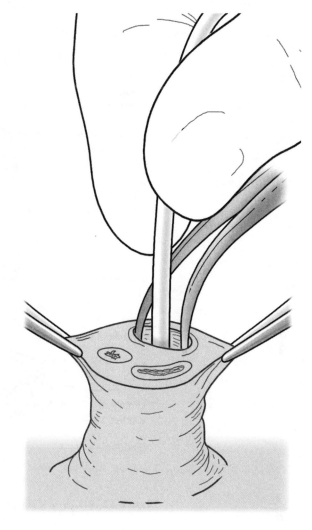

Figure 12–3. *Introduction of catheter.*

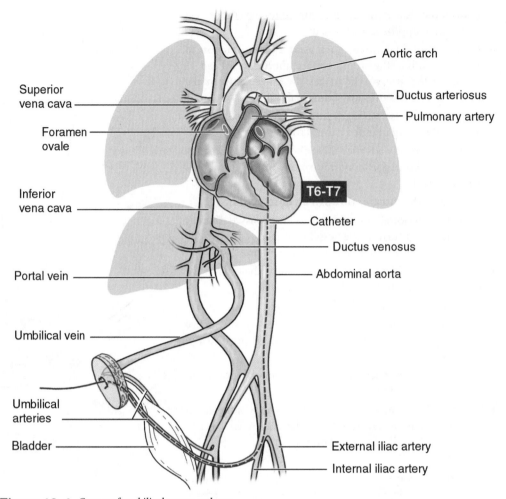

Figure 12–4. *Course of umbilical artery catheter.*

■ Confirmed necrotizing enterocolitis.

• However, in controlled studies, the presence of an umbilical arterial catheter has not been associated with necrotizing enterocolitis.

• The catheter should always be removed if there are signs of necrotizing enterocolitis.

Embolic and Thrombotic Complications

■ Renal infarction causing hypertension.

■ Ileofemoral thrombosis causing loss of limb.

■ Skin sloughing over the buttocks.

■ Embolization to the gut causing localized perforation or necrotizing enterocolitis.

CAVEATS

■ Dilatation of the artery before cannulation contributes greatly to successful cannulation of the umbilical artery.

■ Sometimes the catheter will not pass into the aorta due to arterial spasm or creation of a false passage.

■ Alternatively, the catheter passes into the aorta, but a white/blue leg or blue toes develop due to vasospasm.

• Warm compresses may be applied to the contralateral leg to promote reflex vasodilatation in cases of mild vasospasm.

• However, if severe, or if no improvement is noted, the catheter should be removed.

■ The incidence of the above complications is very low if the catheter is always infused with heparinized solution and always removed when early signs of emboli or vascular compromise are noted.

REFERENCES

MacDonald MG. *Atlas of Procedures in Neonatology.* 3rd ed. Philadelphia: Lippincott Williams and Wilkins; 2002.

Rennie JM, Roberton NRC. *A Manual of Neonatal Intensive Care.* 4th ed. London: Hodder Arnold; 2002.

Speidel B, Fleming P, Henderson J et al. *A Neonatal Vade-Mecum.* 3rd ed. London: Hodder Arnold; 1998.

CHAPTER 13

Umbilical Vein Cannulation

Janine Y. Khan, MD and Robin H. Steinhorn, MD

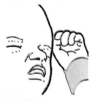
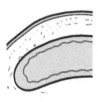
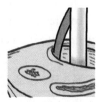

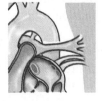

INDICATIONS

- Emergency vascular access for fluid and medications.
- Administration of high glucose concentration and total parenteral nutrition.
- Central venous pressure monitoring.
- Exchange transfusion.

CONTRAINDICATIONS

Absolute

- Omphalitis.
- Abdominal wall defects (eg, omphalocele, gastroschisis).
- Necrotizing enterocolitis.
- Umbilical surgery.
- Peritonitis.

EQUIPMENT

- Sterile catheter.
  - Use 3.5F catheter for patients weighing < 1500 g.
  - Use 5F catheter for patients weighing > 1500 g.
- Sterile umbilical catheter tray includes the following:
  - Sterile drapes.
  - Povidone-iodine swabs.
  - Umbilical tie.
  - Toothed iris forceps.
  - 2 curved non-toothed hemostats.
  - Suture scissors.
  - Small needle holder.
  - 3-0 silk suture on small curved needle.
  - 3-way stopcock with Luer-Lok.
  - 3-mL and 1-mL syringes with needles.
  - 2 × 2 gauze.
  - 4 × 4 gauze.
  - Saline solution with heparin 1 unit/mL.

RISKS

- Although serious complications have been reported from venous catheterization, very few are seen in practice if adequate precautions are observed.
- The risk of infection is minimized by placing the catheter under sterile conditions and using a sterile technique for blood sampling from the catheter.
- Catheters should be removed after 7 days of use to further decrease the chance of infection.
- Hemorrhage may occur if the catheter inadvertently becomes disconnected or dislodged; however, this is avoided by maintaining exposure of the umbilical site at all times in an isolette or radiant warmer, together with constant nursing supervision.
- Embolization and thrombosis can occur.

PEARLS AND TIPS

- Position the catheter tip away from the origin of hepatic vessels, portal vein, and foramen ovale; the tip should lie in the inferior vena cava just below its junction with the right atrium.
- **Never force the catheter past an obstruction.**
- Once secured, never advance nonsterile portions of the catheter into the vessel. If the catheter needs to be advanced, it should be replaced.
- Avoid hypertonic infusions when catheter tip is not in the inferior vena cava.
- Do not leave the catheter open to the atmosphere due to the danger of air embolus.
- Always confirm catheter position on radiograph before use. The only exception is when an umbilical venous catheter is inserted for resuscitation in the delivery room; in this case a low-lying catheter should be used.

PATIENT PREPARATION

- Place the infant on a radiant warmer.
- Place chest leads for continuous cardiorespiratory monitoring and a sensor for pulse oximetry monitoring throughout the procedure.
- Measure the distance from the tip of the shoulder and umbilicus and calculate the length of catheter insertion needed.
  - $^2/_3$ of shoulder-umbilical cord distance.
  - $^1/_2$ of UAC line calculation.

PATIENT POSITIONING

- Place the infant in the supine position, and secure the upper and lower extremities (Figure 13–1).

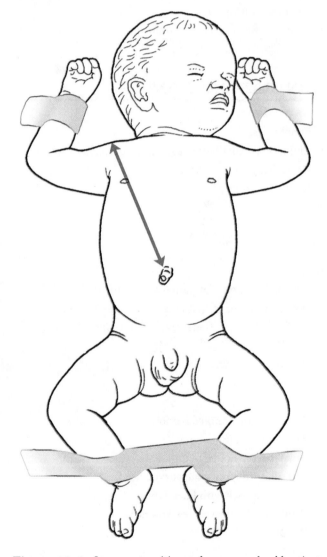

Figure 13–1. *Secure extremities and measure shoulder tip to umbilicus.*

ANATOMY REVIEW

- In the full-term infant, the umbilical vein is approximately 2–3 cm long. It is directed cephalad and usually lies to the right of the umbilicus.
- The umbilical vein gives off several large intrahepatic branches directly to the liver before joining the left branch of the portal vein.
- The ductus venosus arises from the left branch of the portal vein and becomes a continuation of the umbilical vein.
  - It is located in the groove between the right and left lobes of the liver at the level of the 9th–10th thoracic vertebrae.
  - It terminates in the inferior vena cava along with hepatic veins.

PROCEDURE

- Carefully clean the cord and surrounding skin with povidone-iodine and alcohol solutions.
- Place an umbilical tie at the base of the umbilicus to control bleeding.
- Drape the infant with sterile drapes with head and feet visible.
- Cut the cord horizontally with a scalpel, approximately 1–2 cm above the skin.
- Identify vessels—usually 2 arteries and 1 vein. The vein is a large, thin-walled gaping vessel lying superiorly (Figure 13–2).
- Grasp the umbilical stump on either side with the curved hemostats (Figure 13–3).
- Remove visible clots in the lumen with a forceps.
- Gently insert the tip of the iris forceps into the lumen of the vein and dilate as needed. In general, minimal dilation is needed.
- Insert the heparinized saline-filled catheter attached to a stopcock and syringe into the vessel while applying gentle traction on the cord.
- Advance in a cephalad direction to the estimated catheter length (Figure 13–4).
- Aspirate gently. If there is smooth blood flow, secure in place and obtain chest and abdominal radiographs to verify position.

MONITORING

- The ideal location of the tip of the umbilical catheter is T9–10, just above the right hemidiaphragm and below the heart.
- On a radiograph, the catheter will lie to the right of the vertebral column in the inferior vena cava.

COMPLICATIONS

- Hemorrhage from displacement of the catheter or perforation of the umbilical artery.

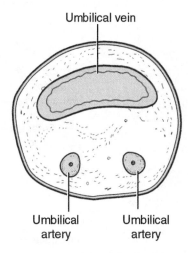

Figure 13–2. *Cross sectional view of umbilical arteries and vein.*

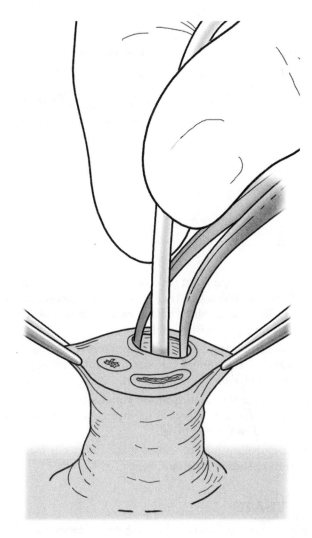

Figure 13–3. *Introduction of catheter.*

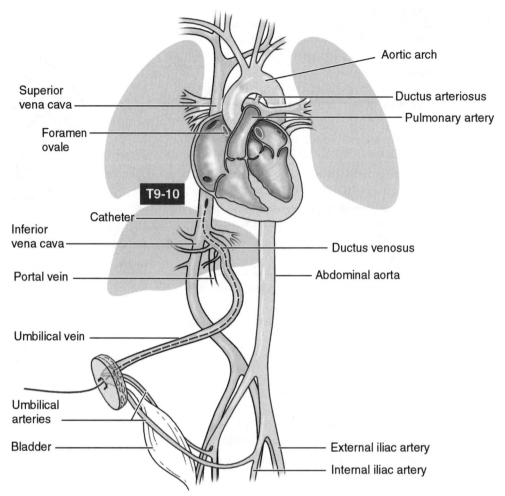

Figure 13–4. *Course of umbilical venous catheter.*

- There is a significant risk of infection. Portal venous thrombophlebitis can later lead to portal hypertension; therefore, the umbilical venous catheter should be left in place for the shortest possible time.
- Catheter malpositioned in heart or great vessels may lead to cardiac arrhythmias, cardiac tamponade, cardiac perforation, or thrombotic endocarditis.
- Catheter malpositioned in the portal system may cause hepatic necrosis, especially if hypertonic solutions are infused into the liver tissue.
- Air embolism may be caused if the catheter is inadvertently opened to the atmosphere.

CAVEATS

- If the catheter meets resistance before achieving its estimated distance, it has most likely entered the portal system or an intrahepatic branch of the umbilical vein.

- During resuscitation in the delivery room, radiographic confirmation of catheter placement is usually not possible; therefore, always dilute medications and infusions.
- Always check the position of the catheter tip before exchange transfusion. The tip should not be in the portal system or intrahepatic venous branch.

REFERENCES

MacDonald MG. *Atlas of Procedures in Neonatology.* 3rd ed. Philadelphia: Lippincott Williams and Wilkins; 2002.

Rennie JM, Roberton NRC. *A Manual of Neonatal Intensive Care.* 4th ed. London: Hodder Arnold; 2002.

Speidel B, Fleming P, Henderson J et al. *A Neonatal Vade-Mecum.* 3rd ed. London: Hodder Arnold; 1998.

[PART II]

PROCEDURES BY ORGAN SYSTEM

[CHAPTER 14]

Sedation and Pain Management

Stephen Crotty, MD

INDICATIONS

- Cases that require a relatively motionless child in order to provide adequate working conditions.
- Invasive procedures, such as laceration repair, lumbar puncture, and orthopedic procedures.
- Diagnostic imaging studies.
- Due to the risk of oversedation or an allergic response to a sedative, sedation is indicated only if absolutely necessary.

CONTRAINDICATIONS

- History of an allergy or other untoward reaction to previous sedation attempts.
- Facial dysmorphism or deformity or anatomic variation that would make maintaining airway competency difficult (ie, Pierre Robin syndrome or Goldenhar syndrome). In these cases, consultation with an anesthesiologist is warranted.
- The presence of upper respiratory infection.
  - Although not an absolute contraindication, sedation should be approached with caution.
  - In a patient with clear lung fields but rhinorrhea, glycopyrrolate or atropine can be used prior to sedation to aid in drying secretions.
- The presence of lower airway symptoms, such as wheezing.
  - For nonemergent sedations, rescheduling should be strongly considered.
  - For emergent sedations, pretreatment with nebulized albuterol and use of ketamine should be considered.

EQUIPMENT

- Vital signs must be assessed before, during, and after the sedation process.
- Pulse oximetry should be recorded regularly.
  - Derangements in pulse oximetry may be the first sign of a problem, perhaps stemming from hypoventilation or laryngospasm.

[▪ ▪ ▪]

- Although there are few absolute contraindications, the points presented here are important to consider when weighing the risks and benefits of the sedation procedure.

- Capnography, while not widely used, had been studied recently as an adjuvant in monitoring patients during sedation.
  - There is some evidence that elevation of carbon dioxide as measured by inline capnography may be a reliable early indicator of respiratory compromise from oversedation.

RISKS

- Loss of airway patency; if unrecognized, hypoventilation or upper airway obstruction can lead to hypoxemia and respiratory arrest.
- Circulatory collapse can be induced by peripheral vasodilation and direct myocardial effects of some drugs.
- Potential for aspiration is increased with deep sedation because the gag reflex is lost.
- Allergic reactions are uncommon but do occur. The physician must be able to quickly diagnose and intervene if anaphylaxis begins.

PEARLS AND TIPS

- Terms such as "conscious sedation" and "twilight sleep" are misleading as any degree of sedation has potential to change to deep anesthesia and must be approached with this in mind.
- Practitioners who sedate patients must be skilled in advanced airway management, pediatric advanced life support, and in assessment of patients for changing levels of sedative effects.
- Trained support staff and resuscitation equipment and drugs must also be immediately available.
- Sedation should be initiated in a controlled environment. No sedation medications should be given by the parents on the way to the hospital or office, as was once common.

PATIENT PREPARATION

- Although complications from sedation are infrequent, the physician must be prepared for any clinical situation.
- In addition to being prepared for airway and cardiovascular emergencies, the qualified sedation practitioner must supervise or perform the following:
  - Adequate presedation clinical evaluation.
  - Formulation of a sedation plan.
  - Adequate monitoring during and after the sedation process.
  - Documentation, including details of drug administration, monitoring record, and occurrence of any complications (eg, airway obstruction, emesis, allergic reactions, paradoxical reactions to sedatives).
  - Fulfillment of preestablished criteria before discharge from a monitoring environment.
  - Appropriate management of pain.

Presedation Evaluation

- A thorough presedation evaluation is necessary before any drug administration. This screening process concentrates on past and current medical conditions, previous reactions to sedatives or to general anesthetics, and known drug allergies.
- A history of snoring, mouth breathing, asthma, or recent upper respiratory tract infections suggests possible airway obstruction or increased secretions.
- A history of difficult intubations or sleep apnea may require referral for consultation with an anesthesiologist or otolaryngologist (or both) prior to the procedure.
- A focused inspection of the airway must explore potential airway difficulties due to adenotonsillar hypertrophy, micrognathia, or other abnormal airway anatomy.
- The cardiovascular assessment should elicit information about the following:
  - Congenital heart defects.
  - Heart murmurs.
  - Presence of a pacemaker.
  - Previous cardiovascular surgical procedures.
  - Cyanosis.
  - Fatigue.
  - Failure of growth.
- Neurologic evaluation includes notation of shunts, neurologic abnormalities, and seizure disorder.
- Important gastrointestinal issues to address are reflux and liver disease.
- Compromise of renal function and the frequency of dialysis should be noted.
- Exposure to infectious diseases should be recorded.
- The presence of an organ transplant must be documented.
- Finally, endocrine screening must evaluate the possibility of diabetes and questions should be asked about pituitary and thyroid dysfunction.
  - Patients with pituitary dysfunction routinely are given stress-dose corticosteroids prior to sedation under the guidance of an endocrinologist.
- The patient's fasting status should be reviewed before drug administration.
  - Children aged younger than 6 months should not ingest milk or solids for 4 hours before elective sedation.
  - Children older than 6 months should not ingest milk for 6 hours before elective sedation.
- Clear liquids may be given up to 2 hours prior to sedation in all age groups.
- Patients at risk for regurgitation or aspiration (eg, children with known reflux or extreme obesity) may benefit from prolonged fasting or pharmacologic therapy to reduce gastric volume and acidity.

- Hydration with intravenous fluids is often necessary after prolonged fasting, particularly in young infants.
- In an emergency department, waiting many hours prior to sedation may not be an option.
- Although fasting is preferred, there is little evidence to show patients who have not fasted have worse outcomes, such as aspiration, than those who fasted.

PROCEDURE

Sedation Options for Painful Procedures

A. KETAMINE

- Onset of sedation and analgesia is extremely rapid (as little as 30 seconds).
- Duration ranges from 15 minutes to 30 minutes.
- Ketamine produces a trance-like state that is quite distinct from the sleep state induced by other agents.
- Nystagmus, open blank staring eyes, and purposeless occasional jerking movement all occur with ketamine sedation.
- The myoclonic jerking may necessitate an alternate drug choice if the patient must remain absolutely motionless for the procedure.
- Nausea and vomiting, which occurs in approximately 20% of children, can be attenuated by concurrent administration with midazolam.
- Emergence reactions (hallucinations) occur significantly more frequently in adults than in children.
- Atropine or glycopyrrolate is given with ketamine to diminish the hypersalivation induced by ketamine and minimize the potential that such secretions trigger laryngospasm.
- Ketamine also has potent bronchodilatory effects that might make it a useful choice for sedating asthmatic patients.
- Ketamine should not be used in patients with significant eye injuries or acute neurologic injuries because it can increase intraocular and intracranial pressures.

B. OPIOIDS

- Morphine and fentanyl are the opioids most commonly used as adjuncts to relieve pain during the sedation process.
- The side effects associated with meperidine have virtually eliminated its use in pediatric sedation.
- For painful procedures that last 30 minutes or longer, morphine is often combined with a benzodiazepine; for shorter procedures, fentanyl is used instead of morphine.
- Adverse effects of narcotic administration include chest wall rigidity, respiratory suppression or arrest, and nausea.

- One benefit to using opioids for sedation is that naloxone can be used to reverse their effects.
  - Naloxone works quickly, but has a shorter duration than the narcotics.
  - Therefore, you must be prepared to continue to administer naloxone and to observe the patient to prevent an adverse outcome.

Sedation Options for Nonpainful Procedures

A. BENZODIAZEPINES

- Midazolam and diazepam are the most commonly administered benzodiazepines for pediatric sedation.
- Midazolam is often combined with other medications, as described for the management of painful procedures.
  - It has a rapid onset and duration.
  - It can be given orally, intranasally, intramuscularly, or intravenously, providing the practitioner with multiple routes of administration.
  - Midazolam may produce retrograde and anterograde amnesia, which can be helpful for painful or anxiety-provoking procedures.
- Diazepam, which has a longer duration than midazolam (1 hour or more), is used less frequently for sedation in children.
- Diazepam is quite useful for treating muscle spasms, such as torticollis or those experienced by patients with cerebral palsy.
- Benzodiazepine administration can produce respiratory depression and paradoxical reactions that include extreme agitation and confusion.
- Benzodiazepine drug effects can be reversed with administration of flumazenil, which displaces benzodiazepines from the GABA receptor.
- The duration of flumazenil is shorter than that of the benzodiazepines, necessitating prolonged observation of the patient and possible repeated doses.
- Children who have been taking benzodiazepines long term are at risk for having seizures when flumazenil is given to them.

B. BARBITURATES

- Pentobarbital is commonly used as a sedative for long nonpainful procedures, such as a magnetic resonance imaging scan or bone scan.
- Ideal working conditions are obtained within 5 minutes of drug administration and often can be maintained for up to 1 hour.
- Thiopental can be used for studies of short duration.
  - Thiopental offers some advantages to patients with increased intracranial pressure, since it produces a dose-

dependent depression of cerebral metabolism, cerebral blood flow, and intracranial pressure.

- The quick duration of thiopental's effect is the result of redistribution of the drug as the drug's half-life is actually quite long.

- Extended postprocedural observation may be required when multiple doses of thiopental have been given.

- Side effects of thiopental administration include histamine release, which may be a relative contraindication for its use in asthma patients.

■ All barbiturates can cause profound hypotension via venodilation, direct myocardial depression, and depression of the baroreflex mechanism.

■ The patient's family should be informed about emergence reactions that may occur after sedation with barbiturates.

■ Such reactions occur fairly frequently in children and can be quite alarming to the unprepared family.

■ The signs of an emergence reaction are extreme agitation, inconsolable crying or screaming, and often kicking and punching.

■ It is important to counsel the family that their child cannot respond to reasoning during an emergence reaction.

■ The goals of managing such reactions are to keep the patient safe and to treat the reaction, if possible.

■ Treatment decision is based on whether the patient is in the midst of a reaction or if it has gone on for several minutes and appears to be ending.

■ Administration of midazolam, meperidine, physostigmine, or even oral caffeine (eg, soft drink) has been shown to be beneficial.

■ Emergence reactions may be attenuated or even avoided by administration of benzodiazepines with barbiturates.

C. Chloral Hydrate

■ This drug may be used effectively in infants and toddlers for brief procedures.

■ Chloral hydrate may be given by mouth or per rectum.

■ Onset is within 15 minutes and duration can be as long as 2 hours.

■ The half-life of the drug is long, which may necessitate longer observation and may prevent the patient from safely undergoing sedation within the next 24 hours if additional studies are needed.

■ Side effects include respiratory depression and hypoxia.

■ Despite its broad use, and the widespread belief that it is a very safe drug, chloral hydrate has been associated with deaths.

D. Etomidate

■ Etomidate, like ketamine, induces a trance-like state.

■ Etomidate acts as a sedative-hypnotic, though it lacks any analgesic properties.

■ Etomidate is used both in rapid-sequence intubation and in procedural sedation, such as fracture reductions.

■ Side effects include transient hypoventilation or apnea, pain at site of injection, or myoclonus.

■ Etomidate-induced myoclonus can look like seizure activity.

■ When etomidate is administered with a benzodiazepine, myoclonus can be decreased or eliminated.

■ Unlike ketamine, no increase in intracranial pressure is noted with etomidate.

MONITORING

■ The recovery area must contain monitoring and resuscitation equipment equivalent to that available and used during the sedation process.

■ Oxygen saturation and heart rate need to be continuously monitored for at least 15 minutes *after* the patient reaches appropriate discharge criteria.

■ Patients should be observed for at least 2 hours following administration of reversal agents, since the half-life of the reversal agent is generally less than that of the sedating agents being reversed.

■ Infants younger than 3 months and preterm infants younger than 60 weeks of postconceptional age may require an extended period of observation even after apparent recovery due to the risk of apnea.

■ For the purposes of initiating monitoring and for providing the necessary personnel, all patients should be considered deeply sedated until they have demonstrated a stable lesser level of sedation.

■ Patients who fulfill moderate sedation criteria may then be monitored at that level of intensity until they recover.

■ The sedation team members must be aware that a patient may regress to a deeper level of sedation without warning, and monitoring is essential.

COMPLICATIONS

■ Increased sleeping, irritability, and decreased appetite are common after sedation.

■ Head position during transport home in a car seat must be adjusted to ensure a patent airway if the patient falls asleep.

■ Resumption of food intake should be done slowly because residual dizziness may lead to an upset stomach. It is best to begin with sips of clear liquids followed by a small meal of light foods.

■ Parents need to be well informed about what to expect during the hours after their child has been sedated. Parents should also be prepared for the possibility of admission to the hospital if their child does not meet the criteria for discharge.

■ While postsedation admission to the hospital is rare, it is certainly required when the child is overly sleepy or when severe nausea and vomiting develop.

—————————————{ ■■■ }——————————————

■ Postsedation guidelines given to the family should describe the symptoms requiring parents to contact their physician or the physician at the facility who administered the sedatives or to call 911.

REFERENCES

American Academy of Pediatrics, Committee on Drugs: Guidelines for monitoring and management of pediatric patients during and after sedation for diagnostic and therapeutic procedures. *Pediatrics.* 1992;89:1110–1115.

American Society of Anesthesiologists Task Force on Sedation and Analgesia by Non-Anesthesiologists. Practice guidelines for sedation and analgesia by non-anesthesiologists. *Anesthesiology.* 2002;96:1004–1017.

Collins VJ. Barbiturate intravenous anesthetic agents: thiopental. In: *Principles of Anesthesiology: General and Regional Anesthesia.* 3rd ed. Philadelphia: Lea and Febiger; 1993:665–671.

Committee on Drugs. American Academy of Pediatrics. Guidelines for monitoring and management of pediatric patients during and after sedation for diagnostic and therapeutic procedures: addendum. *Pediatrics.* 2002;110:836–838.

D'Agostino J, Terndrup TE. Comparative review of the adverse effects of sedatives used in children undergoing outpatient procedures. *Drug Saf.* 1996;14:146–157.

Fragen RJ, Avram MJ. Barbiturates. In: Miller RD, ed. *Anesthesia.* 3rd ed. New York: Churchill Livingstone; 1980:225–243.

Helmers JH, Adam AA, Giezen J. Pain and myoclonus during induction with etomidate. A double-blind, controlled evaluation of the influence of droperidol and fentanyl. *Acta Anaesthesiol Belg.* 1981;32:141–147.

Jastak JT, Pallasch T. Death after chloral hydrate sedation: report of case. *J Am Dent Assoc.* 1988;116:345.

Joint Commission on Accreditation of Healthcare Organizations. Standards for operative or other high-risk procedures and/or the administration of moderate or deep sedation or anesthesia. Revisions to Overview, PC.13.20 for 2004 Comprehensive Accreditation Manual for Hospitals: The Official Handbook (CAMH), 2004 Feb.

Malviya S, Voepel-Lewis T, Prochaska G, Tait AR. Prolonged recovery and delayed side effects of sedation for diagnostic imaging studies in children. *Pediatrics.* 2000;105:E42.

Modica PA, Tempelhoff R. Intracranial pressure during induction of anaesthesia and tracheal intubation with etomidate-induced EEG burst suppression. *Can J Anaesth.* 1992;39:236–241.

Pena BMG, Krauss B. Pediatric sedation: seeing patients safely through. *Contemp Pediatr.* 2000;8:42.

Roback MG, Bajaj L, Wathen JE, Bothner J. Preprocedural fasting and adverse events in procedural sedation and analgesia in a pediatric emergency department: are they related? *Ann Emerg Med.* 2004;44:454–459.

Sacchetti A, Schafermeyer R, Geradi M et al. Pediatric analgesia and sedation. *Ann Emerg Med.* 1994;23:237–250.

Wathen JE, Roback MG, Mackenzie T, Bothner JP. Does midazolam alter the clinical effects of intravenous ketamine sedation in children? A double-blind, randomized, controlled, emergency department trial. *Ann Emerg Med.* 2000;36:579–588.

Yldzdas D, Yapcoglu H, Ylmaz HL. The value of capnography during sedation or sedation/analgesia in pediatric minor procedures. *Pediatr Emerg Care.* 2004;20:162–165.

CHAPTER 15

Intramuscular, Subcutaneous, and Intradermal Injections

Renee Dietz, RN and Sandra M. Sanguino, MD, MPH

INTRAMUSCULAR INJECTION

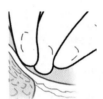
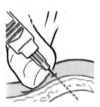
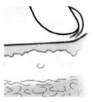

INDICATIONS

- Administration of medications or immunizations.
- Immunizations commonly administered intramuscularly include the following:
  - Diphtheria.
  - Tetanus and pertussis.
  - *Haemophilus influenzae* type b.
  - Hepatitis A.
  - Hepatitis B.
  - Pneumococcal conjugate.
  - Influenza.

CONTRAINDICATIONS

Relative

- Known bleeding disorder or thrombocytopenia.
- Erythema or swelling at the injection site.

EQUIPMENT

- Alcohol wipe.
- Gauze pad.
- Syringe with medication or immunization.
- Appropriate size needle.
- Bandage.

RISKS

- Pain, swelling, bleeding, or infection at the injection site.

PEARLS AND TIPS

- It may be necessary to enlist the help of a second person to hold the child.

PATIENT PREPARATION

- Position the child and assess the injection site.
- Clean the injection site with an alcohol wipe.

ANATOMY REVIEW

- In infants and toddlers, it is recommended that intramuscular injections be given in the middle one-third of the lateral aspect of the vastus lateralis muscle (anterolateral upper thigh).
- In older children, intramuscular injections are given in the deltoid muscle.
- The ventrogluteal site can be used in children over age 2. This site is used less commonly because of the risk of nerve damage.

PROCEDURE

- Pinch muscle and quickly insert 1-inch 23- or 25-gauge needle at a 90-degree angle (Figure 15–1).
- Larger adolescents and adults may require the use of a 1.5-inch needle.
- Aspirate to check for possible blood vessel entry.
  - Aspirate for at least 5 seconds.
  - This ensures that the needle is not in a small blood vessel.
  - If blood is obtained, withdraw the needle, discard the medication and syringe, and start again.
- If blood is not obtained, slowly inject the medication.
- Do not recap the needle.
- Dispose of the needle in the proper container.
- Apply pressure to the injection site with a gauze pad.
- Apply bandage and comfort the child.

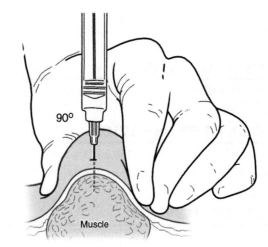

Figure 15–1. *Intramuscular injection.*

MONITORING

- Watch the patient for any reaction to the medication.

COMPLICATIONS

- Bleeding, pain, or swelling at the injection site.

SUBCUTANEOUS INJECTION

INDICATIONS

- Administration of medications or immunizations.
- Immunizations commonly administered subcutaneously include the following:
  - Inactivated polio.
  - Measles, mumps, and rubella.

CONTRAINDICATIONS

Relative

■ Erythema or swelling at the injection site.

EQUIPMENT

■ Alcohol wipe.
■ Gauze pad.
■ Syringe with medication or immunization.
■ Appropriate size needle.
■ Bandage.

RISKS

■ Pain, swelling, bleeding or infection at the injection site.
■ Lipohypertrophy or lipoatrophy may develop after repeated injections.

PEARLS AND TIPS

■ A second person may be necessary to help hold the child.

PATIENT PREPARATION

■ Position the child and assess the injection site.
■ Clean the injection site with an alcohol wipe.

ANATOMY REVIEW

■ In infants and toddlers, it is recommended that subcutaneous injections be given in the outer aspect of the upper thigh.
■ For older children, the upper outer arm is the preferred spot.

PROCEDURE

■ Gently pinch the skin at the injection site.
■ Insert a 25- or 27-gauge $^5/_8$-inch needle into the subcutaneous layer.
■ The needle should be directed at a 45-degree angle (Figure 15–2).
■ Aspirate to check for entry into a blood vessel.
■ If blood is obtained, withdraw the needle, discard the medication and syringe, and start again.
■ If blood is not obtained, slowly inject the medication.
■ Do not recap the needle.
■ Dispose of the needle in the proper container.
■ Apply pressure to the injection site with a gauze pad.
■ Apply bandage and comfort the child.

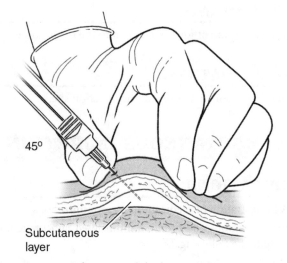

45°

Subcutaneous layer

Figure 15–2. *Subcutaneous injection.*

MONITORING

- Watch the patient for any reaction to the medication.

COMPLICATIONS

- Bleeding, pain, or swelling at the injection site.

INTRADERMAL INJECTION

INDICATIONS

- Medication administration.
- Placement of a tuberculosis skin test (purified protein derivative [PPD]).

CONTRAINDICATIONS

- Erythema at the proposed injection site.

EQUIPMENT

- Alcohol wipe.
- Gauze pad.
- Syringe with medication or immunization.
- Appropriate size needle.

RISKS

- Pain, swelling, bleeding, or infection at the injection site.

PEARLS AND TIPS

- A second person may be necessary to help hold the child.

PATIENT PREPARATION

- Locate the injection site.
- Clean the site with an alcohol wipe.

ANATOMY REVIEW

- The most common site for intradermal injections is the inner lower arm.
- Other possible sites include the upper chest and the back (between the scapulae).

PROCEDURE

- Hold the skin tautly with the syringe bevel up at a 15-degree angle to the skin.
- Use a 0.5-inch 27-gauge needle.

- Insert the needle just below the surface of the skin of the forearm (Figure 15–3).
- The needle should go through the epidermis into the dermis.
- Slowly inject the fluid.
- The medication should form a small bleb under the skin.
- Do not recap the needle.
- Dispose of the needle in the proper container.

MONITORING

- Watch the patient for any reaction to the medication.

COMPLICATIONS

- Bleeding, pain, or swelling at the injection site.

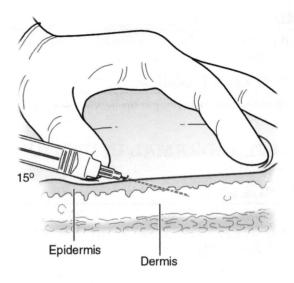

Figure 15–3. *Intradermal injection.*

REFERENCES

Siberry G, Iannone R. *The Harriet Lane Handbook: A Manual for Pediatric House Officers.* 15th ed. St. Louis: Mosby; 2000:66.

Section 2: Respiratory System

CHAPTER 16

Inhalation Medications

Adrienne Prestridge, MD

INDICATIONS

- Administration of medication to the lungs.

CONTRAINDICATIONS

Absolute

- Allergic reaction to medication.

Relative

- Anatomic abnormalities that cause increasing symptoms with treatment.

EQUIPMENT

- Nebulizer and compressor.
- Metered-dose inhaler with spacer.
- Dry powder inhaler (Figure 16–1).

RISKS

- Bronchoconstriction secondary to preservative (most solutions are now preservative free).
- Tachycardia.
- Arrhythmia (supraventricular tachycardia).
- Agitation.
- Oral candidiasis.

PEARLS AND TIPS

- If used correctly, each method of delivery of inhalation medications is equally effective.
- When using a nebulizer, when mist starts sputtering, tapping on cup allows for aerosolization of remainder of medicine.
- Effective administration involves transport of medication to the lower airways.
- The medication must be aerosolized and inhaled to facilitate delivery.

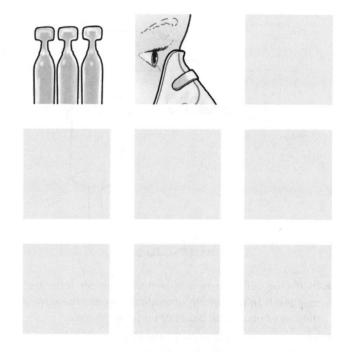

- Risks are related to medication rather than delivery method.

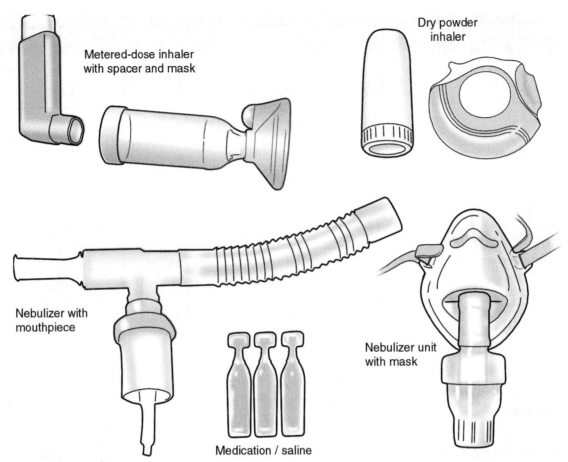

Figure 16-1. *Equipment.*

- Ineffective aerosolization as well as improper technique may result in disposition of medication onto the skin of the face or on the soft palate or posterior pharynx.
- In some younger children, the use of a spacer with a mask may allow more effective delivery than a spacer with a mouthpiece.

PATIENT PREPARATION

- Most children who require inhalation medication for wheezing will be stable.
- Children with severe bronchospasm or hypoxia should be placed on a cardiac monitor and pulse oximeter. They should be allowed to sit in a position of comfort, preferably upright.

PATIENT POSITIONING

- Sitting upright is preferred.
- Young children should be held by their caregivers.

ANATOMY REVIEW

- Effective administration involves transport of medication to the lower airways.

- The medication must be aerosolized and inhaled to facilitate delivery.
- Ineffective aerosolization as well as improper technique may result in disposition of medication onto the skin of the face, or on the soft palate or posterior pharynx.

PROCEDURE

Nebulizer

- Provide power to the compressor of the nebulizer machine (electric or battery).
- Attach oxygen tubing to the compressor and attach the nebulizer cup to the free end of the oxygen tubing.
- Open the top of the nebulizer cup by twisting and lifting the cap, pour medication into the cup, and reattach the top.
- Have patient put mouthpiece in mouth with seal made by lips, or if using mask, place it on patient's face (Figure 16–2).
- Turn the machine on.
- Instruct the patient to take slow deep breaths until the mist stops.

Metered-Dose Inhaler and Spacer Device

- Shake the inhaler.
- Remove the cap and attach it to the spacer device.
- Have the patient exhale completely.
- Place the mouthpiece of the spacer into the mouth and make a seal with the lips.
- If using a mask, apply it to the patient's face.
- Spray 1 puff from the inhaler into the spacer and have the patient breathe deeply and slowly.
  - 4–5 breaths for young children.
  - A single large breath held for 10 seconds for older children.
- Wait 1 minute and repeat with the second puff.

Dry Powder Inhaler

- Open inhaler (lever to slide open or cap to remove).
- Hold it in a horizontal position.
- Patient should inhale and exhale fully, put mouth on inhaler, inhale slowly and fully, and hold breath to count of 10.
- Close inhaler.

MONITORING

- No specific monitoring is needed for the routine use of inhalation medications.
- For children in acute respiratory distress, symptoms (ie, respiratory rate, wheezing, retractions) should be assessed before and after the administration of medication.

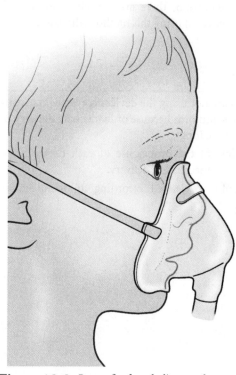

Figure 16–2. *Proper fit of a nebulizer mask.*

COMPLICATIONS

■ While the complication of the procedure is the failure to deliver the medication, there are complications of the medications delivered using this method (discussed in the Risks section).

CAVEATS

■ Patients who are not using the devices correctly may continue to have symptoms because of inadequate delivery of medication to the lungs.

■ Routine review of the proper use of each device helps ensure adequate medication delivery.

■ Devices should be cleaned according to manufacturer suggestions.

FOLLOW-UP

■ The management plan is dictated by the illness necessitating the use of inhalation medications.

■ For children with acute wheezing, follow-up should be 1–7 days after the intervention.

■ For those with stable disease, follow-up every 3–6 months is adequate.

REFERENCES

Rubin BK, Fink JB. The delivery of inhaled medication to the young child. *Pediatr Clin North Am.* 2003;50:717–731.

CHAPTER 17

Tracheostomy Tube Placement

Adrienne Prestridge, MD

INDICATIONS

- Routine replacement (usually once a week).
- Emergent replacement (occlusion with secretions, mucous plug, foreign body, or accidental dislodgment).

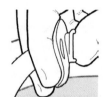

CONTRAINDICATIONS

Absolute

- Insufficient training in procedure. (Children with tracheostomies should never be left in the care of someone who is not trained in replacement of a tracheostomy.)

EQUIPMENT

- Suction catheters.
- Sterile gloves.
- Suction machine.
- Saline bullets.
- 5-mL syringe to deflate balloon, if applicable.
- Tracheostomy ties.
- Scissors.
- New tracheostomy tube of appropriate size (1 of same size and 1 size smaller).
- Lubrication (water soluble).
- Oxygen with tubing.
- Resuscitation bag.

RISKS

- Inability to establish a new airway.
- Perforation of airway.
- Bleeding.
- Infection.

PEARLS AND TIPS

- If replacement is emergent and no new tracheostomy tubes of appropriate size are available, an endotracheal tube of the same size can be used as a temporary airway.
- Once the endotracheal tube is inserted, the old tracheostomy tube can be cleaned and replaced.
- Size of tracheostomy tube is embossed on wings of tracheostomy tube.
- Suctioning of the tracheostomy is only to clear the tube itself.
- The suction catheter should not extend beyond the end of the tracheostomy tube. (Aggressive deep suctioning can lead to granulation tissue in the airway.)
- If unable to insert same size tracheostomy tube, use 1 size smaller.

PATIENT PREPARATION

- Explain the procedure in a developmentally appropriate manner before and during the procedure to help the patient remain calm; many patients are familiar and comfortable with the routine replacement of their tracheostomy tubes.

PATIENT POSITIONING

- A shoulder roll helps extend the neck for improved visualization.

PROCEDURE

- If nonemergent replacement, prepare all equipment prior to beginning procedure.
  - Place tracheostomy ties on new tracheostomy.
  - Lubricate new tracheostomy.
  - Prepare suctioning equipment.
  - Prepare resuscitation bag.
- Suction tracheostomy tube.
  - Give several positive pressure breaths with resuscitation bag (use 100% oxygen, if available).
  - With sterile gloves on, insert appropriate suction catheter (without suction applied) into tracheostomy tube. (**Do not insert past end of tracheostomy tube.**)
  - Once at desired depth, occlude suction port to begin suction.
  - Remove suction catheter while applying suction and twist catheter in fingers to allow sweep of sides of tracheostomy tube.
  - Give several positive pressure breaths with resuscitation bag (use 100% oxygen, if available).
  - Repeat as needed to clear tracheostomy tube.

- A few drops of saline may need to be instilled before positive pressure breaths to loosen secretions and facilitate removal.
- If tracheostomy tube has balloon, attach syringe to bulb and withdraw air.
- Remove tracheostomy ties while holding current tracheostomy tube in place.
- Remove tracheostomy tube.
- Immediately replace new tracheostomy tube into existing tract.
- Insert straight and then curve gently posteriorly and distally (Figure 17–1). **Do not force.**
- Hold tracheostomy tube in place with fingers.
- Remove stylet.
- Provide positive pressure breaths with 100% oxygen.
- Check for equal breath sounds bilaterally.
- Replace tracheostomy ties.
- If tracheostomy tube has balloon, fill with same amount of air that was removed.

MONITORING

- Assess respiratory status (eg, respiratory rate, retractions, breath sounds, pulse oximetry) before, during, and after procedure.

COMPLICATIONS

- Inability to establish an airway.
- Inability to replace same size tracheostomy tube.
- Bleeding.
- Infection (if not done with sterile technique).
- Trauma to trachea.

CAVEATS

- Established tracheostomy tubes should be replaced on a routine basis, usually once a week, by trained caregivers.
- Tubes should be replaced using a 2-person technique unless of an emergent nature. Two caregivers ensure the patient has an adequate airway at all times.
- Anytime a patient with a tracheostomy tube is in respiratory distress, which does not improve with suctioning, an emergent tracheostomy tube change should be performed because there may be a plug at the end of the tube obstructing air exchange.
- Even if the patient is able to be ventilated using a resuscitation bag and a suction catheter can be inserted, a mucous plug can act in a ball-valve fashion to obstruct the tracheostomy tube.

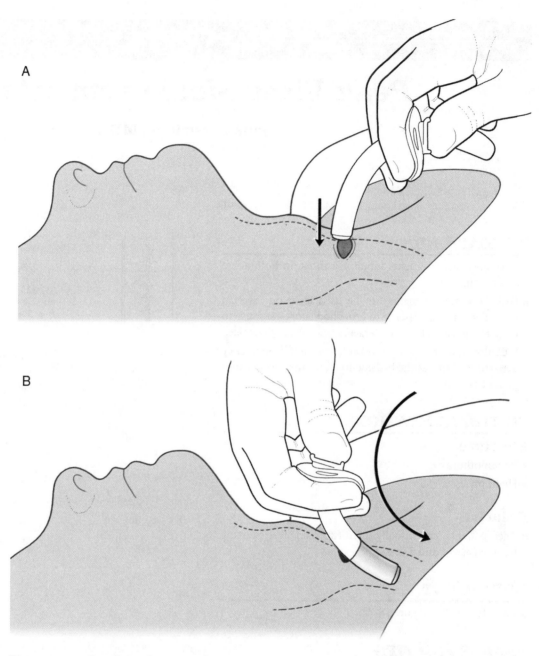

Figure 17–1. *Inserting tracheostomy tube.*

FOLLOW-UP

- If a smaller size tracheostomy tube or endotracheal tube was used during replacement, the appropriate size tube should be inserted as soon as possible to allow adequate aeration and ventilation.

REFERENCES

Fiske E. Effective strategies to prepare infants and families for home tracheostomy care. *Adv Neonatal Care.* 2004;4:42–53.

Heffner JE. Tracheostomy management in the chronically ventilated patient. *Clin Chest Med.* 2001;22:55–69.

Mirza S, Cameron DS. The tracheostomy tube change: a review of techniques. *Hosp Med.* 2001;62:158–163.

CHAPTER 18

Peak Flow Measurements

Adrienne Prestridge, MD

INDICATIONS

- Peak flow measurements monitor asthma, in both acute and chronic cases.
- Peak flow measurements can be used to assess severity, diurnal variation, response to bronchodilators, response to triggers (eg, viral illnesses, allergens), and effect of exercise.
- Peak flow monitoring is useful at home, in the emergency department, and at the bedside to assess the severity of a patient's asthma.

CONTRAINDICATIONS

Absolute

- Pneumothorax.
- Hemoptysis.

Relative

- Age; patients can usually perform maneuver starting between ages 4 and 5 years.

EQUIPMENT

- Peak flow meter (Figure 18–1).

PEARLS AND TIPS

- Peak flows are highly variable and effort dependent.
- Measurements can vary from 1 peak flow meter to the next. (It is important to use same meter each time.)
- Peak flows change as patient gets taller.
- Diurnal variation occurs—as much as 25–30% in children.
- Measurement of peak flows is mainly determined by resistance in large airways; therefore, peak flow measurement is insensitive to small airways resistance, which is most often affected in asthma.

PATIENT PREPARATION

- Explain procedure in a developmentally appropriate manner before and during procedure.

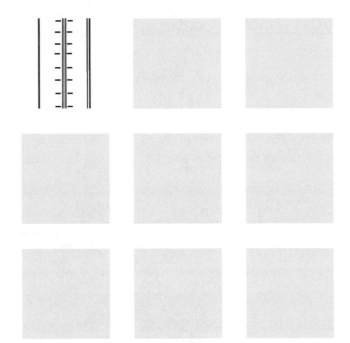

- Coach the patient for optimal effort to ensure acceptable results.

PATIENT POSITIONING

- Patient should be sitting upright or standing with erect posture.

PROCEDURE

- Return indicator/arrow on peak flow meter to zero.
- Hold peak flow horizontal.
- Take a deep full breath in (to total lung capacity).
- Place mouth on peak flow meter and make a seal with lips.
- Exhale hard and fast.
- Read number from indicator/arrow.
- Repeat 2 more times.
- Record best of 3 efforts.

INTERPRETATION AND MONITORING

- Patients should determine their baseline and personal best peak flow measurement.
- To obtain baseline, have patient perform maneuver 3 times in morning and 3 times at night for 2 weeks and maintain a record.
- Personal best is the highest of these values over these 2 weeks.
- Normal peak flow values are greater than 80% of the personal best, with mild values being 50–80% and critical values < 50% of personal best.
- Predicted nomograms are also available based on patient height.
- Response to various triggers and exercise can be defined as a decrease in peak flow of 15%, whereas a positive response to bronchodilator therapy is an increase of 15% in peak flow.
- Awareness of patient effort dependence and variations assists in making clinical decisions based on peak flow measurements.

CAVEAT

- The most significant limitation is that this test is effort dependent.

FOLLOW-UP

- Routine review of technique, establishment of new personal best peak flows, and appropriate asthma action plan for alterations in peak flow should be used to maximize the benefit of peak flow use.

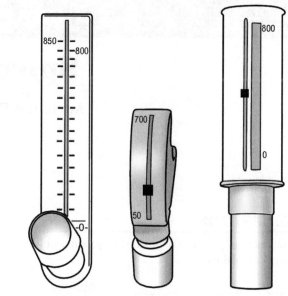

Figure 18–1. *Peak flow meters.*

REFERENCES

Boggs PB, Wheeler D, Washburne WF et al. Peak expiratory flow rate control chart in asthma care: chart construction and use in asthma care. *Ann Allergy Asthma Immunol.* 1998; 81:552–562.

Brand PL, Roorda RJ. Usefulness of monitoring lung function in asthma. *Arch Dis Child.* 2003;88:1021–1025.

Gibson PG, Wlodarczyk J, Hensley MJ et al. Using quality-control analysis of peak expiratory flow recordings to guide therapy for asthma. *Ann Intern Med.* 1995;123:488–492.

CHAPTER 19

Spirometry

Adrienne Prestridge, MD

INDICATIONS

- Assessment of pulmonary function in patients with respiratory complaints.

CONTRAINDICATIONS

Absolute

- Pneumothorax.
- Hemoptysis.

Relative

- Age; patients can usually perform maneuver starting between ages 4 and 5 years.

EQUIPMENT

- Spirometer.
- Individual mouthpieces.
- Nose clips.

RISKS

- Pneumothorax (rare).

PEARLS AND TIPS

- Adequate height, as measured with a stadiometer, is crucial to ensure utilization of appropriate predicted values.
- A positive response to bronchodilator testing is defined as a 12% increase in the forced expiratory volume in 1 second (FEV_1).

PATIENT PREPARATION

- Explain the procedure in a developmentally appropriate manner before and during procedure.
- Coach the patient for optimal effort to ensure acceptable results.
- In older patients, it is ideal to recommend no smoking for 24 hours prior to testing.

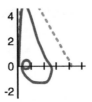

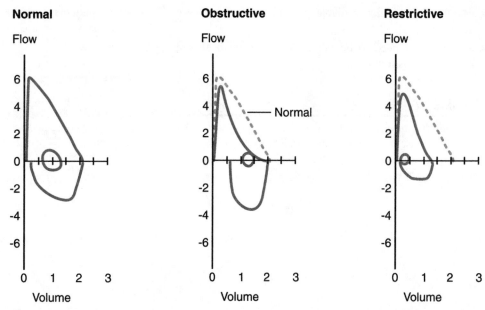

Figure 19–1. *Flow-volume loops showing normal pulmonary function as well as obstructive and restrictive lung disease.*

■ If assessing response to a bronchodilator, any bronchodilator medications should not be used for at least 8 hours before testing.

PATIENT POSITIONING

■ Patient should be sitting upright or standing tall.

PROCEDURE

■ Place nose clips on patient.

■ Patient makes a seal with lips around mouthpiece.

■ Ensure tongue does not block opening.

■ Have the patient breathe comfortably for 3 breaths (tidal breathing).

■ At end exhalation, have patient take fast breath in to fill lungs completely (to total lung capacity).

■ At top of inspiration, have patient exhale fast and hard and keep exhaling for 6 seconds or until flow plateaus.

■ At end of exhalation, inhale to fill lungs completely (total lung capacity).

■ Maneuver should be repeated to obtain 3 tests that are acceptable and reproducible.

INTERPRETATION AND MONITORING

■ A test must first be considered acceptable and reproducible.

■ A test is acceptable if it fulfills the following criteria:
  • No cough or glottic closure in first second of exhalation.
  • No leaks or obstruction of mouthpiece.

• Adequate start of test without hesitation.

• Full exhalation of 6 seconds or until plateau of volume.

• No early termination of test.

■ Reproducibility in children can be defined as the values of the forced vital capacity (FVC) and FEV_1 being within 5% on 3 acceptable maneuvers.

■ Obstructive lung disease is determined by a combination of the following:
  • Decreased flows (FEV_1, FVC, mid-range flows).
  • Scooped appearance to the flow volume curve (Figure 19–1).
  • Decreased FEV_1/FVC ratio.

■ Restrictive lung disease is suggested by a decreased FEV_1 and FVC and a normal or decreased FEV_1/FVC ratio (see Figure 19–1).

■ In order to adequately determine restrictive lung disease, full pulmonary function tests should be obtained to include lung volumes.

CAVEATS

■ Spirometry alone may not give a complete assessment of the patient's lung status; however, it is an excellent initial test.

■ It is crucial the test be done correctly because inadequately performed tests that are interpreted can lead to inappropriate management decisions.

■ Many young patients are unable to perform spirometry on initial attempts; these should not be interpreted if not performed correctly; however, these attempts are useful to have the patient become acquainted with the maneuvers.

■ Many commercially available portable spirometers are available.

■ All machines need to be calibrated routinely to ensure adequate measurements.

FOLLOW-UP

■ Spirometry should be performed when a patient is healthy so that a baseline can be obtained. The test can then be used to determine the severity of a respiratory illness.

■ Many patients will be unable to perform adequate spirometry if they are coughing.

REFERENCES

Brand PL, Roorda RJ. Usefulness of monitoring lung function in asthma. *Arch Dis Child.* 2003;88:1021–1025.

Mintz M. Asthma update: part I. Diagnosis, monitoring, and prevention of disease progression. *Am Fam Physician.* 2004; 70:893–898.

CHAPTER 20

Thoracentesis

Adrienne Prestridge, MD

INDICATIONS

- Therapeutic drainage of pleural effusion in patient with respiratory compromise when fluid is unlikely to reaccumulate.
- Diagnostic evaluation of pleural effusion of unknown etiology.
- Therapeutic removal of small pneumothorax.

CONTRAINDICATIONS

Relative

- Skin infection (eg, herpes zoster) at site of insertion.
- Bleeding diathesis, anticoagulant therapy.
- Mechanical ventilation.

EQUIPMENT

- Sterile gloves, mask, and gown.
- Iodinated skin preparation with sterile sponges.
- Sterile towels.
- Local anesthetic (1% lidocaine without epinephrine).
- 5-mL syringe with 25-gauge needle.
- 18-gauge 2-inch needle.
- 18–20-gauge angiocatheter.
- Collection basin.
- 3-way stopcock.
- 20–60-mL syringe.

RISKS

- Bleeding.
- Laceration of lung or other underlying tissues.
- Potential for need to remove additional fluid or air at a later time.
- If fluid or air is likely to reaccumulate, then tube thoracostomy is indicated.

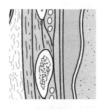
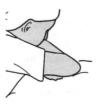
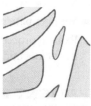

PEARLS AND TIPS

- In a cooperative child, the procedure does not take more than 10–15 minutes.
- Use lateral decubitus film to determine whether pleural effusion is free-flowing fluid or loculated.
- Insert needle over top of rib since the neurovascular bundle is under the rib (see Figure 20–1).

PATIENT PREPARATION

- Patient should have intravenous access.
- Oxygen should be available.
- Monitor oxygen saturation with pulse oximetry.
- Younger patients may need sedation for procedure.
- Explain procedure in a developmentally appropriate manner before and during procedure.

PATIENT POSITIONING

- Pleural effusion.
  - Sitting upright with arms supported on table in front of patient (see Figure 20–2).
  - Lying in lateral decubitus position with effusion side down.
- Pneumothorax: Supine with head of bed up 30 degrees.

ANATOMY REVIEW

- Neurovascular bundle is on the caudad edge of the rib (Figure 20–1).

PROCEDURE

Locate Effusion

- Chest radiograph.
- Manual percussion to find onset of dullness.
  - Ideal location is 1–2 cm (about 1 intercostal space) below onset of dullness.
  - Effusion is usually accessible via the sixth or seventh intercostal space just distal to the scapular tip in the midscapular line or posterior axillary line (Figure 20–2).
  - If pneumothorax is present, it is usually accessible via the second intercostal space anterior (Figure 20–3).
- Ultrasonogram marked location.
  - Mark location of effusion with the patient in the same position as necessary for procedure.
  - If possible, do not move patient after marking the location because the fluid may shift.

Prepare Sterile Field

- Cleanse area in sterile fashion.
- Drape surrounding area with sterile towels.

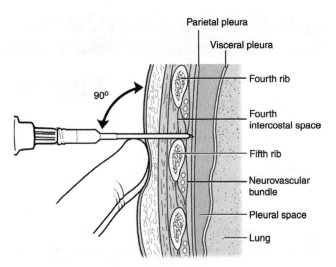

Figure 20–1. *Anatomy of the neurovascular bundle.*

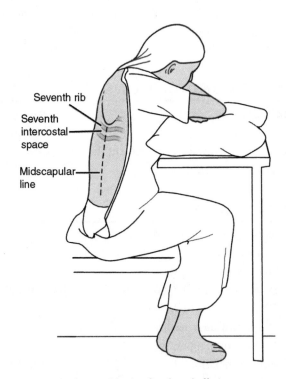

Figure 20–2. *Patient positioning for pleural effusion.*

Numb the Area

- Use a 25-gauge needle and 5-mL syringe to infiltrate the skin and make a wheal under the skin.
- Change needle to 18 gauge with 2-inch needle.
- Going over top of sixth rib, infiltrate through wheal, over top of rib to anesthetize the periosteum, and into pleural space.
  - Be sure to aspirate first, and know when you are in the pleural space.
  - The parietal pleura needs to be anesthetized, but, to avoid a puncture of the lung, do not advance the needle further.
  - When in the pleural space, a "pop" may be felt and fluid or air will enter syringe.

Removal of Pleural Effusion for Diagnostic Evaluation

- Remove lidocaine syringe and needle to outside the pleural space, with needle still inserted but outside the pleural space; replace syringe with empty 20–60-mL syringe.
  - Reinsert needle into pleural space while applying gentle negative pressure on syringe.
  - When in pleural space, a "pop" may be felt and fluid or air will enter syringe.
- Remove effusion into syringe.
- Remove needle and apply bandage to area.

Therapeutic Removal of Pleural Effusion

- Completely remove needle and syringe filled with lidocaine.
- Insert angiocatheter into same track and enter pleural space while applying gentle negative pressure.
  - When in pleural space, a "pop" may be felt and fluid or air will enter syringe.
- Remove inner needle, leaving catheter in place.
  - Ensure that the stopcock is closed to pleural space and chest wall or place a finger over the end of catheter to avoid introducing air into chest wall and creating a pneumothorax.
- Withdraw fluid.
  - Withdraw syringe full of fluid, close stopcock to chest wall and pleural space and drain into collection basin.
  - Repeat withdrawal of fluid until desired amount has been removed.
- Remove angiocatheter and apply bandage to area.

INTERPRETATION AND MONITORING

- The following laboratory tests should be done on the fluid obtained during thoracentesis:
  - Protein levels.

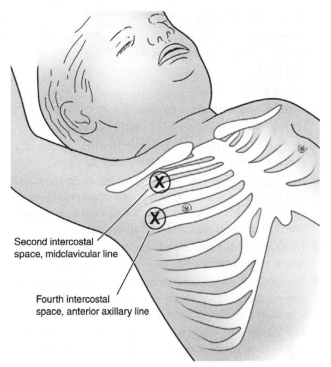

Second intercostal space, midclavicular line

Fourth intercostal space, anterior axillary line

Figure 20–3. *Patient positioning for pneumothorax.*

- Lactic acid dehydrogenase levels.
- Glucose levels.
- Blood cell count and differential.
- pH levels.
- Gram stain.
- Aerobic and anaerobic culture.
- Other cultures as indicated (eg, viral, mycoplasma, fungal).

■ Analysis of these factors helps determine whether the effusion is a transudate or an exudate (Table 20–1).

■ Transudative effusions occur when the hydrostatic and oncotic pressures favor filtration over absorption and are most often caused by systemic causes, such as congestive heart failure, nephritis, and hypoalbuminemia.

■ Treatment of the underlying cause will allow for resolution of the effusion.

■ Exudative effusions occur when there is a change in capillary permeability or block of lymphatic drainage, often secondary to inflammation or malignancy.

■ The differential diagnosis for an exudative effusion is extensive and further evaluation should be pursued.

COMPLICATIONS

■ Pneumothorax.
■ Bleeding: from intercostal vessel creating subcutaneous hematoma or hemothorax.
■ Hypoxia.
■ Pulmonary edema.
■ Puncture of liver or spleen.
■ Infection.
■ Laceration of lung.

CAVEATS

■ Younger children may require sedation for the procedure to be performed.
■ Most cases of pleural effusions in children are caused by infections.
■ Thoracentesis prior to initiation of antibiotic treatment allows for culture to guide antibiotic options.
■ Therapeutic removal of fluid in a patient with respiratory distress can also be useful in patients in whom the effusion is not likely to reaccumulate.

FOLLOW-UP

■ Obtain chest radiograph to ensure no pneumothorax.

Table 20–1. Characteristics of fluid that help determine whether the effusion is transudative or exudative.

Characteristic	Transudate	Exudate
Appearance	Clear or straw colored	Clear, milky, turbid, bloody
Odor	Odorless	Possible malodor
Specific gravity	< 1.016	> 1.016
pH	Normal	Normal or acidic
Glucose levels	> 60 mL/dL	< 60 mL/dL
Protein levels	< 3 g/dL	> 3 g/dL
Pleural protein: serum protein ratio[a]	< 0.5	> 0.5
LDH[a]	< Two-thirds upper limit normal of serum	> Two-thirds upper limit normal of serum
Pleural LDH: serum LDH ratio[a]	> 0.6	< 0.6
Red blood cell count	< 100,000/mcL	> 100,000/mcL
White blood cell count	< 1000/mcL	> 1000/mcL

[a]Light's criteria.
LDH, lactic dehydrogenase.

REFERENCES

Lewis RA, Feigin RD. Current issues in the diagnosis and management of pediatric empyema. *Semin Pediatr Infect Dis.* 2002;13:280–288.

Light RW. Clinical practice. Pleural effusion. *N Engl J Med.* 2002;346:1971–1977.

Light RW. *Pleural Diseases.* 4th ed. Baltimore: Lippincott Williams and Wilkins; 2001.

Light RW, Lee YCG. *Textbook of Pleural Diseases.* London: Hodder Arnold; 2003.

CHAPTER 21

Chest Tube Insertion

Adrienne Prestridge, MD

INDICATIONS

- Prolonged drainage of air or fluid (eg, empyema, hemothorax) from the pleural space.
- Definitive treatment of a tension pneumothorax (after needle decompression).

CONTRAINDICATIONS

Relative

- Bleeding diathesis.
- Mechanical ventilation.
- Presence of adhesions: may require pleurodesis.

EQUIPMENT

- Sterile gloves, mask, and gown.
- Iodinated skin preparation with sterile sponges.
- Sterile towels.
- Local anesthetic (1% lidocaine without epinephrine).
- 5-mL syringe with 25-gauge needle.
- 18-gauge 2-inch needle.
- #10 scalpel with handle.
- Chest tube and Kelly clamp for large bore insertion.
- Pleurevac or other drainage system, including all connectors necessary to connect to chest tube and to suction.
- Suction.
- Needle holder.
- Suture scissors.
- 2-0 silk suture.
- 4 × 4 gauze.
- Transparent occlusive dressing.

RISKS

- Bleeding.
- Infection.

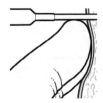
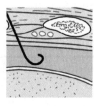

- Pain.
- Pneumothorax.
- Puncture of organ (ie, lung, liver, spleen).

PATIENT PREPARATION

- Patient should have intravenous access.
- Oxygen should be available.
- Monitor oxygen saturation with pulse oximetry.
- Younger patients may need sedation or anesthesia for procedure, especially with large bore chest tube insertion.
- Explain procedure in a developmentally appropriate manner before and during procedure.

PATIENT POSITIONING

- Patient lying on bed with head of table elevated 30 degrees with arm above head.

ANATOMY REVIEW

- Neurovascular bundle is under the rib (Figure 21–1).

PROCEDURE

Prepare Sterile Field

- Cleanse area in sterile fashion.
- Drape surrounding area with sterile towels.

Numb the Area

- Use 25-gauge needle and 5-mL syringe to infiltrate skin and make wheal under skin.
- Change needle to 18 gauge with 2-inch needle.
- Infiltrate through wheal, over top of rib, to anesthetize the periosteum, and into pleural space.
  - Be sure to aspirate first, and know when you are in the pleural space.
  - The pleura needs to be anesthetized, but, to avoid a puncture of the lung, do not advance the needle further.

Insertion of Chest Tube by Seldinger Technique

- Remove syringe from needle (Figure 21–2A).
- Pass guidewire through needle into pleural space (Figure 21–2B).
- Remove needle (while always maintaining a hold on the guidewire).
- Make small incision at site of insertion (large enough to pass chest tube) (Figure 21–2C).

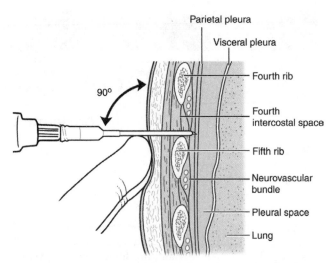

Figure 21–1. *Anatomy of the neurovascular bundle.*

- The fifth or sixth intercostals space in the anterior axillary line is the target for numbing the area.

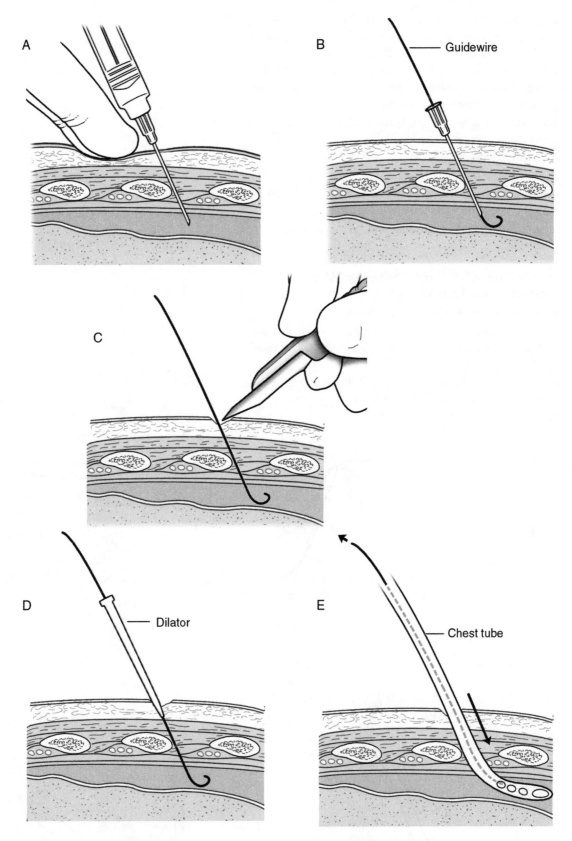

Figure 21–2. *Inserting chest tube using Seldinger technique (patient's head is to the right in this figure).*

- Starting with smallest dilator, insert dilator over guidewire using a twisting motion (while always maintaining a hold on the guidewire) (Figure 21–2D).
- Repeat with larger dilators over guidewire until track is large enough to easily pass chest tube (while always maintaining a hold on the guidewire).
- Insert chest tube over guidewire until all port holes are within the pleural space (Figure 21–2E).
- Remove guidewire.
- Suture chest tube to chest wall.
- Connect tube to drainage device with suction at 15–20 cm H_2O.
- Apply sterile 4 × 4 dressing and transparent occlusive dressing.

Insertion of Chest Tube by Blunt Dissection Technique

- Remove needle used for local anesthesia
- Using scalpel make ~1–2-cm incision through the skin and subcutaneous tissue (large enough to pass chest tube) (Figure 21–3A).
- Insert Kelly clamp and tunnel up 2 intercostal spaces in the subcutaneous space (Figure 21–3B).

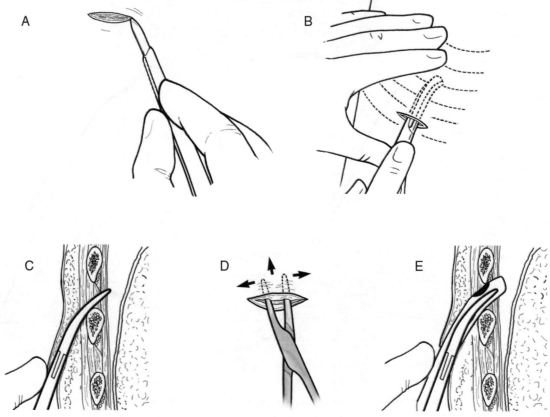

Figure 21–3. *Inserting chest tube using blunt dissection technique.*

- Push through the intercostal muscle superior to the rib with the Kelly clamp and enter the pleural space; air or fluid may rush out (Figure 21–3C).
- Spread the clamp to widen the area to allow for the chest tube (Figure 21–3D).
- Remove clamp.
- Insert gloved finger into tract and ensure correct location and lyse any adhesions.
- Using the Kelly clamp attached to the chest tube as a guide, insert the chest tube into the pleural space (Figure 21–3E).
  - If to drain air, guide anterior and superior (turning the clamp so that the curve is upward will assist with this guidance).
  - If to drain fluid, guide posterior and inferior (turning the clamp so that the curve is down will assist with this guidance).
- Advance chest tube until all ports are within the pleural space.
- Suture chest tube to chest wall.
- Connect tube to drainage device with suction at 15–20 cm H_2O.
- Apply sterile 4 × 4 dressing and transparent occlusive dressing.

INTERPRETATION AND MONITORING

- The following laboratory tests should be done on the fluid obtained from the effusion:
  - Protein levels.
  - Lactic acid dehydrogenase levels.
  - Glucose levels.
  - Blood cell count and differential.
  - pH levels.
  - Gram stain.
  - Aerobic and anaerobic culture.
  - Other cultures as indicated (eg, viral, mycoplasma, fungal).
- Monitoring the drainage system after insertion of the chest tube allows you to assess function and determine appropriate timing of removal.
- In the standard Pleurevac system, there is colored fluid that demonstrates both the amount of suction being applied and allows assessment for air leaks.
- If air bubbles are seen in this chamber, there is an air leak in the system. Although this could be from a broncho-pleural fistula, it can also be due to a side port being outside the chest wall or air entering the system through insecurely attached tubing.
- The patency of the chest tube can be assessed by fluctuation of the colored fluid with inspiration and expiration by the patient.
  - If the fluid does not fluctuate, then there may be a kink in the tubing or a clot in the tubing.

- The other side of the drainage device will collect the draining fluid.
- The appearance and amount of the fluid should be assessed routinely.
- Most often, placing a mark on the outside of the container with a date and time helps determine the amount of fluid that is draining.
- Normal pleural fluid production in an adult is about 10–15 mL/d. Normal values for children are not available, but expectations proportionately extrapolated from adult values are typically used.
- Knowing the normal values allows assessment of when the fluid has slowed down in drainage and removal of the tube can be considered.
- An intermediary step is to place the patient to water seal (no suction being applied) and monitor for drainage.
- If there continues to be no drainage, then the tube can be clamped off (no drainage allowed even to gravity).
- Chest radiograph evaluation after each of these steps allows for determination of reaccumulated fluid.
- If fluid reaccumulates at any point, continue suction drainage.
- If no accumulation occurs, then the tube may be removed.
  - To remove the tube, undo the dressing and remove the suture.
  - Use petroleum-impregnated gauze and hold over tube insertion site.
  - While the patient performs a Valsalva maneuver, quickly withdraw the tube and cover insertion site with gauze.
  - Cover petroleum gauze with bandage.

COMPLICATIONS

- Improper position, such as placement into subcutaneous tissue or peritoneal space; tube should not be encroaching on mediastinum.
- Pneumothorax.
- Bleeding from intercostal vessel creating subcutaneous hematoma or hemothorax.
- Puncture of liver or spleen.
- Infection.
- Laceration of lung.

CAVEATS

- Once it is determined from chest radiograph that a patient has a pleural effusion, the consideration for a thoracentesis versus chest tube placement must be decided.
- If the fluid is likely to reaccumulate, then a chest tube is indicated.
- Lateral decubitus films help determine whether the fluid is free-flowing or loculated.

■ If the fluid is loculated, the chest tube may only be able to drain the area of tube placement and pleurodesis and removal of adhesions by a surgeon may be necessary.

FOLLOW-UP

■ Obtain chest radiograph to ensure correct placement.

REFERENCES

Lewis RA, Feigin RD. Current issues in the diagnosis and management of pediatric empyema. *Semin Pediatr Infect Dis.* 2002;13:280–288.

Light RW. Clinical practice. Pleural effusion. *N Engl J Med.* 2002;346:1971–1977.

Light RW. *Pleural Diseases.* 4th ed. Baltimore: Lippincott Williams and Wilkins; 2001.

Light RW, Lee YCG. *Textbook of Pleural Diseases.* London: Hodder Arnold; 2003.

CHAPTER 22

Pericardiocentesis

Stephen Pophal, MD

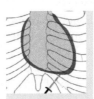

INDICATIONS

- Therapeutic: Impending cardiac tamponade.
- Diagnostic.
  - Infectious pericarditis.
  - Rule out an oncologic process.
- Compromise in the patient's hemodynamic status.

CONTRAINDICATIONS

Relative

- A blood dyscrasia in which a patient may have a significant bleeding complication.
- A cutaneous infection in the area of the most feasible sights for pericardiocentesis.
- A significantly elevated diaphragm, a grossly enlarged liver, or profound ascites, which all change the standard landmarks of inserting the pericardiocentesis needle in the subxiphoid area.
- Under such circumstances, use the intercostal approach.

EQUIPMENT

- Povidone-iodine or equivalent sterilization substrate to cleanse the subxiphoid area.
- 1% or 2% lidocaine or xylocaine.
- 25-gauge, 1.5-inch-long needle.
- 16- or 18-gauge needle, ≥ 1.5 inch.
- Floppy tip wire that can be introduced through the needle.
- Pigtail catheter with multiple side holes as well as an end hole.
- Scalpel.
- 3-way stopcock.
- 30-mL or 60-mL syringe and suture kit.
- ECG monitor, pulse oximeter, and blood pressure cuff.

RISKS

- Infection and bleeding can be minimized with proper technique.

- Pneumothorax (unusual).
- Laceration of the liver (unusual).
- Coronary injury (unusual).
- Cardiac perforation (unusual).

PEARLS AND TIPS

- Ideally, a patient should be continuously monitored with echocardiography and fluoroscopy in an interventional radiology or cardiac catheterization laboratory.
- Frequently, this is not an option, and bedside pericardiocentesis without portable fluoroscopy is performed. In this circumstance, the patient should be sedated.
- Respiratory and hemodynamic status should be monitored by assistants, so that the physician can concentrate on performing the pericardiocentesis.

PATIENT PREPARATION

- Prepare and drape the subxiphoid area in the usual sterile fashion.
- If the subxiphoid approach might be difficult (due to an unusually located heart or elevated diaphragm), consider preparing the left sternal border.
- All equipment should be readily available and an assistant should be available to help with manipulation of needles, wires, and catheters.

PATIENT POSITIONING

- Supine position, with 10–30 degrees of reverse Trendelenburg.
- Occasionally, the partially sitting position may be required or beneficial.
  - Makes an orthopneic patient more comfortable.
  - May allow for most of the pericardial fluid to position inferiorly or closer to the drainage site.

PROCEDURE

- Prepare the subxiphoid area and left sternal border.
- Administer 1% or 2% lidocaine approximately 0.5–1 cm below the left costoxiphoid angle using a 25- or 27-gauge 1.5-inch-long needle.
  - Infiltration of the lidocaine should be superficial as well as deep, pushing the needle superiorly, posteriorly, and leftward.
  - Withdraw fluid each time the needle is passed deeper within the skin and subcutaneous tissues.
- To allow for easier passage of the needle, precut the skin with the scalpel before introducing the 16- or 18-gauge 1.5-inch to 2.5-inch needle.

- Insert the larger needle at an approximate 30–45-degree angle with the abdomen with constant negative pressure on the syringe.
- Monitor ECG very carefully for evidence of dysrhythmias or ST segment changes (evidence of coronary or myocardial injury).
- Slowly insert the needle until fluid is withdrawn.
  - Suspect cardiac perforation is the fluid is grossly bloody.
  - Serous fluid confirms that the needle has passed into the pericardial space.
  - It is not unusual to feel the needle pass through the pericardium.
- Fix the needle into position once pericardial fluid is extracted.
- Pass the floppy tip wire through the needle with the intent of passing the wire deep within the pericardium and into the posterior pericardial space (Figure 22–1).
- Because the wire may irritate the epicardium, ventricular ectopy is not uncommon.
- Once the wire is secured deep within the pericardium, remove the needle.
- Make a larger incision in the skin adjacent to the wires so that the catheter can be inserted.
- Insert the soft-tipped multiple sidehole or pigtail catheter over the wire and secure it in the posterior pericardial space.
- Connect the catheter to a 3-way stopcock, and fluid should be extracted slowly, monitoring for blood pressure and ectopy.
- Continuous echocardiographic monitoring is useful for location of the wire and catheter as well as for monitoring adequate extraction of pericardial fluid.
- Once catheter position is confirmed, the catheter should be secured with sutures and the entire site covered sterilely to minimize infection.

INTERPRETATION AND MONITORING

- Send pericardial fluid for cell count, protein, glucose, lactic dehydrogenase, cytology as well as all other studies for infectious agents.
- Normal pericardial fluid is clear to straw colored, scant (< 50 mL) with < 500 white blood cells/mcL.
- An elevated white blood cell count suggests either an infectious or inflammatory process.
- Protein, glucose, and lactic dehydrogenase can be helpful in differentiating a transudate from an exudate.
- Metastasis to the pericardial space or pericardial tumors are frequently exudative, with abnormalities seen on cytology.
- Monitor the patient closely for rhythm disturbances and unstable blood pressure.

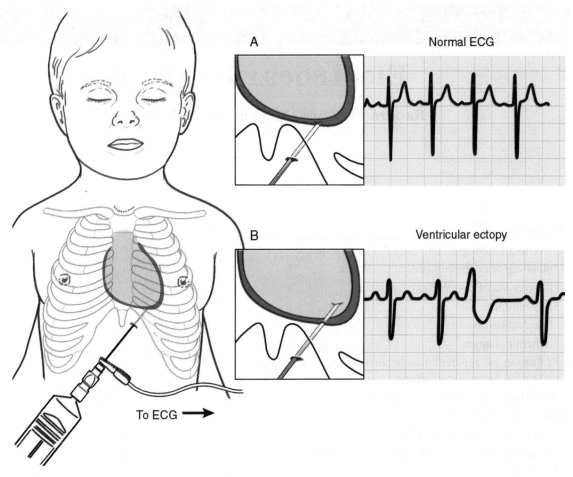

Figure 22-1. *Pericardiocentesis may trigger ventricular ectopy.*

■ Patients may require fluid resuscitation if large amounts of fluid are extracted from the pericardial space.
  • Remove the fluid slowly.
  • Replace with isotonic fluid, if possible.
  • Large children with nephrotic syndrome can have as much as 1–2 L of pericardial fluid and be relatively asymptomatic.

COMPLICATIONS

■ Compromise in the hemodynamic status.
■ Bleeding.
  • Can be superficial and easily controlled with pressure.
  • Deeper bleeding from either a liver or splenic injury may be less obvious and more difficult to control.
■ A coronary injury is rare but potentially catastrophic (as is a cardiac perforation). These require emergent intervention by a cardiac surgeon.

■ Arrhythmias are typically transient and can be managed by repositioning the needle, wire, or catheter.
■ Occasionally, more persistent rhythm disturbances occur that require antiarrhythmic therapies.
■ A pneumoperitoneum or small pneumothorax requires careful monitoring but can be self-limited.
■ Pneumopericardium should resolve as long as the pericardiocentesis catheter is secure, in proper position, and connected to negative pressure.

REFERENCES

Chang A, Hanley F, Wernosky G, Wessel D. *Pediatric Cardiac Intensive Care.* Philadelphia: Williams & Wilkins; 1998.

Neches W, Park S, Zuberbuhler J. *Perspectives in Pediatric Cardiology.* Vol 3. Pediatric Cardiac Catheterization. Futura Publishing Company, Inc; 1991

Zahn E, Houde C, Benson L, et al. Percutaneous pericardial catheter drainage in childhood. *Am J Cardiol.* 1992;70:678–680.

CHAPTER 23

Electrocardiography

Kendra M. Ward, MD and Barbara J. Deal, MD

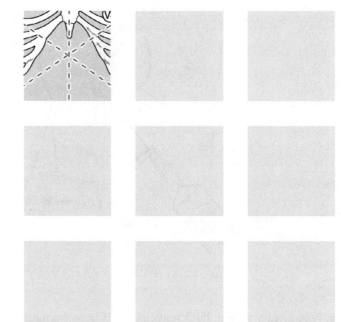

INDICATIONS

- Screening for congenital or acquired heart disease.
- Follow-up of established cardiac disorders:
  - Progression of chamber enlargement.
  - Hypertrophy.
  - Conduction disorders.
  - Ischemic changes.
- Evaluation of apparent life-threatening event, syncope, chest pain, or new-onset seizure.
- Arrhythmia detection and evaluation.
- Evaluation of conduction disorder.
- Monitoring cardiac effects of medication.
- Evaluation for appropriate pacemaker or defibrillator function.
- Evaluation of cardiac effects of electrolyte or metabolic abnormalities.

CONTRAINDICATIONS

- Disorders that limit access to skin of chest wall, such as thoracic wound.
- Extensive bandages over chest.
- Third-degree skin burns.

EQUIPMENT

- ECG machine, leads.
- Electrode stickers; pediatric patches are best.
- Alcohol pads to clean skin.

RISKS

- Improper electrical grounding may deliver electrical shock; extremely rare.

PEARLS AND TIPS

- Improper lead positioning is a major source of abnormal tracings.
  - Results in repeat ECGs or unnecessary further testing.
  - As many as 15–20% of pediatric ECGs performed in emergency departments or intensive care units show improper lead placement.
- The most common recording error is limb lead reversal.
  - **White** electrode should be on **right** arm.
  - **Black** electrode should be on **left** arm.
- Automated ECG interpretations that read "left atrial rhythm" usually reflect limb lead reversal.
- Negative P, QRS, and T waves in leads I and aVL are another indicator of lead reversal.
- Make sure the initial recording is at the appropriate speed: 25 mm per second, and appropriate gain: 10 mm per mV.
- Eliminating as much patient movement as possible is essential; blowing bubbles over young children often allows time for recording without movement.

PATIENT PREPARATION

- Clean the area with alcohol swab.
- Skin must be clean and dry.
- Leads cannot be placed over bandages: either reposition bandage or omit lead.

PATIENT POSITIONING

- Supine position is essential.
- Some patients have T wave changes in upright positions, and decubitus positioning may slightly alter the location of the heart relative to the ECG leads.

ANATOMY REVIEW

- Lead placement is important and must be consistent.
- Inappropriate placement of limb or precordial leads results in interpretation errors, including hypertrophy or infarct patterns.
- Figure 23–1 shows placement of leads.
  - RA: Right forearm, distal to insertion of deltoid muscle.
  - LA: Left forearm, distal to insertion of deltoid muscle.
  - RL: Right leg.
  - LL: Left leg.
  - V1: Fourth intercostal space, right sternal edge.
  - V2: Fourth intercostal space, left sternal edge.
  - V3: Halfway between V2 and V4.
  - V4: Fifth intercostal space, midclavicular line.

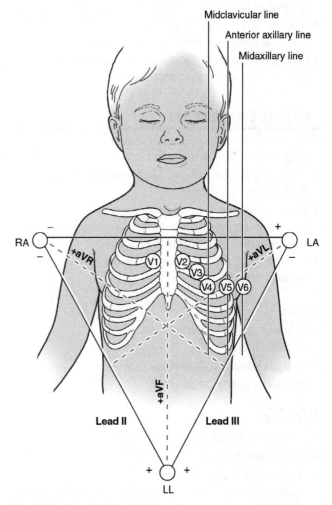

Figure 23–1. *Lead positioning.*

• V5: Same level as V4 on anterior axillary line.

• V6: Same level as V4 on midaxillary line.

PROCEDURE

■ Place electrode stickers appropriately.

■ Attach the leads, with careful attention to limb lead placement.

■ Enter the patient data into the ECG machine. ECGs without name, age, and date cannot be officially interpreted.

■ Select gain and paper speed (standard speed 25 mm per second and standard gain 10 mm per mV).

■ Use standard settings initially.

■ Modify gain as needed.

■ Select the type of tracing desired.

• 12-lead ECG.

• 12-lead rhythm strip.

• 3-lead rhythm strip.

■ Ensure the patient is still and the tracing is stable on the monitor of the ECG machine.

■ Once there is no artifact, record.

■ Inspect the tracing before disconnecting the leads.

■ If no additional tracings are needed, disconnect the leads and remove the electrode stickers.

INTERPRETATION

■ To avoid missing important information, interpret ECGs consistently and systematically.

■ Knowledge of the patient's age is essential because standards are age-dependent.

■ ECGs in children should be interpreted by clinicians specifically trained in pediatrics because of the significant age-related differences from adult ECGs.

■ Evaluate **rate, rhythm, axis, intervals, hypertrophy, ST segments.**

Rate

■ Normal rates are age-dependent.

• Infants: 100–170 bpm.

• Young children: 80–140 bpm.

• Adolescents: 60–100 bpm.

Rhythm

■ Analyze P/QRS relationship and consistency.

■ Atrial rhythm.

• P wave before each QRS.

• Sinus P wave has normal axis (upright in leads I and aVF).

• Usually normal PR interval.

■ Junctional rhythm.

• P waves during or after QRS.

• Usually narrow QRS complexes.

■ Ventricular.

• Usually wide QRS complexes, although several simultaneous leads may be needed to determine QRS duration.

• Preceding upright P wave with 1:1 P/QRS relationship should not be present.

■ Atrioventricular (AV) dissociation.

• Consider conduction abnormality or accelerated junctional or ventricular rhythm.

P Wave Axis

■ Normal P wave axis is upright in leads I and aVL.

■ Left atrial rhythm, or limb lead reversal, shows negative P wave in leads I and aVL.

■ Low atrial rhythm shows negative P wave in inferior leads: II, III, aVF.

QRS Axis

■ Normal frontal QRS axis is age-dependent.

■ Neonates have relatively rightward QRS axis (+40 to +180 degrees), which gradually shifts toward left with age.

■ Left axis deviation or superior axis (0 to −90 degrees) in neonate is highly suggestive of congenital heart disease, particularly among infants with Down syndrome.

■ Left axis deviation or superior axis is also associated with the following:

• AV septal defects (primum atrial septal defects).

• Tricuspid atresia.

• Underdevelopment of right ventricle.

• Left ventricular hypertrophy.

• Preexcitation.

■ Right axis deviation is suggestive of right ventricular hypertrophy or underdevelopment of left ventricle.

PR Intervals

■ Measured from onset of P wave to onset of QRS.

■ Normal PR interval is age-dependent, usually < 160 msec in young children.

A. First-Degree AV Block

■ PR interval greater than expected for age.

■ Associated with atrial septal defects, rheumatic fever, ectopic atrial rhythms.

B. Second-Degree AV Block

■ Type I (Wenckebach).

- Successive PR lengthening until atrial impulse is not conducted (generally does not progress).
  - May be normal variant, particularly during sleep.
- Type II.
  - Nonconducted atrial impulse without progressive PR lengthening.
  - Not commonly seen.
  - Not usually considered a normal variant.

C. THIRD-DEGREE AV BLOCK

- Failure of an atrial impulse to be conducted to the ventricles.
- Never a normal variant but needs to be differentiated from accelerated junctional or ventricular rhythms.
- Congenital form associated with autoimmune disorders or complex congenital heart disease.
- Acquired form secondary to surgical repair of congenital heart disease.
- Congenitally corrected transposition of the great arteries.
- Myocarditis.
- Lyme disease.

QRS Duration

- Reflects ventricular depolarization.
- Normal.
  - Less than 90 msec in infants and young children.
  - Less than 100 msec in older children.
- Prolonged QRS duration for age reflects right or left ventricular conduction delay or block (> 120 msec in adults).
- Right ventricular conduction delay may be associated with atrial septal defects.
- Right bundle branch block is seen after surgical repair of some forms of congenital heart disease, especially tetralogy of Fallot.
- Left bundle branch block is rare and usually associated with surgical repair of lesions obstructing left ventricular outflow tract or with significant cardiomyopathy.

QT Interval

- Measured from onset of QRS to end of T wave.
- Reflects ventricular depolarization and repolarization.
- The normal QT interval of 400 msec is based on a heart rate of 60 bpm.
- Rate-corrected QT interval = QTc.
- Bazett's correction: Measured QT interval/square root of RR interval.
- Normal QTc.
  - < 460 msec for females.
  - < 450 msec for males.

- A prolonged QT interval increases the risk for potentially life-threatening arrhythmias and may result in the long QT syndrome (a cardiac ion channelopathy) or as an acquired abnormality from drug, electrolyte, or nervous system disorders.
- Patients with seizures, syncope, or hearing loss should be screened for QT abnormalities.
- A prolonged QT interval may require cardiac consultation.
- QT prolongation may be intermittent; therefore, a normal QT interval does not preclude the presence of long QT syndrome.

Atrial Enlargement

A. RIGHT ATRIAL ENLARGEMENT

- Tall pointed P waves.
- Amplitude > 2.5 mm.
- Best seen in leads II, III, V1.
- Associated with the following:
  - Atrial septal defects.
  - Right ventricular hypertension.
  - Pulmonary disease.
  - Cardiomyopathy.

B. LEFT ATRIAL ENLARGEMENT

- Increased P wave duration (> 90–100 msec).
- Biphasic P wave in V1 with deep negative component.
- Associated with large left to right shunts and mitral valve disease.

C. BIATRIAL ENLARGEMENT

- Increased amplitude and duration.
- Associated with large left to right shunts and ventricular hypertrophy as well as cardiomyopathy.

Ventricular Hypertrophy

- ECG diagnosis of hypertrophy is sensitive but not specific, resulting in frequent overinterpretation of hypertrophy.
- Thin chest wall, anemia, volume overload, and athletic training may contribute to ECG appearance of ventricular hypertrophy.

A. LEFT VENTRICULAR HYPERTROPHY

- Voltage criteria include tall R waves in left precordial leads V5–V6 > 98 percentile for age, or deep S waves in V1–V2.
- Sum of R wave in V6 and S wave in V1 or V2 > 98 percentile for age.
- Deep Q waves in inferior limb leads or left precordial leads.

- Seen with the following conditions:
  - Patent ductus arteriosus.
  - Lesions obstructing left ventricular outflow tract, such as aortic stenosis or coarctation.
  - Hypertension.
  - Sickle cell anemia.
  - Cardiomyopathy.

B. RIGHT VENTRICULAR HYPERTROPHY

- Voltage criteria include increased R wave amplitude in right precordial leads V1–V2 > 98 percentile for age.
- A Q wave in V1 is never normal and suggests right ventricular hypertrophy or ventricular inversion.
- Upright T wave in right precordial leads after the first week of life, and before "adult" ECG pattern is achieved, indicates right ventricular hypertrophy.
- Deep S wave amplitude in V6 suggests right ventricular hypertrophy; usually > 7 mm.
- An rSr′ pattern is a common normal variant in children; however, a tall R′ is not normal.
- Seen when lesions obstruct right ventricular outflow tract, such as in cases of pulmonic stenosis and tetralogy of Fallot.

C. BIVENTRICULAR HYPERTROPHY

- Voltage criteria for both right and left ventricular hypertrophy.
- Katz-Wachtel criteria for biventricular hypertrophy: Large combined voltages of R + S wave amplitude in V4 > 60 mm.
- Associated with the following:
  - Large patent ductus arteriosus.
  - Large ventricular septal defects.
  - AV septal defects.
  - Truncus arteriosus.
  - Single ventricle.
  - Cardiomyopathy.

ST Changes

- Normal ST segment horizontal, isoelectric.
- Can be normal to have 1 mm elevation or depression of ST segment in limb leads.
- Left precordial leads may have up to 2-mm elevation or depression of ST segment.
- Beware of calling ST changes normal if they are a change from a previous ECG or if the patient has chest pain or other cardiac symptoms.
- J point elevation is a normal finding.
- ST changes can be seen in the following:
  - Myocardial ischemia.
  - Myocarditis.
  - Pericarditis.

ARRHYTHMIA DETECTION

Rate: Too Fast or Too Slow?

- Bradycardia may reflect the following:
  - Sinus node dysfunction (either intrinsic or, more often, secondary to systemic disorders).
  - Blocked premature atrial beats.
  - Conduction disorders.
- Tachycardia may be due to the following:
  - Sinus tachycardia associated with fever, sepsis, anemia, or hemodynamic stress.
  - Pathologic rhythm (eg, supraventricular, junctional, or ventricular).

Rhythm: Regular or Irregular?

- Irregular rhythms include the following:
  - Sinus arrhythmia (very common in young children).
  - Sinus node dysfunction.
  - Premature beats.
  - Atrial fibrillation.
  - Ventricular fibrillation.

QRS Complex: Wide or Narrow?

- Wide QRS rhythms are seen in the following:
  - Supraventricular tachycardia with bundle branch block.
  - Supraventricular tachycardia conducted via an accessory connection.
  - Profound electrolyte abnormalities (hyperkalemia).
  - Drug intoxication (digoxin).
  - Toxic ingestions (yew berry).
  - Ventricular tachycardia.

What Is the P/QRS Relationship?

- 1:1 P/QRS ratio.
  - If P wave precedes QRS with constant PR interval, consider sinus or atrial rhythm.
  - Analyze P wave morphology to distinguish between these rhythms.
  - If QRS precedes P wave, consider ventricular or junctional rhythm, or reciprocating rhythms with retrograde conduction to atria (supraventricular tachycardia).
- If there are more P waves than QRS complexes, consider atrial arrhythmia (ie, atrial flutter, atrial tachycardia).
- If there are more QRS complexes than P waves, consider junctional or ventricular rhythm.

• Abnormal potassium levels.

• Digitalis.

• Left ventricular hypertrophy with "strain."

• Central nervous system pathology.

Preexcitation

■ Short PR interval in sinus rhythm, associated with a slurred upstroke to QRS (delta wave).

■ The term "Wolff-Parkinson-White syndrome" refers to the association of preexcitation pattern on ECG with supraventricular tachycardia.

■ Left axis deviation or the absence of a Q wave in V6 may be subtle indicators of preexcitation.

■ Preexcitation may be intermittent, and it may be associated with the development of supraventricular tachycardia in about 30–35% of cases.

■ Due to the small but present risk of life-threatening arrhythmias as the initial symptomatic event with preexcitation, patients with this finding on ECG should be referred for cardiac consultation.

COMPLICATIONS

■ Rare.

■ Incorrect set-up or equipment malfunction may result in an ECG that is misinterpreted, resulting in additional (unnecessary) testing.

FOLLOW-UP

■ Depends on the reason the test was obtained, the patients' clinical status, and the ECG findings.

■ Patients with abnormal ECGs should be referred to a pediatric cardiologist; the timing of referral depends on both the ECG finding and the clinical context.

REFERENCES

Deal BJ, Johnsrude CL, Buck SH. *Pediatric ECG Interpretation: An Illustrative Guide*. Futura, Blackwell Publishing; 2004.

Park MK, Guntheroth WG. *How to Read Pediatric ECGs*. 3rd edition. St. Louis: Mosby-Year Book; 1992.

CHAPTER 24

Blood Pressure Management

Rae-Ellen W. Kavey, MD

INDICATIONS

- All children aged 3 years or older who are seen in any medical setting should have their blood pressure (BP) measured.
- BP is a primary measure of cardiac output in acute assessment of any potentially compromised patient.
- BP change over time allows monitoring of changing hemodynamic status and of response to intervention.
- In critical care settings, BP is best monitored by arterial line, since peripheral measures can be inaccurate when cardiac output is compromised.

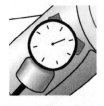

CONTRAINDICATIONS

Relative

- BP measurement is not recommended as a routine in well children less than 3 years of age.
- However, specific conditions signal the need for BP determination beginning in infancy and include the following:
  - History of prematurity, very low birth weight, or any problem requiring neonatal intensive care.
  - Congenital heart disease (repaired or unoperated).
  - Recurrent urinary tract infections, hematuria, or proteinuria.
  - Renal or urologic disease.
  - Family history of renal disease.
  - Solid organ transplant, malignancy, or bone marrow transplant.
  - Treatment with drugs known to raise BP.
  - Systemic illnesses associated with hypertension.
  - Increased intracranial pressure.

EQUIPMENT

- BP should be measured using a standard clinical sphygmomanometer on the upper right arm and a stethoscope over the brachial artery pulse, just below the cuff.

- Automated oscillometric BP devices are convenient and reduce observer error, but they do not provide exactly comparable results to the auscultatory method.
  - However, because of their ease of use, these devices are valuable as a screening method and in intensive care settings.
  - Abnormal readings must be confirmed by auscultation.
- Correct BP measurement requires a cuff size appropriate to the size of the child; this means a range of sizes, including a large adult cuff and thigh cuff, must always be available.
- An appropriate cuff meets the following criteria:
  - Height of the inflatable bladder is at least 40% of the arm circumference at a point midway between the olecranon and the acromion.
  - Bladder length should cover > 80% of the arm's circumference (bladder width-to-length ratio ≥ 1:2).
- Practically speaking, this means the cuff selected must be large enough to cover the majority of the upper arm with just room for the head of the stethoscope in the cubital fossa (Figure 24–1).

PEARLS AND TIPS

- Whenever upper extremity hypertension is diagnosed, lower extremity BPs and pulses should be obtained and compared to exclude the possibility of coarctation of the aorta, which is the most commonly missed congenital heart diagnosis.
- In children over 10 years of age, white coat hypertension is increasingly common.
  - It is defined as elevated BP in medical settings but normal pressure at all other times.
  - This can be diagnosed by the use of ambulatory BP monitoring, which allows computation of mean wake and sleep pressures for comparison with published norms for age/gender/height.

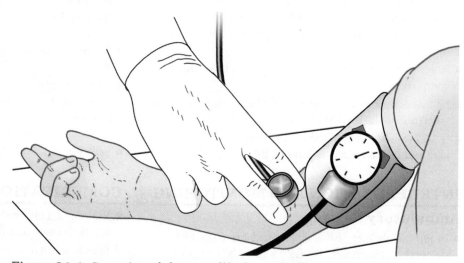

Figure 24–1. *Proper size and placement of blood pressure cuff.*

- In the presence of hypertension, left ventricular mass is increased; this measurement, obtained by echocardiography, is very useful in determining when to initiate therapy in children with high BP.
- Through the efforts of the NIH-based Working Group on High Blood Pressure in Children and Adolescents, there is now a large national database of normal BP values throughout childhood to allow identification of children with early hypertension.

PATIENT PREPARATION

- To determine usual BP in a nonemergent situation for comparison to norms, the child should ideally have avoided stimulant food or drugs and have been sitting quietly for 5 minutes.

PATIENT POSITIONING

- In the nonemergent setting, the child should be seated with the back supported, feet on the floor, and right arm supported with the cubital fossa at heart level.
- In critical care settings, consistency in position of the patient, the limb in which BP is measured and the technique of measurement should be maintained to optimize detection of physiologic change.

PROCEDURE

- Cuff pressure should be pumped up to above anticipated systolic BP, then slowly and consistently deflated while listening with the bell of the stethoscope over the brachial artery pulse in the cubital fossa.
- Systolic BP is the onset of the tapping sound of arterial flow, the first Korotkoff sound (K1).
- In acute care settings where Korotkoff sounds may be difficult to appreciate, a Doppler probe over the brachial or radial pulse can optimize measurement of systolic BP.
- Diastolic BP occurs with the disappearance of Korotkoff sounds (K5).
- In some children, Korotkoff sounds can be heard down to 0 mm Hg.
  - If this occurs, measurement should be repeated with less pressure on the head of the stethoscope.
- If K5 persists down to 0, then K4, muffling of the Korotkoff sounds is recorded as diastolic BP.

INTERPRETATION AND MONITORING
Ambulatory Setting

- In normal children, BP is determined primarily by body size and age; therefore, BP results must be compared to norms for age and height.

- BPs are consistently higher in males beginning in early childhood; therefore, BP results must also be compared to norms for gender.
- Revised BP tables from the 2004 report by the National High Blood Pressure Education Program Working Group on High Blood Pressure in Children and Adolescents include the 50th, 90th, 95th, and 99th percentiles by gender, age, and height.
  - Use standard height charts to determine height percentile.
  - On appropriate gender table, follow the age row across to the intersection with the column for the height percentile for systolic and diastolic BP.
- Classification.
  - BP < 90th percentile is normal.
  - BP between 90th and 95th percentile is prehypertension; repeat BP measurement twice and record the average.
  - In adolescents, BP ≥ 120/80 mm Hg is prehypertension even if < 90th percentile.
  - BP > 95th percentile indicates possible hypertension; see Staging.
- Staging.
  - Stage 1: BP ≤ 99th percentile + 5 mm Hg, repeat BP on 2 more occasions; if high BP is confirmed, begin evaluation.
  - Stage 2: BP > 99th percentile + 5 mm Hg prompts referral for evaluation and therapy.
  - Symptomatic patients require immediate referral and treatment.

Acute Care Setting

- Because BP measurements by cuff and auscultation are unreliable in unstable patients and automated oscillometric methods lack accuracy and reliability, arterial monitoring of BP is preferable.
- In initial assessment of BP, mild to moderate hypotension is diagnosed when systolic BP is 20–30% below normal mean systolic BP for age; severe hypotension is diagnosed when systolic BP is < 30% of normal systolic BP for age.
- In critical care settings, mean BP is often used to monitor BP.
- BP results must always be interpreted in light of all available evidence for cardiac output, including mental status, skin perfusion, and urinary output, since hypotension is the last sign to develop in the failing circulation.
- Sedation can lower BP without compromising perfusion.

COMPLICATIONS

- Prolonged cuff application and inflation can lead to a transient ulnar neuropathy.
- Petechiae can develop below the level of cuff application if initial inflation pressure is too high.

REFERENCES

Adatio I, Cox PN. Invasive and Non-Invasive Monitoring. In: Chang A, Hanley F, Wernovsky G, Wessel DL, eds. *Pediatric Cardiac Intensive Care.* Baltimore: Lippincott Williams and Wilkins; 1998:137–150.

Centers for Disease Control and Prevention, National Center for Health Statistics. 2000 CDC growth charts: United States. Available at: http://www.cdc.gov/growthcharts/.

Lurbe E, Sorof JM, Daniels SR. Clinical and research aspects of ambulatory blood pressure monitoring in children. *J Pediatr.* 2004;144:7–16.

National High Blood Pressure Education Program Working Group on High Blood Pressure in Children and Adolescents. The fourth report on the diagnosis, evaluation, and treatment of high blood pressure in children and adolescents. *Pediatrics.* 2004;114(2 Suppl 4th Report):555–576.

[CHAPTER 25]

Nasogastric Tube Insertion

Boris Sudel, MD and B U.K. Li, MD

INDICATIONS

- Decompression of the upper gastrointestinal tract (eg, pancreatitis, intestinal obstruction).
- Gastric lavage.
- Enteral feeding.

CONTRAINDICATIONS

Absolute

- Unstable airway.
- Intestinal perforation.
- Cervical spine trauma.
- Facial trauma.

Relative

- Coagulopathy (prothrombin time > 18 seconds).
- Thrombocytopenia (platelet count < 100,000/mcL).
- Recent intestinal tract surgery (< 1 month ago).

EQUIPMENT

- Lubricant gel.
- Nasogastric (NG) tube.
  - Larger diameter, polyethylene NG tube for suction and decompression.
  - Smaller diameter, silicone NG tube for enteral feeding.
- Water or normal saline at room temperature.
- Drainage bag or feeding pump.
- 60-mL catheter tip syringe.
- Stethoscope.

RISKS

- Bleeding.
- Perforation.

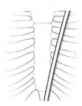
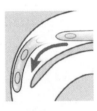

PEARLS AND TIPS

- Measure length of tube insertion by positioning the tube from the nares or mouth to the ear, then to the umbilicus.
- There is also a standard table, which uses height of child.
- If the tube is obstructed, flush first with water; longstanding obstruction may be removed by flushing the tube with caffeinated soda.

PATIENT PREPARATION

- Explain indication and risks to the patient and parents.
- Inform the patient of the intention of the procedure.

PATIENT POSITIONING

- Patient should be sitting.

ANATOMY REVIEW

- Tube position from the nose to the stomach.

PROCEDURE

- Measure the length of insertion from the nares to the ear and to the epigastrium (Figure 25–1); mark it on the tube with an indelible pen.
- Lubricate tube with gel.
- Insert the tube through the nose (Figure 25–2).
- Ask the patient to cooperate by swallowing while the tube is being inserted.
- Advance the tube to the length mark.
- To check position, aspirate tube with 50-mL syringe (Figure 25–3); gastric aspirate (pH = 1–3) confirms positioning in stomach.
- Insert small amount of air (20–30 mL) via NG tube while listening to epigastric area of stomach with stethoscope.
- If unsure about tube placement, verify tube position by obtaining a chest film before starting enteral feeding or drug treatment.
- Secure tube to the face with tape.

MONITORING

- Monitor intake and output volume.
- Evaluate tube position.
- Patient symptoms.

COMPLICATIONS

- Aspiration.
- Infection.

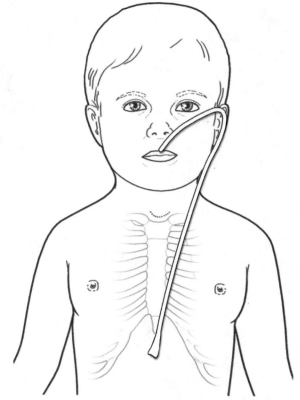

Figure 25–1. *Measuring the length of tube for insertion.*

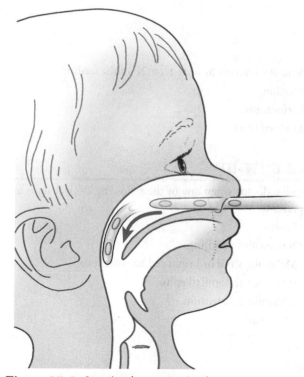

Figure 25–2. *Inserting the nasogastric tube.*

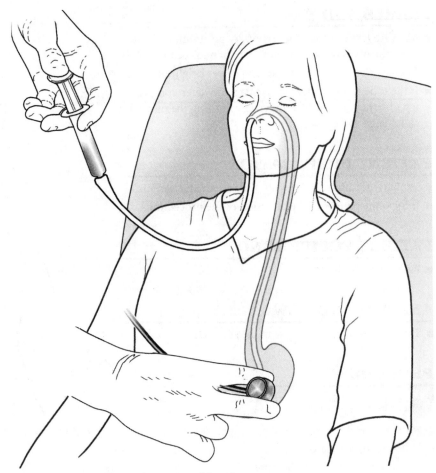

Figure 25–3. *Checking the position of the tube.*

- Sinusitis (caused by long-term NG tube feeding).
- Bleeding.
- Perforation.
- Mucosal tears.

FOLLOW-UP

- Call a doctor when any of the following clinical signs are present:
  - Fever.
  - Nausea and vomiting.
  - Melanotic stool or bright red hematemesis.
  - Persistent abdominal pain.
  - Abdominal distention.
  - Chest pain.

REFERENCES

Arbogast D. Enteral feedings with comfort and safety. *Clin J Oncol Nurs.* 2002;6:275–280.

Gopalan S, Khanna S. Enteral nutrition delivery technique. *Curr Opin Clin Nutr Metab Care.* 2003;6:313–317.

Levy H. Nasogastric and nasoenteric feeding tubes. *Gastrointest Endosc Clin N Am.* 1998;8:529–549.

CHAPTER 26

Gastric Lavage

Boris Sudel, MD and B U.K. Li, MD

INDICATIONS

- Therapeutically: To remove gastric contents after poisoning or drug overdose.
- Diagnostically: To confirm upper gastrointestinal bleeding.

CONTRAINDICATIONS

Absolute

- Unstable airway.
- Intestinal perforation.
- Cervical spine trauma.
- Facial trauma.

Relative

- Coagulopathy (prothrombin time > 18 seconds).
- Thrombocytopenia (platelet count < 100,000/mcL).
- Recent intestinal tract surgery (< 1 month ago).

EQUIPMENT

- Lubricant gel.
- Large bore orogastric tube.
- Terumo 60-mL catheter tip syringe.
- Normal saline at 38 °C.
- Drainage basin.
- Stethoscope.

RISKS

- Perforation.
- Bleeding.

PEARLS AND TIPS

- Measure length of tube insertion by positioning the tube from the nares or mouth to the ear, and to the umbilicus.
- There is also a standard table, which uses height of child.

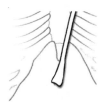
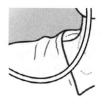

- If the tube is obstructed, flush first with water; longstanding obstruction may be removed by flushing the tube with caffeinated soda.

PATIENT PREPARATION

- Explain indication and risks to the patient and parents.
- Inform the patient of the intention of the procedure.

PATIENT POSITIONING

- Left lateral head-down position with a 20-degree table tilt (Trendelenburg).

ANATOMY REVIEW

- Tube position from the nose to the stomach.

PROCEDURE

- Measure the length of insertion from the mouth to the ear to the epigastrium (Figure 26–1); mark it on the tube with an indelible pen.
- Lubricate tube with gel.
- Insert the tube through the mouth midline after lubrication.
- Ask the patient to cooperate by swallowing while the tube is being inserted.
- Advance the tube to the length mark.
- To check position, aspirate tube with 50-mL catheter tip syringe (Figure 26–2); gastric aspirate confirms positioning in stomach.
- Insert small amount of air (20–30 mL) via orogastric tube while listening to the epigastric area with stethoscope.
- If unsure about tube position, obtain a chest film to confirm tube position.
- Secure tube to the face with tape.
- After insertion of the orogastric tube, begin to irrigate stomach with saline.
- Use 10–15-mL/kg aliquots of warm (38 °C) isotonic saline.
- Lavage should continue until the effluent is clear.
- For diagnostic lavage, notice presence of fresh red blood, blood clots, or coffee ground material to confirm upper gastrointestinal bleeding.
  - At this time, diagnostic lavage should be stopped.
  - Confirm presence of blood with Gastroccult cards.

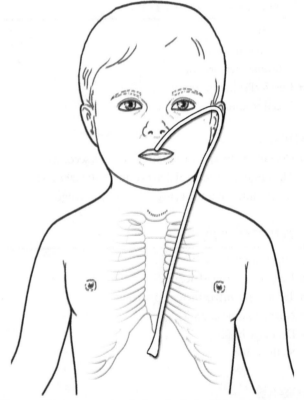

Figure 26–1. *Measuring the length of tube for insertion.*

MONITORING

- Monitor intake and output volume.
- Evaluate tube position.
- Patient symptoms.

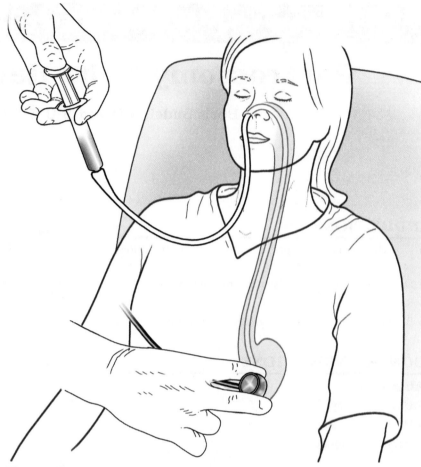

Figure 26–2. *Checking the position of the tube.*

COMPLICATIONS

- Aspiration.
- Bleeding.
- Perforation.
- Mucosal tears.

CAVEATS

- There is no certain evidence that gastric lavage improves clinical outcome, and it can cause significant morbidity.
- In experimental studies, the amount of marker removed by gastric lavage was highly variable and diminished with time.
- Gastric lavage should not be considered unless a patient has ingested a potentially life-threatening amount of a poison and the procedure can be undertaken within 60 minutes of ingestion. Even then, clinical benefit has not been confirmed in controlled studies.

FOLLOW-UP

- Call a doctor when any of the following clinical signs are present:

- Fever.
- Nausea and vomiting.
- Melanotic stool or bright red hematemesis.
- Abdominal pain.
- Abdominal distention.
- Chest pain.

REFERENCES

Bartlett D. The ABCs of gastric decontamination. *J Emerg Nurs.* 2003;29:576–577.

Tucker JR. Indications for, techniques of, complications of, and efficacy of gastric lavage in the treatment of the poisoned child. *Curr Opin Pediatr.* 2000;12:163–165.

Vale JA, Kulig K; American Academy of Clinical Toxicology; European Association of Poisons Centres and Clinical Toxicologists. Position paper: gastric lavage. *J Toxicol Clin Toxicol.* 2004;42:933–943.

CHAPTER 27

Gastrostomy Tube Replacement

Boris Sudel, MD and B U.K. Li, MD

INDICATIONS

- First change should be performed 6–8 weeks after initial gastrostomy tube placement.
- Dislodged gastrostomy tube or gastrostomy button.
- Replacing a gastrostomy button.
- Blocked gastrostomy tube or gastrostomy button.

CONTRAINDICATIONS

Absolute

- Unstable airway.
- Hemodynamically unstable patient.
- Intestinal perforation.

Relative

- Coagulopathy (prothrombin time > 18 seconds).
- Thrombocytopenia (platelet count < 100,000/mcL).
- Recent intestinal tract surgery (< 1 month ago).

EQUIPMENT

- Lubricant gel.
- Gastrostomy catheter.
- Button.
- Normal saline.
- 10-mL syringe.

RISKS

- Bleeding.
- Perforation.

PATIENT PREPARATION

- Explain indication and risks to the patient and parents.
- Inform the patient of the intention of the procedure.

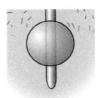

PATIENT POSITIONING

■ Supine.

ANATOMY REVIEW

■ The gastrostomy opening is usually located in the left upper quadrant of the abdomen with the bulb located in the body of the stomach.

PROCEDURE

■ Prepare new tube for insertion.
- • Remove from package.
- • Check balloon integrity by inflating.
- • Deflate and lubricate end with gel.
- • Put stopper in place.
■ Remove old tube.
- • Deflate balloon fully with syringe and pull out firmly.
- • There is usually some resistance caused by the tube cuff.
■ Insert new tube into stoma.
- • If patient is obese, may need to go further.
- • Check old tube shaft measurements before removing.
■ Without moving the tube, inflate balloon fully.
■ Tug on tube to check whether the balloon is inflated and then secure (Figure 27–1).

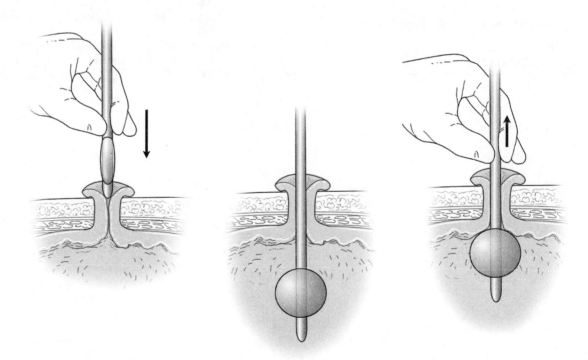

Figure 27–1. *Inserting and positioning gastrostomy tube.*

- While firmly pulling tube upward, push fixation bolster down to the skin so that any in-out movement of the tube is prevented.
- Small amount of slack (~2–5 mm) is advised for comfort and to prevent pressure necrosis.
- Gastric contents will probably now be apparent in the tube.
  - If not, and stoma is new, aspirate tube to check.
  - If stoma is well established (> 3 months) and this is not the first tube change, aspiration test is unnecessary.

Checking the Balloon

- Balloons deflate over time (by osmosis), so contents should be checked monthly (more often leads to increased risk of bursting).
- Withdraw the contents of balloon using a 10-mL syringe; hold the tube in place carefully to avoid displacement.
- Observe amount withdrawn and top up to correct amount.
- Refill balloon with normal saline.
- **Note:** It is wise to push the tube down into the stomach to avoid accidentally pulling it out. (If this happens, simply push the tube back in.)
- **Caution:**
  - You may feel resistance if you are inflating the balloon in the tract. Stop and push in further. Deflate the balloon and reposition the tube.
  - Pushing the tube in too far can place it through the pyloric sphincter into the duodenum. If you inflate the balloon there, the stomach cannot empty, causing excessive billous, formula free vomiting, and tube leakage.

MONITORING

- Assess balloon inflation.

- Evaluate position of the gastrostomy tube for blockage, dislodgment.
- Check the skin for infection or granulation tissue as well as around the tube for leakage.

COMPLICATIONS

- Perforation, creating false tract.
- Pneumoperitoneum.
- Bleeding.
- Infection.

FOLLOW-UP

- Call a doctor when any of the following clinical signs are present:
  - Fever.
  - Nausea and vomiting.
  - Melanotic stool or bright red hematemesis.
  - Abdominal pain.
  - Abdominal distention.

REFERENCES

Arrowsmith H. Nursing management of patients receiving gastrostomy feeding. *Br J Nurs.* 1996;5:268–273.

Kirby DF, Craig RM, Tsang TK, Plotnick BH. Percutaneous endoscopic gastrostomies: a prospective evaluation and review of the literature. *JPEN J Parenter Enteral Nutr.* 1986;10:155–159.

Willwerth BM. Percutaneous endoscopic gastrostomy or skin-level gastrostomy tube replacement. *Pediatr Emerg Care.* 2001;17:55–58.

CHAPTER 28

Paracentesis/Peritoneal Lavage

Boris Sudel, MD and B U.K. Li, MD

INDICATIONS

- Diagnostic sampling of ascitic fluid (eg, internal bleeding following blunt abdominal trauma, chylous ascites after surgery, rule out malignancy, identification of infectious organism in spontaneous bacterial peritonitis).
- Therapeutic removal of the ascitic fluid (eg, chylous ascites, tense ascites, intestinal lymphangiectasia).

CONTRAINDICATIONS

Absolute

- Unstable airway.
- Hemodynamically unstable patient.
- Intestinal perforation.

Relative

- Infection of the abdominal wall.
- Coagulopathy (prothrombin time > 18 seconds).
- Thrombocytopenia (platelet count < 100,000/mcL).
- Recent intestinal tract surgery (< 1 month ago).

EQUIPMENT

- Alcohol swabs, povidone-iodine.
- 23-gauge and 21-gauge needles or angiocatheters with syringes.
- Local anesthetic (eg, 1% lidocaine).
- Large bore needle with plastic catheter.
- Sterile containers for fluid collection.
- Appropriate culture tubes for microorganisms.

RISKS

- Pneumoperitoneum.
- Perforation: Intestine, solid organs.
- Bleeding.
- Infection.

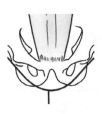

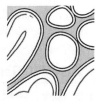

PATIENT PREPARATION

- Explain indication and risks to the patient and parents.
- Inform the patient of the intention of the procedure.

PATIENT POSITIONING

- Supine or side.

ANATOMY REVIEW

- The preferred site is in the midline approximately one-third of the distance from the umbilicus to the symphysis pubis (Figure 28–1).
- In infants, the fluid may bulge laterally, and the paracentesis may be obtained laterally to that point.

PROCEDURE

Paracentesis

- The puncture site should be shaved, if necessary, and cleansed with povidone-iodine.
- Inject local anesthetic, infiltrating the skin first and then penetrating into deeper layers.
- A small 3-mm incision can be made with a scalpel to help insert the needle. Using Z-track technique, insert the tap needle 1–2 inches into the abdomen (Figure 28–2).
- Obtain a sample of fluid or withdraw as much fluid as necessary with a syringe (in case of therapeutic lavage) (Figure 28–3).
- Remove the needle and apply a pressure dressing to the puncture site.
- If an incision was made, it may be closed using 1 or 2 stitches.
- The ascitic fluid removed may be replaced 1:1 with 5% albumin IV.

Diagnostic Peritoneal Lavage

- The puncture site should be shaved, if necessary, and cleaned with povidone-iodine.
- Inject local anesthetic, infiltrating the skin first and then penetrating into deeper layers.
- A small 3-mm incision can be made with a scalpel to help insert the needle.
- Insert the tap needle 1–2 inches into the abdomen.
- Insert a trochar and peritoneal catheter until the peritoneal cavity is reached (the resistance suddenly gives away).
- Remove the trochar and fix the catheter to the skin with a stitch.
- Aspirate.

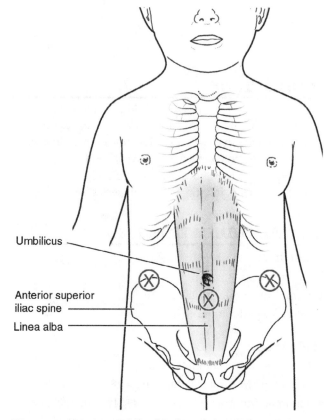

Umbilicus

Anterior superior iliac spine

Linea alba

Figure 28–1. *Anatomic landmarks and sites of entry.*

- Diagnostic peritoneal lavage is usually performed by a surgeon to rule out internal bleeding following trauma.

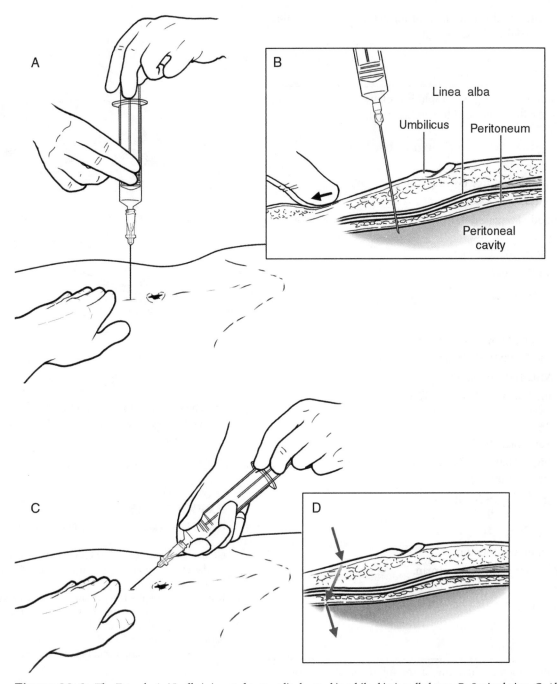

Figure 28–2. *The Z-track.* ***A:*** *Needle is inserted perpendicular to skin while skin is pulled taut.* ***B:*** *Sagittal view.* ***C:*** *Alternatively, needle can be inserted at 45 degrees to skin and aimed caudally.* ***D:*** *Resultant Z-track (arrows).*

■ If no bloody fluid is withdrawn, infuse 20 mL/kg of Ringer's lactate over 5–10 minutes:

- Turn the patient from side to side.
- Siphon the fluid off.
- Inspect for level of turbidity.
- Send fluid to laboratory for red and white blood cell counts, bacterial culture, amylase.

• Ascitic fluid should be sent for cytology, amylase, albumin, triglycerides, and culture.

MONITORING

■ Monitor vital signs (a rapid loss of significant volumes of ascitic fluid may lead to hypotension).

Diagnostic Peritoneal Lavage

A. POSITIVE

■ Aspiration of free flowing blood, or

■ Aspiration of feces, or

■ Bloody lavage fluid, from peritoneal lavage catheter containing:

• RBC > 100,000/mcL.

• WBC > 500/mcL.

• Amylase > 175 IU/dL.

B. INDETERMINATE

■ Serosanguinous lavage fluid:

• RBC 50,000–100,000/mcL.

• WBC 100–500/mcL.

• Amylase > 75 IU/dL, < 175 IU/dL.

C. NEGATIVE

■ Clear lavage fluid:

• RBC < 50,000/mcL.

• WBC < 100/mcL.

• Amylase < 75 IU/dL.

Complications

■ Pneumoperitoneum.

■ Perforation: Intestine, organ.

■ Bleeding.

■ Infection.

FOLLOW-UP

■ Call a doctor when any of the following clinical signs is present:

• Fever.

• Nausea and vomiting.

• Blood in the stool.

• Abdominal pain.

• Abdominal distention.

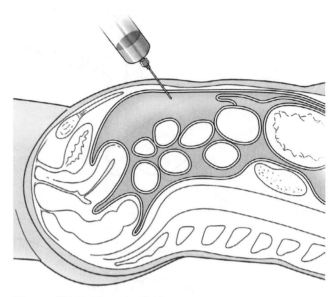

Figure 28–3. *Removing fluid.*

—————————[■ ■ ■]—————————

■ The evidence for visceral blunt trauma with peritoneal lavage is gauged as positive, indeterminate, or negative.

REFERENCES

Gerber DR, Bekes CE. Peritoneal catheterization. *Crit Care Clin.* 1992;8:727–742.

Grabau CM, Crago SF, Hoff LK et al. Performance standards for therapeutic abdominal paracentesis. *Hepatology.* 2004;40: 484–488.

Kramer RE, Sokol RJ, Yerushalmi B et al. Large-volume paracentesis in the management of ascites in children. *J Pediatr Gastroenterol Nutr.* 2001;33:245–249.

Sartori M, Andorno S, Gambaro M et al. Diagnostic paracentesis. A two-step approach. *Ital J Gastroenterol.* 1996;28:81–85.

CHAPTER 29

Hernia Reduction

Marybeth Browne, MD, Anthony Chin, MD, and Marleta Reynolds, MD

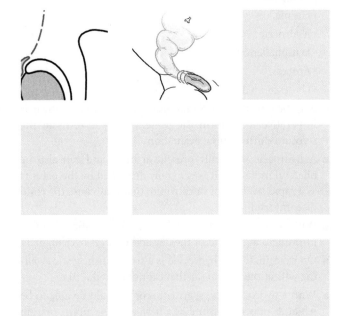

INDICATIONS

- A hernia is a benign process unless the contents within the hernia sac become incarcerated.
- Incarceration is the inability of the hernia's contents to be reduced.
- The risk of incarceration is highest during infancy with a 28–31% incarceration rate before 3 months of age and 15–24% by 6 months of age.
- Although the risk of incarceration gradually decreases with age, the severity of its consequences mandates immediate manual reduction when possible, followed by prompt operative repair.

CONTRAINDICATIONS

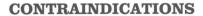

Absolute

- Reduction should not be attempted if there has been bowel compromise or when the patient appears toxic.
- Concern for toxicity should arise when the patient has any of the following:
  - Severe tachycardia.
  - Increased leukocyte count.
  - Bloody stool or positive result on modified guaiac test.
  - Severe pain with palpation.
  - Erythema of the hernia sac.

Relative

- Some surgeons do not advocate manual reduction if the patient has any signs or symptoms of intestinal obstruction.

EQUIPMENT

- Gloves.

RISKS

- There are few risks with manual reduction.
  - However, parents should be informed that once a hernia has been incarcerated, it has a high probability of recurring.

• A hernia will not resolve on its own and operative management will be required in the near future.

■ If sedation is used during the reduction, a parent is required to sign a consent form and be made aware of the risks and benefits that accompany sedation.

■ In addition, a parent should be instructed not to feed the child should the hernia become strangulated or is not reducible and the patient requires emergent operative intervention.

PEARLS AND TIPS

■ The most common differential diagnosis for a bulge in the groin consists of the following:
  • Hernia.
  • Hydrocele.
  • Lymphadenopathy.
  • Abscess.
  • Undescended testis.

■ A testicle in the groin may resemble a hernia; thus, it is imperative to confirm the presence of the testis in the scrotum during initial evaluation.

■ A hydrocele is usually present at birth and can also be bilateral in nature. It is generally described by the parents as a rapid swelling of the scrotum that may cause the child discomfort if tense.

■ With a communicating hydrocele, the swelling is most prominent at the end of the day and reduces over night.

■ On examination, a hydrocele is a soft, bluish, cystic swelling within the scrotal sac that cannot be reduced.

■ With a hydrocele, the spermatic cord should be able to be felt at its upper limits unlike a hernia, whose upper margin is not clearly defined and continues into the internal ring.

■ Transillumination may help differentiate a hernia from a hydrocele.
  • Hernias do not transilluminate as brightly as hydroceles.
  • However, hernias can transilluminate if they are filled with an air-filled loop.

■ Simple hydroceles generally resolve by the age of 1 year and do not require an operation until after this time.

PATIENT PREPARATION AND POSITIONING

■ The child should be examined supine and undressed to observe any asymmetry or obvious masses in the scrotum or groin area.

■ Both testicles should be palpated and identified separately from the mass.

■ Next, the index finger should be placed over the inguinal canal in the attempt to palpate the cord structures.

■ While perpendicular to the inguinal structures, the finger should be rubbed from side to side.

- If the cord structures appear thickened compared with the normal side, this is considered a positive silk glove sign.
  - Ideally, this should feel similar to rubbing 2 pieces of silk together or running your fingers over a plastic baggy that contains a drop of water.
- If there is a good history of a hernia but the physical examination does not demonstrate a bulge, attempts to reproduce the hernia may be accomplished by increasing the intra-abdominal pressure.
  - This can be achieved in infants by holding the patient with legs and arms extended, which will cause some struggle and an increase in intra-abdominal pressure.
  - For older children, a Valsalva maneuver, such as blowing up a balloon or pretending to blow out candles, may be performed.
- It is important to note the extent of the hernia sac and the ease by which it reduces when the child is relaxed.

ANATOMY REVIEW

- The anatomy for the inguinal region is basically that of the adult (Figure 29–1).
- However, the inguinal canal is not completely developed, making it extremely short, and the external ring is placed almost directly over the internal ring.

PROCEDURE

- The patient should be placed supine and allowed to relax.
- If the hernia does not reduce with gentle pressure, consider using mild or conscious sedation. After allowing enough time for the sedation to take effect, attempts are made to align the hernia sac in the inguinal canal.
- When attempting manual reduction, it is important to remember that the inguinal canal is not completely developed, making it extremely short, and the external ring is placed almost directly over the internal ring.
- After alignment, firm, constant, posterior, and upward pressure is applied to the hernia sac with the contralateral hand while guiding the hernia's contents through the internal ring with the ipsilateral hand (Figure 29–2).
- This may take several minutes of constant pressure and several attempts at reduction.
- Placing the patient in the Trendelenburg position, as well as applying an ice pack to the groin area for several minutes prior to manipulation, may help ease the reduction.

COMPLICATIONS

- Manual reduction has few complications.
- However, the physician who performs the reduction should be aware that, with too much force, it is possible to cause a bowel perforation.

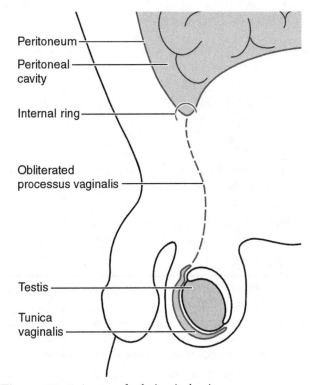

Figure 29–1. *Anatomy for the inguinal region.*

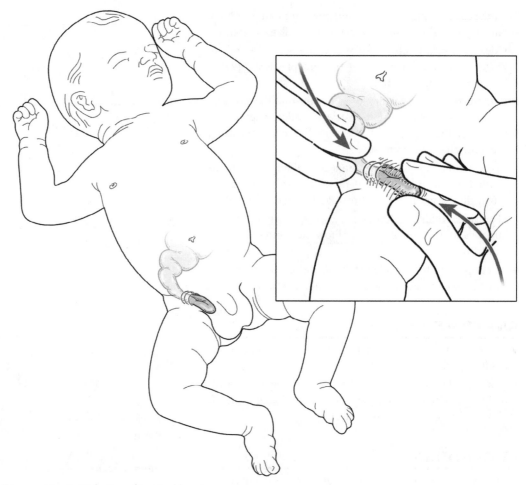

Figure 29–2. *Reduction of inguinal hernia.*

■ There is also the possibility that a piece of strangulated bowel may be reduced together with the hernia sac.

• If this should occur, the patient's symptoms will not resolve.

• Peritonitis may develop, requiring an emergent operation.

CAVEATS

■ Over 80% of incarcerated hernias can be initially reduced with manual reduction.

■ However, because most inguinal hernias do not spontaneously resolve and have a risk of recurrent incarceration or possible strangulation, definitive operative repair is necessary.

■ Most surgeons will attempt operative repair 48 hours after the manual reduction, allowing tissue swelling to resolve prior to the procedure.

FOLLOW-UP

■ A pediatric surgeon should be contacted to arrange for prompt follow-up in all patients with an incarcerated hernia.

■ However, if a patient has signs of intestinal obstruction, toxicity, bowel strangulation, or an incarcerated hernia that cannot be reduced, a pediatric surgeon should be notified immediately and the patient prepared for operative repair.

REFERENCES

Coles J. Operative cure of inguinal hernia in infancy and childhood. *Am J Surg.* 1945;69:366.

D'Agostino J. Common abdominal emergencies in children. *Emerg Med Clin North Am.* 2002;20:139–153.

Grosfeld JL. Current concepts in inguinal hernia in infants and children. *World J Surg.* 1989;13:506–515.

Gross RE. Inguinal Hernia. In Gross RE, ed. *The Surgery of Infancy and Childhood.* Philadelphia: WB Saunders Company; 1953:449–462.

Kapur P, Caty MG, Glick PL. Pediatric hernias and hydroceles. *Pediatr Clin North Am.* 1998;45:773–789.

Ladd WE, Gross RE. *Abdominal Surgery in Infancy and Childhood.* Philadelphia: WB Saunders Company; 1941.

Ziegler MM, Azizkhan RG, Weber TR, eds. Inguinal and Femoral Hernia. In: *Operative Pediatric Surgery.* New York: McGraw-Hill Co; 2003:543–554.

CHAPTER 30

Rectal Prolapse Reduction

Anthony Chin, MD, Marybeth Browne, MD, and Marleta Reynolds, MD

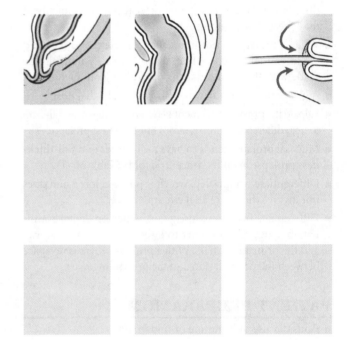

INDICATIONS

- Most cases of rectal prolapse reduce spontaneously.
- Rarely, a surgical procedure may be necessary to correct a full-thickness prolapse.
- Rectal prolapse should be promptly reduced to prevent a sustained prolapse that allows edema to form and potential subsequent venous congestion and thrombosis to develop, which may lead to ulceration of the rectal mucosa with bowel ischemia and infarction.
- A rectal examination needs to be performed to differentiate prolapse from an intussusception or rectal polyp.
- Diagnostic studies are often not necessary, but a proctoscopy, colonoscopy, or barium enema may be indicated when the patient has a history of rectal bleeding.
- Children need to be tested for parasites and cystic fibrosis as well as other causes of anal straining (including neuromuscular problems, proctitis, and inflammatory bowel disease).

CONTRAINDICATIONS

Absolute

- Presence of nonviable bowel or rupture of rectal mucosa.
- Child appears toxic (ie, with fever, tachycardia, or leukocytosis).

Relative

- Uncooperative patient.
- Questionable viability of bowel.
- Mucosal ulceration.
- Recent rectal pull-through procedure.

EQUIPMENT

- Gloves.
- Lubrication.
- Table sugar or salt.
- 6F rectal tube.

RISKS

■ There are very few risks with manual reduction.

■ Parents should be informed that prolapse may recur and instructed on proper technique for reduction.

■ Discuss the potential risk of sedative medication.

■ Recurrent prolapse or a prolapse that is not amenable to manual reduction may require operative intervention.

PEARLS AND TIPS

■ Rectal prolapse commonly presents in children between the ages of 1 and 3 years, with a primary symptom of anal discomfort or prolapse after defecation; occasionally it may present as bleeding.

■ When a prolapse is not immediately present and the child is old enough to cooperate, diagnosis can potentially be made with the child squatting or straining on the toilet.

■ A glycerine suppository may also aid in the diagnosis.

■ Palpate the prolapsed segment between the fingers and thumb to help differentiate mucosa from full-thickness prolapse.

■ Mucosal prolapse tends to have radial folds and full-thickness prolapse exhibits concentric folds (Table 30–1).

■ Differentiate from polyp, which is plum-colored and does not involve the entire anal circumference.

■ Differentiate from intussusception, which on digital examination allows the examiner to insert between the anal wall and the protruding mass. With a prolapse, there is no space between the perianal skin and the protruding mass.

PATIENT PREPARATION

■ Consider use of ketamine or midazolam.

PATIENT POSITIONING

■ Have the patient lie supine in the Trendelenburg position on a padded surface.

■ Elevate the lower extremities and flex the patient's hips.

ANATOMY REVIEW

■ Rectal prolapse occurs with stretching of the pelvic peritoneum, weakening and dilation of the rectal suspension mechanism, and a low resting anal sphincter pressure that may be secondary to protracted straining due to diarrhea and constipation.

■ It may also be attributed to poor posterior rectal fixation, redundant rectosigmoid colon, neurologic diseases, cystic fibrosis, infections, malnutrition, previous surgery, undiagnosed Hirschsprung disease, or imperforate anus.

■ On examination, a mucosal prolapse is described as a swollen rosette of mucosa with radial folds at the anal junction (Figure 30–1).

Table 30–1. Classification of rectal prolapse.

Characteristics	Mucosal Prolapse	Full-thickness Prolapse (Procidentia)
Layers involved	Mucosa only	All layers of the rectum
Physical appearance	Rosette appearing with radial folds at anal junction	Circular folds in prolapsed mucosa May not be seen with significant edema

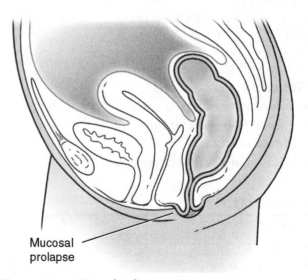

Mucosal prolapse

Figure 30–1. *Mucosal prolapse.*

- A full-thickness prolapse (procidentia), involving all layers of the rectum, has circular folds of prolapsed mucosa (Figure 30–2).

PROCEDURE

- The prolapsed rectum may be reduced with gentle and steady digital pressure.
- The herniated bowel should be grasped with a lubricated glove between fingertips with cephalad pressure applied to the tip of the prolapsed rectum until reduction is complete.
- Firm and steady pressure for several minutes may be necessary in edematous bowel to reduce swelling and allow reduction.
- A digital examination at the end of the procedure is necessary to verify that the reduction is complete.
- Taping of the buttocks has been used in the past but is not always effective.
- If manual reduction is unsuccessful, sedation and perianal field block with local anesthesia may aid in the success of reduction.
- With significant bowel edema, the application of topical sucrose or table salt applied to the prolapsed rectum may decrease edema and allow reduction of herniated bowel.
- It has also been described that use of a soft, lubricated, 6F rectal tube inserted through a segment of prolapsed bowel may help guide reduction (Figure 30–3).
- Reduction is accomplished by pushing the prolapsed segment over the tube.
- If all attempts fail, the prolapse needs to be surgically reduced.
- The parents should be instructed on how to reduce the prolapsed rectum should it occur at home and instructed to call or return to the emergency department if they are unable to reduce the prolapse.
- Surgical consultation should be obtained for the reduction under the following circumstances:
  - Presence of mucosal ulceration.
  - Failure of reduction.
  - Severe pain and discomfort.
  - Patient with history of pull-through procedure for imperforate anus and Hirschsprung disease.

MONITORING

- Monitor patient vital signs if using sedation.

COMPLICATIONS

- Recurrence.
- Mucosal ulceration.
- Necrosis of bowel wall.

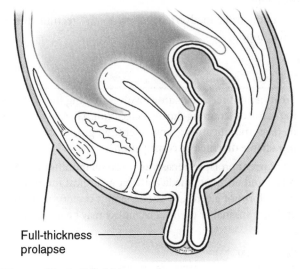

Full-thickness prolapse

Figure 30–2. *Full-thickness prolapse.*

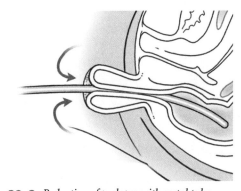

Figure 30–3. *Reduction of prolapse with rectal tube.*

- Bleeding.
- Infection from inadvertent injury to the rectum during reduction.

CAVEATS

- Treatment of rectal prolapse involves treating the underlying cause of straining during defecation. Therapy includes dietary modifications and identifying the cause (eg, intractable diarrhea or constipation).
- If recurrent prolapse persists after several months of appropriate and adequate medical therapy, surgical intervention in the form of a cerclage, sclerotherapy, cauterization therapy, or transanal or perineal rectopexy may be necessary.

FOLLOW-UP

- Instruct parents to notify you if prolapse recurs and is unable to be reduced.

REFERENCES

Bhandarkar DS, Tamhane RG. Reduction of complete rectal prolapse. *Trop Doct.* 1992;22:180.

Coburn WM III, Russell MA, Hofstetter WL. Sucrose as an aid to manual reduction of incarcerated rectal prolapse. *Ann Emerg Med.* 1997;30:347–349.

Corman ML. Rectal prolapse in children. *Dis Colon Rectum.* 1985;28:535–539.

Duhamel J, Pernin P. Anal prolapse in the child. *Ann Gastroenterol Hepatol (Paris).* 1985;21:361–362.

Groff DB, Nagaraj HS. Rectal prolapse in infants and children. *Am J Surg.* 1990;160:531–532.

Siafakas C, Vottler TP, Andersen JM. Rectal prolapse in pediatrics. *Clin Pediatr (Phila).* 1999;38:63–72.

Stafford PW. Other Disorders of the Anus and Rectum, Anorectal Function. In: O'Neil JA et al, eds. *Pediatric Surgery.* 5th edition. St Louis: Mosby; 1998:1449–1460.

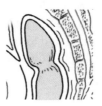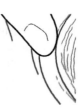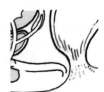
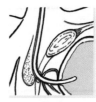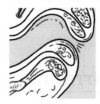

[CHAPTER 31]

Straight Urethral Catheterization

Mark Adler, MD

INDICATIONS

- Diagnostic evaluation.
- Temporary relief of urinary retention.

CONTRAINDICATIONS

Absolute

- Suspected urethral injury (eg, blood at meatus, laceration).
- Unable to identify urethra (eg, labial adhesion).
- Neutropenia.

EQUIPMENT

- Catheter.
  - Feeding tube (4–5F).
  - Urinary catheters (6F and up).
- Sterile collection cup.
- 10% povidone-iodine (or equivalent).
- Castile soap.
- Sterile gloves, drapes, and gauze.
- Lidocaine (2%) anesthetic jelly or water-based lubricant.
- Catheter sizing estimates:
  - Infant: 5F feeding tube or 6F catheter
  - Toddler: 6–8F catheter
  - Older child: 8F catheter
  - Adolescent: 8–10F catheters

RISKS

- Urethral trauma.
  - Hematuria.
  - Pain (common).
- Psychological stress (common, as child is restrained for procedure).
- Catheter mishaps (eg, knot forms in bladder) (very rare).

—[■ ■ ■]—

- All equipment should be latex free. Allergy to latex is common, particularly in certain populations (such as patients with meningomyelocele.)

—[■ ■ ■]—

- Always choose the smallest catheter that will work; a catheter that is too small might kink and one that is too large will cause unnecessary pain.

PEARLS AND TIPS

- Because spontaneous voiding may occur during skin preparation or as the procedure is initiated, have a sterile container available to collect the urine.
- When labial adhesions are present, holding the child in a frog-leg position and rocking the hips back and forth may line up the opening in the adhered labia with the urethral opening.
- Cotton gauze pads are useful to hold the penis or to apply traction to the labia once the skin has been prepared and is slippery.
- Remember that many of the newer, non-latex gloves fit poorly, making holding a slippery skin surface nearly impossible; wear tightly fitting non-latex gloves when possible.
- Although 1 study showed that pain was reduced by applying lidocaine topically **and** injecting anesthetic into the urethra, this does not represent typical use of lidocaine jelly in clinical practice.

PATIENT PREPARATION

- Keep the patient covered until ready to begin.
- Good lighting is helpful.

PATIENT POSITIONING

- The child is placed supine.
- The female patient is placed in the frog-leg position.
- The male patient is placed with legs extended.

ANATOMY REVIEW

- Catheterization requires the passage of a tube through the urethra into the urinary bladder.
- In girls, the urethra is a short tube that opens just rostral to the vaginal introitus and is often obscured in younger girls by vaginal tissue (Figure 31–1).
- A common problem with catheterization of young females results from confusion and erroneous passage of the catheter into the vagina (Figure 31–2).
- In boys, the urethra begins at the meatus and passes down through the penile shaft and into the urinary bladder after passing through the prostate gland (Figure 31–3).
- The prostate and the urethral valves cause some resistance to catheter passage.
- Uncircumcised males have a foreskin that covers the glans completely; this structure must be retracted partially to clean the urethral meatus before catheterization (Figure 31–4).
- Occasionally, a tight phimosis prevents retraction and visualization of the meatus.
- While it is possible to catheterize without visualization, the risk of obtaining a contaminated specimen increases.

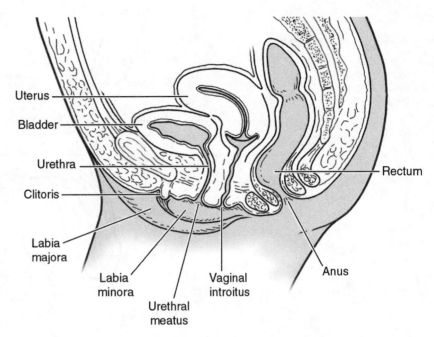

Figure 31–1. *Female genitourinary system.*

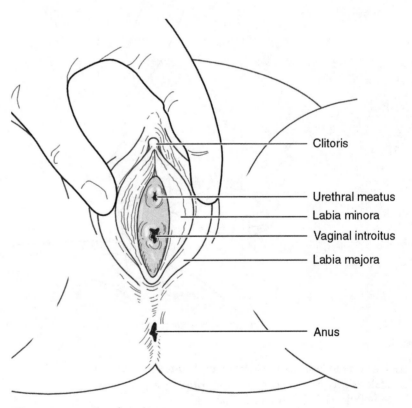

Figure 31–2. *Female perineum.*

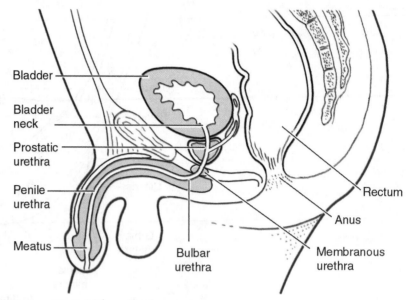

Figure 31–3. *Male genitourinary system.*

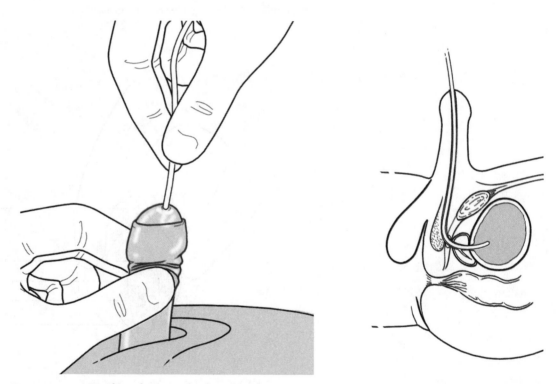

Figure 31–4. *Foreskin reduction and catheter insertion.*

■ Take care to evaluate the location of the urethra in young males since an undiagnosed hypospadias is a possibility, even if the child has been circumcised.

• The urethra in hypospadias can be located anywhere along the caudal aspect of the phallus from the base to just slightly caudal to the normal meatus.

• Significant hypospadias should not be catheterized without urologic evaluation.

PROCEDURE

- Observe sterile procedure.
  - Wear sterile gloves.
  - Use 1 hand to touch the patient if necessary, while keeping the hand with the catheter clean.

Male

A. CIRCUMCISED BOYS

- The glans and the distal phallus are cleaned with a 10% povidone-iodine solution.
- The penis is held gently retracted away from the body in the nondominant hand, with the penis held at about a 90-degree angle to the body.
- The catheter is lubricated with a water-based jelly with or without lidocaine and passed directly through the meatus downward (not angled rostrally).
- Some resistance may be felt at the prostate level, which can be overcome by using steady pressure.
- Do not push and pull the catheter to get it to pass.
- Once urine is visible in the catheter or collection cup, stop advancing the catheter.
- Remove the catheter gently after the sample is obtained.

B. UNCIRCUMCISED BOYS

- The procedure is the same as in circumcised boys, except that the foreskin is prepared first and then the foreskin is retracted just to the point that the meatus is visible. This area is then prepared as well.
- The catheter is inserted in the same fashion as above.
- The foreskin is then returned to the normal position.

Female

- The periurethral area and labia minora and majora are prepared with a 10% povidone-iodine solution.
- The catheter is lubricated with a water-based jelly with or without lidocaine and is passed into the urethra and directed straight downward toward the bed or very slightly rostrally (Figure 31–5).
- In smaller children, vaginal tissue can obscure the urethral opening; this tissue can be moved with a cotton swab.
- The first portion of the urine may be discarded; this is analogous to a mid-stream urine collection. This is only possible if the collection system is not a kit with the collection vial attached to the catheter.
- Applying pressure of the suprapubic area (Credé maneuver) may force out additional urine.
- Remember to remove residual povidone-iodine from the skin.

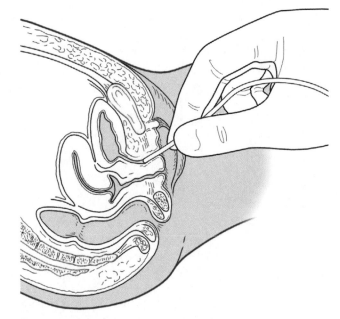

Figure 31–5. *Catheter insertion in female.*

INTERPRETATION AND MONITORING

- Urine obtained via catheter may be evaluated in a number of ways:
  - **Urine dipstick tests** (bedside) are a series of paper squares impregnated with chemical reagents that change color under specific conditions. Be aware that reading the strips beyond the recommended times on the container may lead to false-positive results.
  - **Urinalysis** (formal laboratory testing) is often a combination of the above tests and a microscope examination of the urine. The strict nature of the laboratory procedures yields a more accurate result, even for dipstick test.
  - **Culture** is commonly used to detect bacteria.
  - **Urine** can also be tested for virus (eg, cytomegalovirus) and fungi.
  - **Polymerase chain reaction** is done to test for *Chlamydia trachomatis* and *Neisseria gonorrhoeae*.
  - Urine human chorionic gonadotropin (hCG) is done to detect pregnancy.
  - **Toxicology screen** looks for drugs of abuse or specific substances.
  - **Other** (eg, urine electrolytes, organic acids).

COMPLICATIONS

- Pain.
- Hematuria.
- Dysuria with or without urinary retention.
- Paraphimosis, resulting from failure to reduce the foreskin after the procedure.
- Catheter knot (in infants, caused by advancing small catheters too far, allowing catheter to knot; may require cystoscopy or surgical removal).

FOLLOW-UP

- Dysuria and hematuria complications are transient.
- Infants and toddlers who have dysuria and refuse to void can be placed in a warm bath, which promotes voiding.
- Ongoing symptoms would be unusual and should prompt a new visit and evaluation, with consideration of other causes of the symptoms (eg, inadequate treatment of an infection).

REFERENCES

Dayan PS, Chamberlain JM, Boenning D, Adirim T, Schor JA, Klein BL. A comparison of the initial to the later stream urine in children catheterized to evaluate for a urinary tract infection. *Pediatr Emerg Care.* 2000;16:88–90.

Gerard LL, Cooper CS, Duethman KS, Gordley BM, Kleiber CM. Effectiveness of lidocaine lubricant for discomfort during pediatric urethral catheterization. *J Urol.* 2003;170(2 Pt 1):564–567.

Levison J, Wojtulewicz J. Adventitious knot formation complicating catheterization of the infant bladder. *J Paediatr Child Health.* 2004;40:493–494.

CHAPTER 32

Suprapubic Catheterization

Mark Adler, MD

INDICATIONS

■ Diagnostic evaluation of urine in an infant.

CONTRAINDICATIONS

Absolute

■ Neutropenia.
■ Thrombocytopenia and bleeding disorders.
■ Cellulitis and infection at puncture site.
■ Age greater than 2 years.

Relative

■ Urogenital anomalies.
■ Recent urologic or lower abdominal surgery.

EQUIPMENT

■ 22-gauge, 2–3-cm needle.
■ 3-mL or 5-mL syringe.
■ Sterile collection cup.
■ 10% povidone-iodine (or equivalent).
■ Sterile gloves, drapes, gauze.
■ Topical anesthetic or buffered 1% lidocaine solution, or both.

RISKS

■ Infection (rare).
■ Intestinal perforation (very rare).
■ Failure to obtain urine (success rates vary widely but less successful than catheterization).
■ Psychological stress (common, as child is restrained for procedure).
■ Pain (certain; can be limited somewhat with anesthesia).
■ Hematuria.
  • Microscopic is very common.
  • Macroscopic is uncommon.

■ All equipment should be latex free. Allergy to latex is common, particularly in certain populations (such as patients with meningomyelocele.)

PEARLS AND TIPS

- Appropriate patient restraint is critical to the success of the procedure.
- More than 2 or 3 attempts do not add to success rates.
- Ultrasonography has been reported to increase success rates in some studies.
- Because spontaneous voiding may occur during skin preparation or as the procedure is initiated, have a sterile container available to collect the urine.

PATIENT PREPARATION

- Keep the patient covered until ready to begin.
- Good lighting is helpful.

PATIENT POSITIONING

- The child is placed supine in the frog-leg position.

ANATOMY REVIEW

- The needle is passed through the abdominal wall just rostral to the pelvic rim in the midline.
- The bladder in an infant is located in the abdomen, which allows for direct access to the bladder lumen with a needle. (The bladder in an older child and adult is located in the pelvis.)
- Various methods to improve success have been cited and include the following:
  - Ensuring that time has passed since the last void.
  - Encouraging the child to drink.
  - Percussing the abdomen to ascertain bladder fullness.
  - Obtaining an ultrasonogram. This can be used to ensure bladder fullness or to guide needle insertion.

PROCEDURE

- Observe sterile procedure.
  - Wear sterile gloves.
  - Use 1 hand to touch the patient if necessary, while keeping the hand with the needle clean.
- Strongly consider applying a topical anesthetic before starting the procedure.
- Leaving the topical anesthetic on for a sufficient time period provides a reasonable degree of topical anesthesia.
- Remove the topical anesthetic prior to skin preparation.
- The practice of additional injection of lidocaine varies; the injection represents a separate needle stick and is associated with pain from lidocaine infiltration.
- Apply 10% povidone-iodine solution to the skin surface of the abdomen 1–2 cm above the pubic symphysis.
- Attach the syringe to the needle.

- The provider should be positioned so that the dominant hand can insert the needle through the skin above the pubic symphysis and direct the needle caudad at about 20 degrees from perpendicular (Figure 32–1).
- A lesser angle may be used in very young infants whose bladder is more rostral.
- The skin is penetrated and the needle is advanced into the bladder.
- Slowly advance the needle while aspirating the syringe.
- When urine appears, stop and fill the syringe, then withdraw the needle.
- Clean the skin of residual povidone-iodine.
- Apply a gauze bandage to the needle puncture site.
- If no urine is obtained on the first attempt, change the angle of the needle slightly toward perpendicular and repeat (without coming out of the skin).
- This may be done once or twice (at most). Additional attempts are unlikely to yield urine.
- Consider waiting and repeating or obtaining urine by urethral catheterization.

INTERPRETATION AND MONITORING

- Urine obtained via suprapubic catheter is usually evaluated for infection.
- Other urine tests that do not require sterile urine would likely be obtained via catheter and include the following:
  - **Urine dipstick tests** (bedside) are a series of paper squares impregnated with chemical reagents that change color under specific conditions. Be aware that reading the strips beyond the recommended times on the container may lead to false-positive results.
  - **Urinalysis** (formal laboratory testing) is often a combination of the above tests and a microscope examination of the urine.
  - **Culture** is commonly used to detect bacteria.
  - **Urine** can also be tested for virus (eg, cytomegalovirus) and fungi.

COMPLICATIONS

- Pain.
- Hematuria.
- Intestinal perforation (rarely results in complications or peritonitis).
- Infection of abdominal wall.

CAVEATS

- There are considerable differences of opinion over the role of suprapubic aspiration (SPA) in the evaluation of children with suspected urinary tract infection.

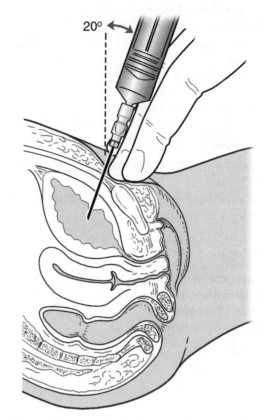

Figure 32–1. *Angle of needle entry (sagittal view).*

■ Advocates argue that SPA carries no risk of contamination when compared with urethral catheterization.

■ Advocates argue that SPA is the first-line test for infants with fever and suspected urinary tract infection so that the consequences of a false-positive urine culture (eg, unnecessary antibiotics, follow-up testing, overlooking another locus of infection) are avoided.

■ The argument against SPA includes the following:

• Procedure is invasive and painful.

• Success rates for obtaining urine are lower for SPA than for catheterization.

• SPA usually requires a physician, whereas catheterization is more often done by nurses.

FOLLOW-UP

■ Clear instructions on caring for the puncture site (ie, watching for redness, pain, and purulent discharge) as well as information about the symptoms of peritonitis should be given to the parents.

REFERENCES

Austin BJ, Bollard C, Gunn TR. Is urethral catheterization a successful alternative to suprapubic aspiration in neonates? *J Paediatr Child Health.* 1999;35:34–36.

Henretig FM, King C. *Textbook of Pediatric Emergency Procedures.* Baltimore, MD: Williams & Wilkins; 1996.

Polnay L, Fraser AM, Lewis JM. Complication of suprapubic bladder aspiration. *Arch Dis Child.* 1975;50:80–81.

Tobiansky R, Evans N. A randomized controlled trial of two methods for collection of sterile urine in neonates. *J Paediatr Child Health.* 1998;34:460–462.

CHAPTER 33

Paraphimosis Reduction

Jennifer Trainor, MD

INDICATIONS

- Reduction of retracted, constricting foreskin.

CONTRAINDICATIONS

Relative

- Recent penile surgery.

EQUIPMENT

- Nonsterile gloves.
- Ice packs.
- 2 × 2 or 4 × 4 gauze.
- Topical anesthetic or buffered 1% lidocaine solution, or both.

RISKS

- Failure of reduction (success rates depend on duration of paraphimosis and degree of edema).
- Psychological stress (common; child is restrained for procedure).
- Pain (certain; can be limited somewhat with anesthesia).
- Cold injury.

PEARLS AND TIPS

- Use gauze to grasp the foreskin.
- If swelling is pronounced, try manual compression prior to reduction.
- Timid attempts at reduction in an effort to reduce pain ultimately result in delayed reduction and increased overall pain.
- If initial attempts are unsuccessful, urgent referral to a urologist is recommended.

PATIENT PREPARATION

- The child is placed supine.

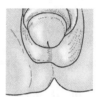
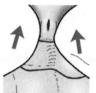

■ Distract the child by having the parent or assistant lean over the examining table, placing his or her body between the child's upper torso and the genital area. This also prevents the child from getting up and allows the parent or assistant to engage the child face to face.

■ Good lighting is helpful.

PATIENT POSITIONING

■ The child is placed supine in the frog-leg position.

■ If the child is uncooperative, his legs and pelvis should also be restrained by an assistant.

ANATOMY REVIEW

■ Figure 33–1A shows a normal penis with foreskin.

■ Early paraphimosis (retracted foreskin) is illustrated in Figure 33–1B.

■ Late paraphimosis (retracted foreskin with significant edema) is shown in Figure 33–1C.

PROCEDURE

■ Consider the use of a dorsal penile block in advance of the procedure, particularly when there is severe edema.

■ With gloved hands, grasp the retracted foreskin between the thumb and the index and middle fingers of each hand.

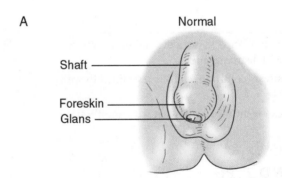

A   Normal

Shaft

Foreskin
Glans

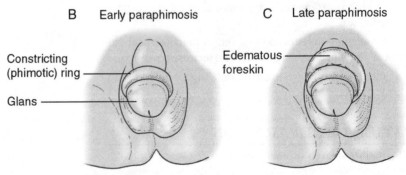

B   Early paraphimosis   C   Late paraphimosis

Constricting (phimotic) ring

Glans

Edematous foreskin

Figure 33–1. *A: Normal penis and foreskin. **B:** Early paraphimosis. **C:** Late paraphimosis.*

- Using a gauze pad to grasp the foreskin improves traction.
- Simultaneously pull the foreskin distally as you compress the glans with both thumbs (Figure 33–2).
- Apply constant and firm pressure.
- When sufficient pressure is applied, the foreskin suddenly reduces, popping over the glans.
- If the initial attempt is unsuccessful, consider manual decompression before subsequent attempts.
- Place your hand around the distal foreskin and glans and apply constant circumferential pressure for approximately 5 minutes.
- Then, attempt reduction again as described above.
- Alternatively, you can apply an ice-water slurry (sealed in either a specimen collection bag or a tied-off glove) to the paraphimotic foreskin and glans.
- You may apply the ice pack for up to 3 minutes at a time, taking care to monitor for cold or pressure injury.
- There is a significant amount of discomfort associated with ice packs, so they may not be tolerated in the absence of a dorsal penile block, especially in young children.

COMPLICATIONS

- Pain.
- Injury to the glans or shaft with overaggressive manipulation.

CAVEATS

- If the simple technique described above in conjunction with decompression fails to reduce the foreskin, the child should be referred to a urologist promptly.
- An unreduced paraphimosis can lead to skin ulceration and necrosis of the distal glans.
- Surgical reduction techniques, such as needle puncture decompression, dorsal slit, or immediate circumcision, are beyond the scope of the general practitioner and should not be performed in the office setting.

FOLLOW-UP

- If there is any breakdown of the surface of the glans or the foreskin, either bacitracin or polymyxin plus bacitracin can be applied until healing is achieved.
- The parents should be instructed to return when new redness or swelling appears or if the swelling fails to resolve within 24 hours.
- Prevention should be stressed.
- The foreskin should always be reduced promptly after retracting it for bathing in order to prevent recurrence.
- Referral to a urologist for consideration of circumcision is strongly suggested, particularly in the older child.

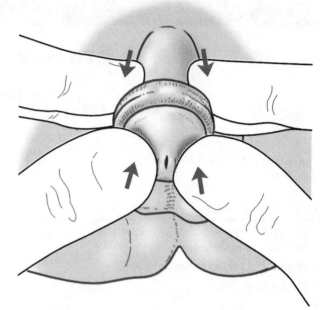

Figure 33–2. *Proper hand positioning for reduction.*

REFERENCES

Henretig FM, King C. *Textbook of Pediatric Emergency Procedures.* Baltimore, MD: Williams & Wilkins; 1996.

[**CHAPTER 34**]

Lumbar Puncture

Joshua Goldstein, MD

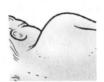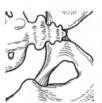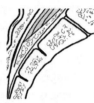

INDICATIONS

- Central nervous system (CNS) infection (viral, fungal, or bacterial) or malignancy.
- Intracranial pressure or pseudotumor.
- Metabolic studies.
- Aminoacidopathies.
- Neurotransmitter disorders.
  - Undiagnosed movement disorders.
  - Undiagnosed infantile or pediatric epilepsy.
- Demyelinating disease (eg, multiple sclerosis).

CONTRAINDICATIONS

Absolute

- CNS herniation.
- Unilateral mass lesion with edema or mass effect.

Relative

- Suspected focal mass lesion.

EQUIPMENT

- Spinal needle: 0.5 inch for neonate, 22 gauge.
- Manometer.
- Sterile collection tubes (sufficient number for studies).
- 3-way stopcock.
- Flexible tubing.

RISKS

- Herniation (extremely rare) is associated with focal structural lesions causing increased intracranial pressure.
- Infection (extremely rare).
- Headache (rare).
- Back pain.

PEARLS AND TIPS

- Placing the patient with the sacral plane vertical is key.
- The head of the patient should be on your nondominant side. (Left-handed physicians should place the patient in the left lateral decubitus position.)
- Use your nondominant thumb to palpate the spinous process of L4 and put your index finger on the iliac crest.
- Use your dominant hand to manipulate the needle.
- If positioning is felt to be correct, try rotating the needle 90 degrees.
- If cerebrospinal fluid (CSF) flows slowly, be patient.

PATIENT PREPARATION

- Sterile technique.
- Povidone-iodine preparation.
- Sterile drape with fenestration over midlumbar spine.
- Sedation, if needed.
- Connect 3-way stopcock to flexible tubing and manometer at 90 degrees from each other.
- Free end of tubing will connect to hub of needle.

PATIENT POSITIONING

- Lateral decubitus position.
- Back arched in extreme lordosis.
- Spine should be as perfectly horizontal as possible.
- Sacral plane should be as vertical as possible (Figure 34–1).

ANATOMY REVIEW

- Spinous process of L4 is on line drawn between iliac crests.
- Cauda equina is in midlumbar region.
- Spinous processes are angled inferiorly (caudally).

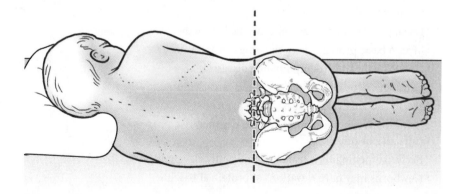

Figure 34–1. *Lateral decubitus position.*

PROCEDURE

- Palpate for L4 spinous process using iliac crests as landmarks (Figure 34–2).
- Place lumbar puncture needle between interspaces L4–5.
- Angle the needle tip approximately 15–30 degrees from perpendicular to plane of back in rostral direction, aiming toward umbilicus (Figure 34–3).
- Needle remains fixed in horizontal plane to back.
- Advance needle slowly until light resistance (a pop) is felt.
- Remove stylet and check for CSF flow.
- If no CSF flows, continue to advance the needle slowly.
- If CSF flows, connect flexible tubing to hub of lumbar puncture needle.
- Allow CSF to flow through tubing into manometer.
- Hold base of manometer and stopcock at level of heart.
- Straighten the patient's back and legs.
- When CSF stops advancing along manometer, measure opening pressure at meniscus.
- Collect CSF for studies.
- Measure closing pressure, if needed.

INTERPRETATION

- Routine studies include protein, glucose, and cell count and differential.
- Studies are selected on clinical suspicion and indication; examples include the following:
  - Bacterial cultures.
  - Bacterial antigen studies.
  - Viral cultures and studies.
  - Herpes polymerase chain reaction.
  - Fungal cultures.
  - India ink stains.
  - Tuberculosis studies.
  - CSF neurotransmitters (movement disorders and epilepsy).
  - Amino acids (for aminoacidopathies, especially glutaric aciduria).
  - Lactate (mitochondrial and energy metabolism disorders).
  - Myelin basic protein (demyelinating diseases).
  - Oligoclonal bands (demyelinating diseases).
  - Cytology (neoplasm, usually requires larger volume).
- Protein (normal values are based on age):
  - Elevations suggest inflammatory or degenerative process (infective or other).
  - Bacterial meningitis is usually significantly elevated.
  - Newborns may have elevations of protein at baseline.
- Leukocytes (normal is 0):
  - Elevations suggest inflammatory process (often infective).

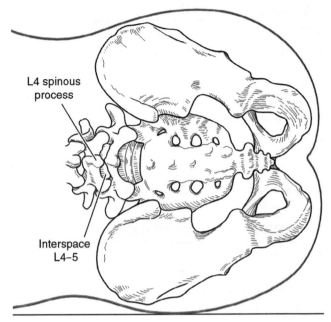

Figure 34–2. *Use iliac crests as landmarks to palpate L4 spinous process.*

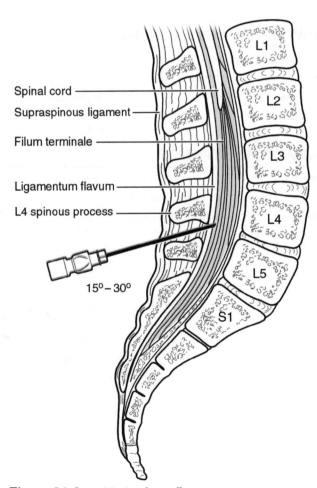

Figure 34–3. *Positioning the needle.*

- Elevations of polymorphonuclear leukocytes suggest acute bacterial infection.
- Elevations of lymphocytes suggest viral infection.
- Erythrocytes (normal is 0):
  - Hemorrhage (not etiologically specific, acute or subacute).
  - Hemorrhagic infection (herpes).
  - Evaluate spun sample for hemochromatosis (subacute hemorrhage).
- Glucose (normal is approximately two-thirds of serum):
  - Decrease in CSF glucose is highly suggestive of active bacterial infection.
  - Decrease in CSF glucose also seen in glucose transporter defect (epilepsy).
- Opening pressure (normal is < 20 cm H_2O):
  - Direct measure of intrathecal pressure and indirect measure of intracranial pressure.
  - Patient must be relaxed and back and legs are extended.

CAVEATS

- Traumatic lumbar punctures should be considered when erythrocytes are present; however, the possibility of hemorrhage should not be discounted, and the presence of hemochromatosis (see above) must be identified.
- In traumatic lumbar punctures, there can be 700–1000 erythrocytes for every 1 leukocyte; more leukocytes suggest an inflammatory or an infective process.
- A test for herpes simplex virus should be strongly considered when patients who have seizures also have fever.
- The usefulness of a brain image (ie, computed tomography or magnetic resonance imaging) prior to lumbar puncture is somewhat controversial, but most practitioners do not routinely recommend an imaging study in the absence of either history or physical findings suggestive of focal structural lesion.
- The risks of a lumbar puncture are extremely low; thus, lumbar puncture should be performed when ambiguity exists.

COMPLICATIONS

- Cerebral herniation.
- Infection.
- Headache.
- Back pain.

FOLLOW-UP

- Sterile dressing.
- Older adolescents should rest in bed for 1–3 hours.

REFERENCES

Boon JM, Abrahams PH, Meiring JH, Welch T. Lumbar puncture: anatomical review of a clinical skill. *Clin Anat.* 2004;17: 544–553.

Janssens E, Aerssens P, Alliet P, Gillis P, Raes M. Post-dural puncture headaches in children. A literature review. *Eur J Pediatr.* 2003;162:117–121.

Oliver WJ, Shope TC, Kuhns LR. Fatal lumbar puncture: fact versus fiction—an approach to a clinical dilemma. *Pediatrics.* 2003;112(3 Pt 1):e174–176.

Roos KL. Lumbar puncture. *Semin Neurol.* 2003;23:105–114.

[CHAPTER 35]

Nail Trephination

Mark Adler, MD

INDICATIONS

- Subungual hematoma with pain.
- Some experts suggest that nail removal and repair should be prompted by the percentage of nailbed involved (eg, greater than 25–50%), but this is not supported in the literature.

CONTRAINDICATIONS

- Procedure is limited to simple hematomas, not complex crush injuries with associated fractures or nailbed injuries.
- Immunosuppression.
- Do not trephinate artificial acrylic nails using cautery (flammable).
- Do not prepare the nail with alcohol (also flammable).

EQUIPMENT

- 10% povidone-iodine (or equivalent).
- Sterile gloves and gauze.
- Single-use, disposable electrocautery device (sterile) is preferred.
- A needle or metal paperclip heated in a flame is an alternative to electrocautery. A metal paperclip is preferred because it is blunt and will do less damage if inserted too far.
- Another alternative is to use either an #11 blade or 18- or 20-gauge needle in a twisting motion to drill the nail.

RISKS

- Infection (very rare).
- Pain (if done correctly, procedure should provide pain *relief*).
- Nail deformity (rare, and associated with more complex injuries).

PEARLS AND TIPS

- Immobilization is important for young children; movement during the procedure can lead to injury to the nailbed or fingertip.

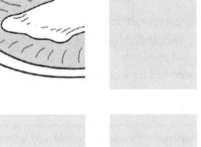

- Hide the cautery device from view of the young child until just before the procedure. Explain the procedure to older children, emphasizing that holding still will prevent pain.
- Do not mistake the pain of an underlying fractured phalanx for the pain of a hematoma.
- Obtain a radiograph if indicated by history or examination.
- Consider nail removal or specialist consultation for management and follow-up when any of the following is present:
  - The nail or nailbed is disrupted.
  - There is a displaced fracture of the phalanx.
  - There is substantial periungual blood (suggesting eponychial injury).

PATIENT PREPARATION

- Prepare the nail with a 10% povidone-iodine solution.

PATIENT POSITIONING

- Place the hand on a sterile surface.

ANATOMY REVIEW

- The nail is firmly adherent to the underlying nailbed (Figure 35–1).
- A hematoma in this space that cannot drain spontaneously causes pain that is sometimes severe.
- The nail itself is insensate, but the nailbed is very sensitive.
- The key to a pain-free procedure is to puncture the nail without entering the nailbed.

PROCEDURE

- With the hand properly positioned and immobilized (if necessary), the cautery device is heated and then applied to the nail in the center of the hematoma area.
- Little or no pressure is required to penetrate the nail, particularly in small children with thin nails.
- Immediately upon entering the subungual space, blood will escape and a sizzling sound will be heard (from the blood hitting the cautery blade).
- Immediately withdraw the blade.
- Slight pressure will express more of the remaining fluid.
- Older hematomas may no longer be liquid and will not drain; however, if pain is present, there is no harm in attempting the procedure even in delayed presentations.
- While a digital block would be effective, this procedure requires at least 2 needle sticks for the infiltration of lidocaine. This is a painful procedure itself and for most trephination attempts would be unnecessary.

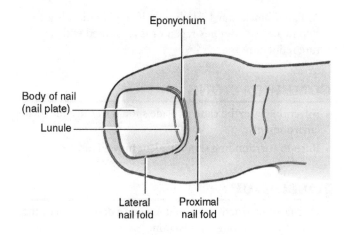

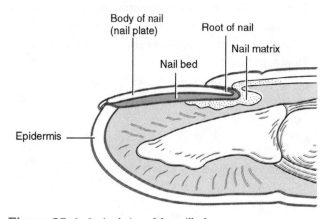

Figure 35–1. *Sagittal view of the nailbed.*

■ A digital block may be indicated if trephination is a first step in a more complex repair or is associated with a fracture reduction.

COMPLICATIONS

■ Infection (rare; the cautery blade should sterilize the local environment).

■ Burn to surrounding skin if patient moves (rare).

FOLLOW-UP

■ Discharge instructions should include a description of the signs and symptoms of infection.

■ Patients and parents should be warned of the following:

• The hematoma may reaccumulate.

• The nail may fall off and may grow back with an abnormal appearance.

REFERENCES

Pirzada A, Waseem M. Subungual hematoma. *Pediatr Rev.* 2004;25:369.

Roberts JR, Hedges JR, Chanmugam AS. *Clinical Procedures in Emergency Medicine.* 4th ed. Philadelphia: WB Saunders; 2004.

Roser SE, Gellman H. Comparison of nail bed repair versus nail trephination for subungual hematomas in children. *J Hand Surg [Am].* 1999;24:1166–1170.

Seaberg DC, Angelos WJ, Paris PM. Treatment of subungual hematomas with nail trephination: a prospective study. *Am J Emerg Med.* 1991;9:209–210.

CHAPTER 36

Ingrown Toenail Treatment

Lina AbuJamra, MD

INDICATIONS

- Pain relief.
- Management of infection.
- Prevention of recurrence.

Specific Indications for Surgical Treatment

- Stage I.
  - Description: Focal pain, erythema, and swelling at lateral margin of the nailbed.
  - Treatment: Conservative management.
- Stage II.
  - Description: Worsening inflammation and infection and formation of purulent granulation tissue.
  - Treatment: Conservative management or angular nail resection with debridement.
- Stage III.
  - Description: Chronic and severe disease state with lateral wall hypertrophy.
  - Treatment: Partial nail resection or total nail avulsion.

CONTRAINDICATIONS

Relative

- Underlying conditions that could complicate wound healing (eg, immunosuppression, diabetes). Referral to specialty clinics may be appropriate for patients with such conditions.

EQUIPMENT

- 1–2% lidocaine without epinephrine.
- Alcohol pads.
- 10% povidone-iodine/antiseptic cleanser.
- Syringe with 25- or 27-gauge needle.
- Digital tourniquet.
- Sterile gauze (4 × 4).

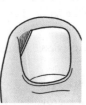

- Sterile towel and drapes.
- Sterile cotton or petrolatum gauze.
- Nail cutter or splitter.
- Hemostats.
- Scissors.
- Antibacterial ointment.
- Silver nitrate sticks.
- Nail file.
- Scalpel #11.

RISKS

- Bleeding, which can be reduced by the use of a tourniquet for hemostasis.
- Pain, which can be alleviated by using a digital block for anesthesia.
- Recurrence of ingrown toenail.
- Absent or abnormal regrowth of the nail, resulting from aggressive debridement.

PEARLS AND TIPS

- Use a tourniquet around the affected toe to provide additional hemostasis.
- Choose conservative treatment with oral antibiotics and warm soaks whenever possible.
- Instruct the parents about maintaining good foot hygiene (eg, trimming the nail transversely) and advise that the child wear loose footwear as much as possible.

PATIENT PREPARATION

- Obtain informed consent from the parents or guardian after a full explanation of the procedure.

PATIENT POSITIONING

- Child should sit or lie down in a comfortable position with the legs elevated to allow easy access to the affected toenail.

ANATOMY REVIEW

- Figure 36–1 shows the sagittal view of the nailbed.

PROCEDURE

Stage 1 Disease (Most Children)

- Wash the nail groove in usual sterile fashion using 10% povidone-iodine solution.
- Soak the foot in warm water.

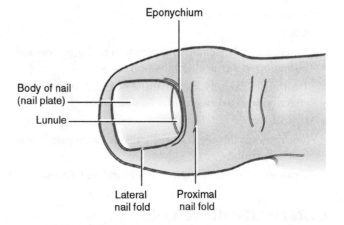

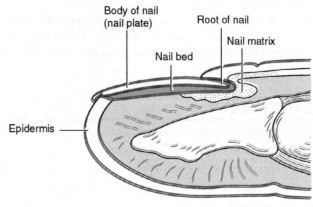

Figure 36–1. *Sagittal view of the nailbed.*

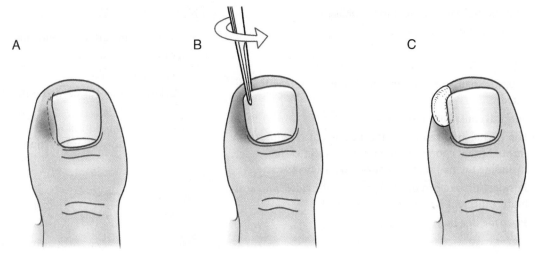

Figure 36–2. *Lifting nail edge to manage stage 1 disease.*

- Elevate the corner of the nail.
- Demonstrate proper nail-trimming technique.
- Prescribe topical or oral antibiotics.

Stage I (Severe)

- For patients with more significant disease, anesthetize the area using a digital nerve block (see Chapter 55).
- Prepare a limited sterile field using 10% povidone-iodine solution and sterile towels.
- Place a digital tourniquet at the base of the toe to prevent excessive bleeding during the procedure.
- Lift the affected nail edge out of the nail groove and rotate it away from the nail fold (Figure 36–2).
- Remove purulent tissue from nail groove with curettage and debridement.
- Apply silver nitrate to granulation tissue.
- File nail as needed, and place a small piece of cotton or petrolatum gauze under the nail edge.
- Gauze may be replaced daily.
- Keep the gauze under the nail for 3–6 weeks or until the nail grows beyond the distal aspect of the nail fold.
- Instruct the patient (and parents) to soak the foot daily in warm water soaks and to maintain strict foot hygiene.

Stage II Disease

- Excise the affected nail in a triangular wedge to a point one-third to two-thirds the distance from the eponychium (Figure 36–3).
- Remove the wedge.
- File the remaining nail edge with a nail file to facilitate smooth regrowth.
- Remove purulent tissue from the nail groove with curettage and debridement.

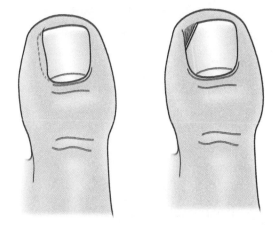

Figure 36–3. *Triangular wedge resection to manage stage 2 disease.*

■ Apply antibiotic ointment to the nailbed.

■ Place a bulky dressing.

Stage III Disease

■ A partial nail resection or complete nail removal is indicated.

■ Surgical consultation is advised.

■ For partial nail resection, the nail is cut longitudinally through the eponychium and the resected nail edge, including the nail root, is removed with a hemostat.

■ Purulent tissue from the nail groove is debrided, and antibiotic ointment is applied to the nailbed.

■ Place toe in a bulky dressing.

COMPLICATIONS

■ Bleeding (very rare).

■ Bacteremia (very rare).

■ Worsening infection or cellulitis (very rare).

■ Abnormal or absent regrowth of the nail (very rare).

■ Recurrence (10–30% of cases).

■ Injury to the neurovascular bundle related to the digital block (very rare).

FOLLOW-UP

■ Home care includes the following:

 • Loose fitting shoes.

 • Daily warm soaks.

 • Packing changes as needed until the nail extends beyond the nail fold.

■ The patient should follow up within 48 hours so that the toe can be assessed for infection.

REFERENCES

Heifetz CJ. Ingrown toe nail. A clinical study. *Am J Surg.* 1937; 38:298.

Murray WR. Management of ingrowing toenail. *Br J Surg.* 1989; 76:883–884.

Platt SL, Foltin GL. Ingrown Toenail Repair. In: Henretig FM, King C, eds. *Textbook of Pediatric Emergency Procedures.* Baltimore: Williams and Wilkins; 1997:1217–1222.

Reijnen JA, Goris RJ. Conservative treatment of ingrowing toenails. *Br J Surg.* 1989;76:955–957.

Silverman RA. Diseases of the nails in infants and children. *Adv Dermatol.* 1990;5:153–170.

Zuber TJ, Pfenninger JL. Management of ingrown toenails. *Am Fam Physician.* 1995;52:181–190.

CHAPTER 37

Molluscum Contagiosum:
Cantharidin Therapy

Sarah Chamlin, MD

INDICATIONS

■ Parent's or child's desire for office-based treatment.

CONTRAINDICATIONS

Absolute

■ Molluscum in facial, genital, or perianal area.

Relative

■ Previous cantharidin application with severe blistering.

EQUIPMENT

■ Cantharidin 0.9% in flexible collodion.
■ Blunt-ended wooden applicator.

RISKS

■ Pain.
■ Blistering.
■ Secondary infection.
■ Temporary hyperpigmentation or hypopigmentation.

PEARLS AND TIPS

■ Inflamed lesions should not be treated because they are resolving spontaneously.
■ If inflamed lesions are treated, they may blister more severely than uninflamed lesions.
■ Excoriated lesions do not need treatment. The central molluscum body has likely been mechanically removed.

PATIENT PREPARATION

■ Patient and parent education is crucial for a successful relationship with families of children with molluscum.
■ Although molluscum contagiosum is a self-resolving infection, parents may demand treatment.

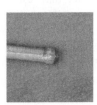

- If a physician defers treatment of a few molluscum and numerous lesions later develop, the parents may "blame" this often unpreventable spread on the physician.
- Treatment does not prevent transmission or the development of new lesions.
- An initial trial of treatment of a few lesions may be helpful in demonstrating the sequelae of therapy.

PATIENT POSITIONING

- The patient should be comfortable and hold still for this therapy because moving may cause cantharidin to be applied in unintended locations and blistering may result.

PROCEDURE

- Apply a small amount of cantharidin to the applicator and transfer this to the molluscum lesion (Figure 37–1).
- Minimize contact with surrounding normal skin.
- Ensure complete drying before the patient moves or dresses.
- Treat a maximum of 20–30 lesions per visit.
- Have the child bathe 4–6 hours after application.
  - The treated areas can be washed with a soft washcloth and mild soap.
  - If child experiences blistering, discomfort, or burning within the first 4 hours, the areas should be gently washed sooner.
  - Scrubbing of treated areas is not necessary and should be discouraged.

COMPLICATIONS

- The blister that occurs with cantharidin therapy may be painful.
  - Apply antibiotic ointment to the areas twice daily until the blisters resolve.
  - Acetaminophen or ibuprofen can be given for pain.
- Scarring, hyperpigmentation or hypopigmentation, and secondary bacterial infection may occur.

FOLLOW-UP

- Follow-up is suggested in 2–4 weeks to treat new lesions.

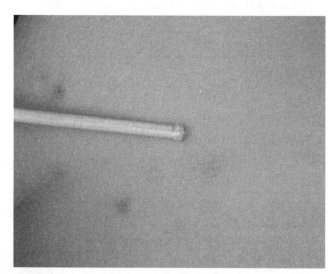

Figure 37–1. *Treating a molluscum lesion with cantharidin on applicator.*

REFERENCE

Silverberg NB, Sidbury R, Mancini AJ. Childhood molluscum contagiosum: experience with cantharidin therapy in 300 patients. *J Am Acad Dermatol.* 2000;43:503–507.

CHAPTER 38

Common Warts: Cryotherapy

Sarah Chamlin, MD

INDICATIONS

- Parent's or child's desire for office-based treatment.

CONTRAINDICATIONS

Relative

- Child unable to undergo painful procedure.
- Some physicians consider verruca in a periungual location a contraindication to destructive therapies (nail matrix damage may occur and result in permanent nail dystrophy).
- History of keloidal scarring.

EQUIPMENT

- Dipstick method.
  - Liquid nitrogen (–195.8 °C).
  - Cotton-tipped applicators.
  - Cotton balls.
  - Styrofoam cup.
  - Extra cotton can be rolled onto cotton-tipped applicators.
- Spray devices
  - Cryospray canister filled with liquid nitrogen.
  - Children may be afraid of these spray canisters and often have less anxiety with the dipstick method.

RISKS

- Treatment causes blistering and rarely scarring.
- Temporary hyperpigmentation or hypopigmentation.
- Hypertrophic or keloidal scarring is rare.

PEARLS AND TIPS

- Pretreatment of the area with paring or salicylic acid may decrease the wart hyperkeratosis and increase the treatment success rate.
- Pretreat for pain with acetaminophen or ibuprofen 1 hour before the procedure.
- The goal of treatment is tissue destruction through skin blistering.

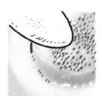

PATIENT PREPARATION

- For the first week, there will be a blister that may be hemorrhagic that turns into a scab or crust, which comes off in approximately 2 weeks. The area can be cleaned with soap and water and covered with a topical antibiotic ointment and a bandage.
- There are no limitations on physical activity unless pain results from the activities.
- Acetaminophen may be required for the first 1–2 days after treatment for discomfort.
- Several treatments are often needed.

PATIENT POSITIONING

- Patient should be positioned so that physician has close access to lesions.
- Good lighting is helpful.

PROCEDURE

- Cotton-tipped applicators should be placed in a cup of liquid nitrogen until thoroughly soaked.
- Apply to wart until white frost develops approximately 2 mm around the wart (Figure 38–1).
  - A freeze-thaw cycle (time when wart becomes frozen white until return of pink skin) of 20–30 seconds is suggested.
  - Wart should be kept frosted for 10–15 seconds to obtain a 20 second freeze-thaw.
- Freeze-thaw times from spray devices are the same as for the cotton applicators.
- An adequate freeze-thaw time is easy to estimate with time and experience.

COMPLICATIONS

- Pain is expected and can be treated with acetaminophen or ibuprofen.
- Although rare, secondary bacterial infection of the blistered area can occur.

CAVEATS

- Most young children will not tolerate the discomfort of this therapy.
- Over-the-counter topical salicylic acid products with or without tape occlusion can be used if cryotherapy is not tolerated.

FOLLOW-UP

- Treatment can be repeated approximately every 3 weeks when the old blister peels off.

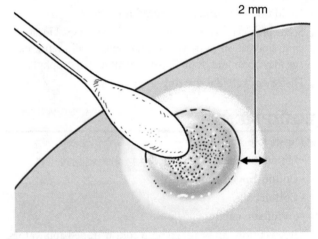

Figure 38–1. *Application of liquid nitrogen to wart.*

REFERENCES

Graham GF. Cryosurgery. In: Robinson JK, Arndt KA, LeBoit P, Wintroub BU. *Atlas of Cutaneous Surgery.* Philadelphia: WB Saunders Company; 1996:53–59.

CHAPTER 39

Mineral Oil Preparation: Diagnosing Scabies

Sarah Chamlin, MD

INDICATIONS

- Suspected *Sarcoptes scabiei* infestation; the diagnosis should be verified because it is often overdiagnosed.

EQUIPMENT

- Glass microscope slide.
- Mineral oil.
- Cotton-tipped applicator.
- Microscope.
- #15 scalpel blade or other device to scrape skin.

RISKS

- Minimal discomfort and bleeding with vigorous scraping.

PEARLS AND TIPS

- Scrape burrows or unexcoriated papules.
- The highest yield of mites, eggs, or fecal pellets is from the burrows, which are most commonly found on hands or feet.
- If many family members have lesions, perform the scraping on the parents, who are often more cooperative and less fearful than infants or young children.
- Treatment includes eradication of the mites on the patient, treatment of associated problems (pruritus, scabietic nodules), treatment of personal contacts, and destruction of the mite in the patient's surroundings.

PATIENT PREPARATION

- Parents and patients should be aware that scraping may cause minimal bleeding and mild discomfort.

PATIENT POSITIONING

- Patient should be positioned in good lighting with access to lesion to be tested.

PROCEDURE

■ Drop mineral oil on to a sterile blade or the lesion itself with a cotton-tipped applicator.

■ Vigorously scrape the lesion 5–6 times until it is unroofed. This may produce bleeding.

■ Collect material from as many lesions as possible, preferably from burrows.

■ Transfer material from each lesion to the slide, add a few more drops of mineral oil, and cover with the coverslip (Figure 39–1).

INTERPRETATION AND MONITORING

■ Scan slide on low-power objective.

■ Diagnosis is made by seeing the mite itself (0.2–0.4 mm in size), mite parts, eggs (oval and one-tenth the size of the mite), egg cases, or golden-brown fecal pellets (scybala).

■ Feces and eggs are easier to find than mites. Feces often occur in clumps.

■ Air bubbles (usually round) are an artifact that can be mistaken for eggs. Gently press on coverslip to dislodge these.

FOLLOW-UP

■ If treated adequately, follow-up is not indicated.

■ Pruritus may persist for weeks or months in patients even after adequate therapy.

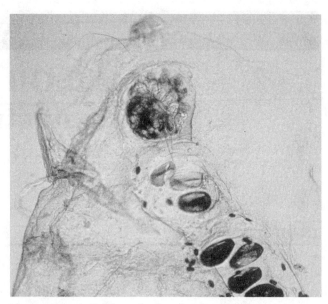

Figure 39–1. *Scabies under the microscope.*

REFERENCES

Cunningham BB, Wagner AM. Diagnostic and therapeutic procedures. In: Eichenfield LF, Frieden IJ, Esterly NB. *Textbook of Neonatal Dermatology.* Philadelphia: WB Saunders Company; 2001:77.

Rasmussen JE. Body lice, head lice, pubic lice and scabies. In: Arndt KA, LeBoit P, Robinson JK, Wintroub BU, eds. *Cutaneous Medicine and Surgery.* Philadelphia: WB Saunders Company; 1996:1195–1199.

CHAPTER 40

KOH Preparation

Sarah Chamlin, MD

INDICATIONS

- Suspected fungal or candidal infection.

EQUIPMENT

- Glass microscope slide and coverslip.
- 10–20% potassium hydroxide (KOH).
- Microscope.
- #15 scalpel blade or other device to scrape skin (edge of microscope slide, cytobrush, or foman blade).
- Matches.

RISKS

- Minimal discomfort and bleeding with aggressive scraping.

PEARLS AND TIPS

- This technique is most commonly used in diagnosing tinea corporis or tinea pedis.
- Although a lower sensitivity is found with this diagnostic test for tinea capitis, spores within hair shafts can be visualized in "black dot" type.
- Samples should be collected from the advancing edge or margins of skin lesions with the edge of a scalpel.
  - In children, use the dull edge if they are moving or use a cytobrush.
  - The foman blade, a 2-sided, spatula-type instrument, is less likely to cut the skin of a moving infant.
- Shavings of nails left in KOH for several hours may assist in diagnosis of onychomycosis.
- KOH is used to digest the proteins, lipids, and epithelial debris in the specimen.
- Gentle cleaning of the area to be tested with an alcohol wipe before this examination may remove confusing oil drops and excess debris from the slide.

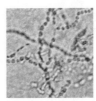

PATIENT PREPARATION

■ Parents and patients should be aware that scraping may cause minimal bleeding and mild discomfort.

PATIENT POSITIONING

■ Patient should be positioned in good lighting with access to lesion to be tested.

PROCEDURE

■ Obtain a skin or nail specimen with gentle scraping of the areas to be tested.

■ Place scale, roof of vesicle, or nail shavings on a glass slide.

■ Scrape with the edge of the #15 blade, the edge of a glass microscope slide, or a foman blade.

■ Apply 1–2 drops of KOH over the specimen.

■ Place a coverslip over specimen and press firmly.

■ Consider gentle heating of the underside of the slide for 5–10 seconds until the epithelial cells and debris dissipate.

INTERPRETATION AND MONITORING

■ The hyphae can be seen under low power (Figure 40–1), but better observation of both hyphae and spores is obtained by use of a dry high objective with reduced illumination.

■ The juncture lines of epithelial cells may be mistaken for hyphae. Cell walls have irregular linearity.

■ Positive preparations appear as septate and branching hyphae. A positive KOH preparation should reveal definite hyphae traversing epidermal cells.

■ Fabric fibers (usually twisted and uniform) and hairs are larger than hyphae.

■ If a tinea or candidal infection is strongly suspected and this examination is negative, consider performing a culture.

CAVEAT

■ This is a diagnostic examination that is underutilized due to lack of experience with interpretation. The identification of spores and hyphae becomes more straightforward the more often the test is done.

FOLLOW-UP

■ As indicated after appropriate treatment.

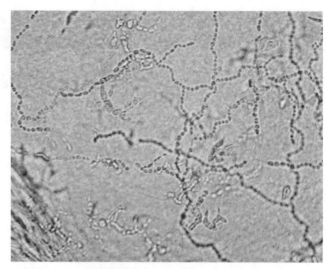

Figure 40–1. *Hyphae under microscope.*

REFERENCE

Cunningham BB, Wagner AM. Diagnostic and therapeutic procedures. In: Eichenfield LF, Frieden IJ, Esterly NB. *Textbook of Neonatal Dermatology.* Philadelphia: WB Saunders Company; 2001:73–74.

CHAPTER 41

Superficial Abscess: Treatment

Lina AbuJamra, MD

INDICATIONS

- Incision and drainage are indicated when a large, localized, and tender collection of pus occurs in the subcutaneous tissues beneath the skin surface.
- When the diagnosis is unclear, needle aspiration may be diagnostic. This is particularly helpful for deeper infections.

CONTRAINDICATIONS

Relative

- Abscesses located in the deep tissues, the hand, or the face.
- Lengthy or painful procedures in young children. Since these may require conscious sedation, they should be performed only if resources for conscious sedation are available.
- Abscesses requiring operative drainage and debridement. These procedures should be performed in the operating area.
- Patients with underlying conditions that may complicate the healing process or require close outpatient follow-up (eg, immunocompromised state or diabetes). Referral to specialty clinics may be appropriate for such patients.

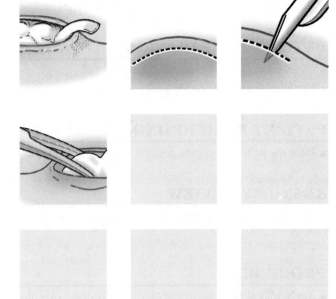

EQUIPMENT

- Mask.
- Sterile gloves.
- Povidone-iodine solution.
- Sterile gauze.
- Sterile dressing and drapes.
- Eutectic mixture of local anesthetics (EMLA/ELAMAX) or 1% lidocaine with epinephrine, or both.
- 25- or 27-gauge needle for lidocaine administration.
- #11 scalpel.
- Curved hemostats.
- Sterile packing material (iodoform gauze).

RISKS

- Bleeding.

■ Pain.

■ Recurrence of the abscess due to inadequate drainage.

PEARLS AND TIPS

■ Be careful not to mistake an abscess for a cellulitis (a diffuse, suppurative inflammation). Needle aspiration can help distinguish them.

■ Make the abscess incision large enough to permit adequate drainage of pus.

■ For very small abscesses, the use of topical local anesthetic ointment may be sufficient for drainage.

■ Take a medical history. Children with cardiac valve disease should receive antibiotic prophylaxis to prevent endocarditis.

PATIENT PREPARATION

■ Clean the area with povidone-iodine.

■ Use lidocaine regionally for local anesthesia.

PATIENT POSITIONING

■ Place the patient in supine position for greatest comfort.

ANATOMY REVIEW

■ The anatomy varies depending on the location of the abscess.

PROCEDURE

■ Apply topical local anesthetic (EMLA/ELAMAX) over the abscess 30 minutes before the procedure. This provides cutaneous anesthesia and often helps begin the drainage process.

■ Put on mask, eye shield, and sterile gloves.

■ Use lidocaine 1% with epinephrine for local anesthesia (Figure 41–1). Infiltrate the dermis overlying the abscess in a linear distribution.

■ Clean the area with povidone-iodine and set up a sterile field.

■ If you are uncertain about the definitive diagnosis of the abscess, use an 18-gauge needle to aspirate the affected area.

■ Using the #11 scalpel, make a linear incision through the skin over the full length of the abscess cavity. Avoid proximate neurovascular structures.

■ Allow the pus to drain from the cavity.

■ Use a sterile gloved finger or hemostats to explore the cavity and break up any loculations of pus.

■ Place sterile packing material into the wound. Use a hemostat to aid in the placement of the packing material (see Figure 41–1).

■ Leave an end of the packing material through the incision site so that it can be easily removed at a later time.

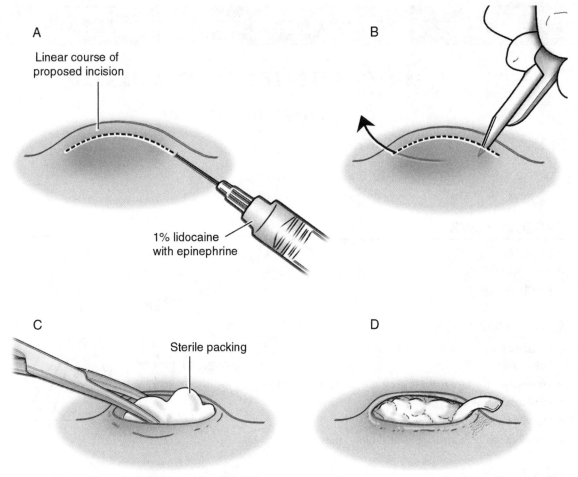

A

Linear course of
proposed incision

1% lidocaine
with epinephrine

B

C

Sterile packing

D

Figure 41–1. *Abscess with incision and sterile packing.*

- Apply a sterile dressing over the wound.
- Follow up within 48 hours for the first dressing change.
  - Remove the dressing and packing material at that time.
  - Examine the wound for reaccumulation of pus.
  - Repack the wound with new sterile packing material.
- Instruct the patient to perform daily dressing changes at home. After a few days, the patient can begin warm soaks before repacking the wound.
- Consider the need for antibiotics.
  - Antibiotics are not necessary in cases of simple abscess drainage in an immunocompetent patient who is not at risk for endocarditis.
  - If antibiotics are used, choose a medication effective against the most likely organisms, which include pyogenic staphylococci, streptococci, and anaerobes.

COMPLICATIONS

- Local spread of infection and cellulitis.
- Bacteremia (especially in patients who are immunocompromised or who have valvular heart disease).
- Bleeding.
- Injury to nerves or vessels.

REFERENCES

Brook I, Feingold S. Aerobic and anaerobic bacteriology of cutaneous abscesses in children. *Pediatrics.* 1981;67:891–895.

Halvorson GD, Halvorson JE, Iserson KV. Abscess incision and drainage in the emergency department. Part I. *J Emerg Med.* 1985;3:227–232.

Llera J, Levy R. Treatment of cutaneous abscess: a double-blind study. *Ann Emerg Med.* 1985;14:15–19.

Meislin H. Cutaneous abscesses—anaerobic and aerobic bacteriology and outpatient management. *Ann Intern Med.* 1977; 87:145–149.

Roberts JR, Hedges JR. *Clinical Procedures in Emergency Medicine.* 2nd ed. Philadelphia: WB Saunders Company; 1991: 591–598.

CHAPTER 42

Lacerations: Suturing

Russell Horowitz, MD

INDICATIONS

- Improve cosmesis.
- Reduce infection.
- Restore function.

CONTRAINDICATIONS

- Wounds on the trunk and torso that are greater than 12 hours old.
- Wounds on the face that are greater than 24 hours old.
- Puncture wounds.
- Heavily contaminated wounds.
- Bites, especially in areas of limited blood flow.

EQUIPMENT

- Sterile gauze.
- Sterile towels, drapes, and gloves.
- Saline.
- Sterile basin.
- Detergent cleanser (Sur-Cleans) or povidone-iodine solution.
- Suture material (Tables 42–1 and 42–2).
- 30–60-mL syringe for irrigation (splash adapter optional).
- Syringe with fine needle (25–30 gauge) for local analgesia infusion.
- Suture scissors.
- Needle holders.
- Forceps with teeth.
- Local anesthetic.

RISKS

- Infection.
- Stitch extrusion.

PEARLS AND TIPS

- Suturing requires a calm and unhurried approach.

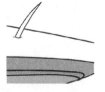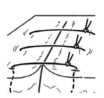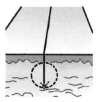
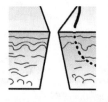

Table 42–1. Surface wound closure guidelines.

Site	Suture Material	Suture Removal
Face	6-0 absorbing or nonabsorbing	5 days
Scalp	5-0 nonabsorbing	7–10 days
Digits	5-0 nonabsorbing	7–10 days
Palms/soles	2-0, 3-0, 4-0 nonabsorbing	7–10 days
Torso	4-0, 5-0 nonabsorbing	7–10 days
Joint	3-0, 4-0, 5-0 nonabsorbing	10–14 days

Table 42–2. Suture material.

Name	Material	Reactivity	Strength	Absorption and Characteristics
Absorbable				
Gut	Monofilament	Severe	Good	7–10 days
Fast absorbing gut	Monofilament heat treated	Moderate	Good	5–7 days
Chromic gut	Monofilament chemically treated	Severe	Good	10–14 days
Polyglycolic acid (Dexon)	Braided	Mild	Very good	60–90 days
Polyglactin 910 (Vicryl)	Braided	Mild	Very good	55–70 days
Polyglecaprone (Monocryl)	Monofilament	Minimal	Very good	90–120 days
Nonabsorbable				
Silk	Braided	Severe	Good	Easy to handle; ties well
Nylon (Ethilon, Dermalon)	Monofilament	Mild	Very good	Slippery; requires many knots
Polypropylene (Prolene)	Monofilament	Minimal	Excellent	Slippery; requires many knots

- The practitioner should be comfortable, since preparation and closure of even small lacerations in children may require more time than initially expected.
- Determine the circumstances and mechanism of injury (eg, blunt or sharp) and risk of contaminants or retained foreign body.
- Obtain past medical history (including allergies, status of tetanus immunization, medication use, and chronic diseases), since specific medications, such as corticosteroids, and conditions, such as diabetes, delay wound healing.

PATIENT POSITIONING

- The patient should be lying flat or sitting.

ANATOMY REVIEW

- Figure 42–1 is a diagram of a skin laceration.

PROCEDURE

- Use universal precautions.
- Document laceration length and depth.
- Assess neurovascular status and investigate for tendon, muscle, or vascular injury.

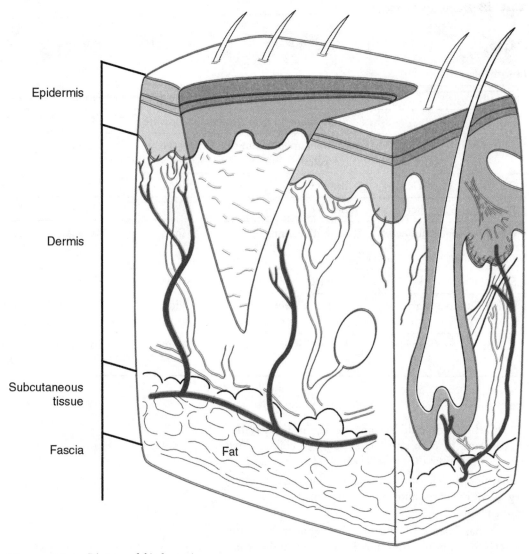

Figure 42–1. *Diagram of skin laceration.*

Epidermis

Dermis

Subcutaneous tissue

Fascia

Fat

- Lidocaine is the most commonly used anesthetic for simple wound repair.
  - Epinephrine may be added to reduce local bleeding but is contraindicated in end organs (eg, penis, toes, fingers, nose, pinnae).
  - Sodium bicarbonate can be combined with lidocaine to reduce pain associated with infusion.
- When administering the anesthetic, proceed in a slow, steady manner because rapid delivery can result in a burning sensation.
- The maximum dose of plain lidocaine is 5 mg/kg. When combined with epinephrine, it is 7 mg/kg.
- Bupivacaine, an alternative to lidocaine, has a much longer duration of action.

- Topical anesthetics such as LET (lidocaine, epinephrine, and tetracaine), which can be infused directly into a wound, are a needleless alternative to lidocaine.
  - Effectiveness requires 10–20 minutes for the medications to absorb.
  - For some procedures, they do not provide sufficient anesthesia alone and are used in combination with injected lidocaine.
- Clean the skin with detergent or povidone-iodine solution.
- Inspect visually for tendon, neurovascular, or deep tissue injury, or the presence of a foreign body.
- A finger may be placed inside the wound to explore the depth of injury.
- Copious irrigation under pressure reduces infection risk.
  - 500–1000 mL (or more) may be needed for large or contaminated wounds.
  - Irrigation should be continued until no contaminants are seen.
- Removal of contaminated, nonviable, or devitalized tissue is done using either a scissors or scalpel.
- Trimming into a lenticular shape allows for simplest wound edge approximation and repair.
- Align appropriate tissue layers to prevent unnecessary scarring.

Skin Sutures

- Select suture appropriate to anatomic location (see Tables 42–1 and 42–2).
- The needle is loaded onto the holder approximately two-thirds of the way from the tip.
- The throw begins in the dermis, passes through an adequate amount of subcutaneous tissue following the natural curvature of the needle, and exits the other side of the wound.
- The exit and entrance points should be equidistant from the wound edge.
- Approximate edges and gently evert the tissue to reduce tension.
- The most commonly used knot is the surgeon's knot.
  - This is accomplished by a double first throw followed by 3 to 4 half-knots using a standard instrument technique.
  - The end-result is a final square knot with sufficient strength to secure the suture (Figure 42–2).
- The suture is then tied and the ends cut at sufficient length to ensure simple removal.
- Suture knots are all aligned away from the wound on 1 side to reduce inflammatory reaction and surface tension at the laceration site (see Figure 42–2).

Deep Sutures

- Select suture (see Table 42–2).

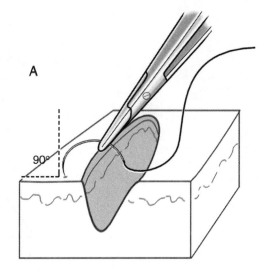

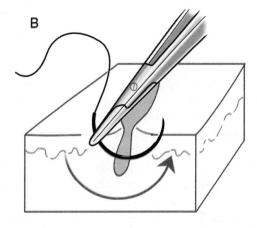

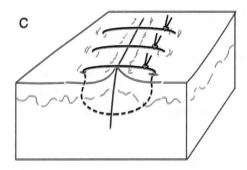

Figure 42–2. *Simple interrupted suture technique.*

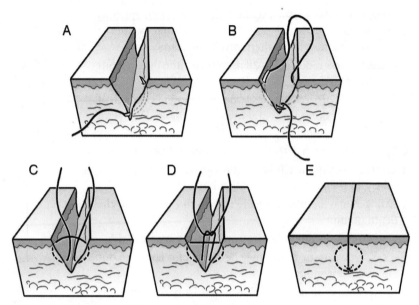

Figure 42–3. *Layered closure.*

- The initial throw begins in the subcutaneous tissue and is brought out in the natural curved path of the needle to the dermal-epidermal junction.
- The needle is then reloaded and inserted superficially into the opposite side and withdrawn in the superficial fascia.
- When the suture is tied, this allows the knot to be buried deep in the wound. The ends are cut short to prevent extrusion (Figure 42–3).
- Deep sutures perform a number of functions, including the following:
  - Reduce surface tension.
  - Reduce dead space, which acts as a potential for abscess and hematoma formation.
  - Restore muscular function in cases of injured muscle.
  - Improve aesthetics by reducing pitting of overlying tissue.
  - Provide additional strength of repair as suture assists in binding tissue.

Mattress Sutures

- These techniques are useful in areas under tension and assist in everting wound edges.
- Their increased strength comes with a risk of ischemia and necrosis of the skin.
- For both horizontal and vertical mattress sutures, the suture passes through the wound twice and finishes on the same side it started from.

A. VERTICAL MATTRESS SUTURES

- This method allows you to close dead space and provide both a deep and skin suture all with 1 tie.

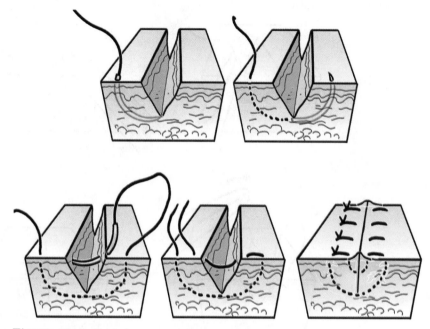

Figure 42–4. *Vertical mattress sutures.*

- The stitch begins slightly further back from the wound edge than the simple interrupted skin suture (Figure 42–4).
- Using a large bite, the needle passes through to the other side.
- It is reloaded and reinserted through the skin closer to the wound edge and passed through to the beginning side.
- The suture is then tied in the customary fashion.

B. Horizontal Mattress Sutures

- The suture is passed from 1 side of the wound to the other.
- It is then reinserted lateral to the exit site and passed back through to the initial side parallel to the first throw of the suture (Figure 42–5).
- It is then tied, which creates a box or square stitch pattern.

COMPLICATIONS

- Scarring.
  - Suturing of wounds helps reduce scarring.
  - Applying modest tension to the skin surface tissue will minimize scarring, but patients and parents should be informed that every wound scars.
- Infection.
  - The skin acts as a barrier against bacteria.
  - Violation of skin may permit entrance of bacteria, and closing of wounds can trap contaminated material and result in infection.

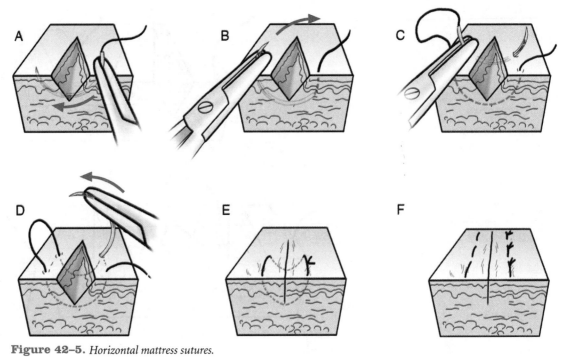

Figure 42–5. *Horizontal mattress sutures.*

■ Wound dehiscence.

　• Despite attention to detail and proper technique, sutures may untie or the wound may open secondary to edema.

REFERENCES

Capellan O, Hollander JE. Management of lacerations in the emergency department. *Emerg Med Clin North Am.* 2003;21: 205–231.

Knapp JF. Updates in wound management for the pediatrician. *Pediatr Clin North Am.* 1999;46:1202–1213.

Marx JA et al, editors. *Rosen's Emergency Medicine: Concepts and Clinical Practice.* 5th ed. St. Louis: Mosby; 2002.

Trott A. *Wounds and Lacerations: Emergency Care and Closure.* 3rd ed. Philadelphia: Mosby; 2005.

Section 8: Ears, Nose, Throat, and Eyes

CHAPTER 43

Otoscopic Examination

Kimberley Dilley, MD, MPH

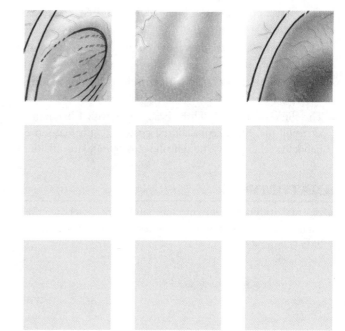

INDICATIONS

- Examination of the tympanic membranes and ear canals is part of routine health maintenance.
- Tympanic membranes should also be visualized with complaint of ear pain, upper respiratory tract infection, or fever.
- Serial examinations are indicated over several months to check for resolution of effusion.
- A complaint of hearing loss should also prompt a careful otoscopic examination.

CONTRAINDICATIONS

Relative

- In the presence of otitis externa, the tympanic membrane will be difficult to visualize because of occlusion with pus.
- Presence of cerumen in the canal may require removal with a curette or irrigation in the office or alternatively use of a cerumen-reducing agent at home with return for reexamination in a few days.

EQUIPMENT

- Otoscope with insufflator attachment.
- Ear curettes.
- Hydrogen peroxide diluted 1:1 with lukewarm water.

RISKS

- If an uncooperative child is not held completely still, there is a risk of laceration to the ear canal.

PEARLS AND TIPS

- While most offices have disposable tips for the otoscope, use of the tips supplied by the manufacturer tend to have a better fit and yield more accurate results on pneumatic otoscopy.

■ A 10-mL syringe with a cut-off angiocatheter plastic tip is useful for instillation of dilute hydrogen peroxide when irrigation is required.

PATIENT PREPARATION

■ Warn the patient that a pressure sensation and possibly pain will be experienced when using the insufflator.

PATIENT POSITIONING

■ Patient must be still for an adequate examination, including visualization of the tympanic membrane and insufflation.

■ There are 2 positioning alternatives for children who need to be held:

• Supine with arms held by parent or an assistant down at the patient's sides.

• Sitting in the parent's lap with arms held to body in bear hug position.

■ The clinician should hold the head steady with 1 hand and also pull the pinna cephalad and posterior with that same hand; the other hand is holding the otoscope and insufflator.

ANATOMY

■ Normal tympanic membrane landmarks include the malleus and incus as well as the pars tensa and pars flaccida (Figure 43–1).

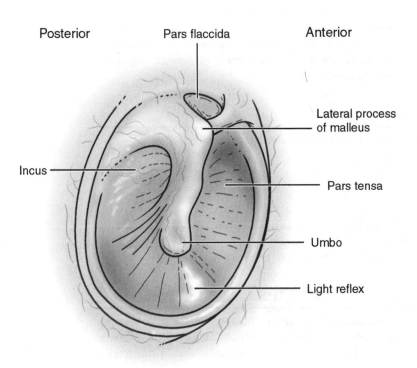

Posterior   Pars flaccida   Anterior

Lateral process of malleus

Incus

Pars tensa

Umbo

Light reflex

Figure 43–1. *Tympanic membrane landmarks.*

■ The light reflex should be sharp on a normal tympanic membrane.

PROCEDURE

■ Using an otoscope, examine the ear canal and remove any occluding cerumen.

■ Choose the appropriately sized ear tip for the patient's ear canal and affix it to the otoscope.

■ Grasp the helix and pull up and back gently to straighten the ear canal.

■ Insert the speculum tip into the entrance of the ear canal to visualize the tympanic membrane.

■ An airtight seal will need to be obtained when performing pneumatic otoscopy.

■ To insufflate, squeeze the bulb to deliver positive pressure against the tympanic membrane while observing for mobility. Also observe for movement when releasing the bulb and generating negative pressure.

INTERPRETATION AND MONITORING

■ Fluid behind the tympanic membrane without evidence of bulging or decreased mobility does not indicate acute otitis media.

■ Acute onset and a bulging or distinctly immobile tympanic membrane in the presence of erythema with pain or fever is diagnostic of acute otitis media (Figure 43–2).

■ Fluid behind the ear with or without immobility without erythema or other signs of acute inflammation is indicative of otitis media with effusion (Figure 43–3), which is not generally treated with antibiotics. Many patients still have effusions up to 3 months after a case of acute otitis media.

COMPLICATIONS

■ Laceration of the ear canal is possible when a patient is difficult to hold.

■ Consider topical antibiotics if laceration is significant; otherwise no management is indicated once hemostasis is ensured.

CAVEATS

■ Tympanometry can also be used to assess for effusions but adds little benefit over pneumatic otoscopy by an experienced examiner.

■ Observation of videotaped pneumatic otoscopy tests yields better sensitivity and specificity for middle ear effusion than observation of a static tympanic membrane, but performance of pneumatic otoscopy on a patient is dependent upon technique.

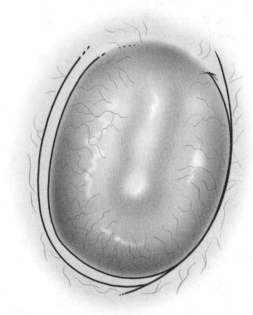

Figure 43–2. *Acute otitis media.*

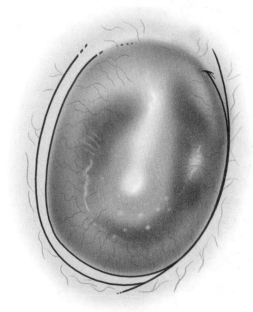

Figure 43–3. *Otitis media with effusion.*

FOLLOW-UP

- Routine follow-up examinations after acute otitis media are not indicated, but when otitis media with effusion is found it should be monitored periodically until resolved.
- If the effusion is not resolved within 3 months, test hearing and consider referral to an otolaryngologist if hearing loss is present.

REFERENCES

American Academy of Family Physicians; American Academy of Otolaryngology-Head and Neck Surgery; American Academy of Pediatrics Subcommittee on Otitis Media With Effusion. Otitis media with effusion. *Pediatrics.* 2004;113:1412–1429.

American Academy of Pediatrics and American Academy of Family Physicians Subcommittee on Management of Acute Otitis Media. Diagnosis and management of acute otitis media. *Pediatrics.* 2004;113:1451–1465.

Behrman RE, Kliegman RM, Jenson HB, eds. *Nelson Textbook of Pediatrics.* 17th ed. Philadelphia: WB Saunders Company; 2004.

Jones WS, Kaleida PH. How helpful is pneumatic otoscopy in improving diagnostic accuracy? *Pediatrics.* 2003;112:510–513.

Rothman R, Owens T, Simel DL. Does this child have acute otitis media? *JAMA.* 2003;290:1633–1640.

Takata GS, Chan LS, Morphew T, Mangione-Smith R, Morton SC, Shekelle P. Evidence assessment of the accuracy of methods of diagnosing middle ear effusion in children with otitis media with effusion. *Pediatrics.* 2003;112:1379–1387.

Wald ER. Acute otitis media: more trouble with the evidence. *Pediatr Infect Dis J.* 2003;22:103–104.

CHAPTER 44

Tympanometry

Alexandra Ryan, MD and Kimberley Dilley, MD, MPH

INDICATIONS

- Tympanometry directly measures the compliance of the tympanic membrane and ossicular chain, estimating middle ear pressure.
- Tympanometry is primarily used to detect the presence of middle ear fluid, enhancing the diagnosis of acute otitis media and otitis media with effusion.
- The procedure is also useful for detecting tympanic membrane perforation, ossicular chain disruption, and the patency of eustachian tubes.
- Tympanometry is commonly performed as part of the early evaluation of hearing loss.

CONTRAINDICATIONS

Absolute

- Age younger than 7 months. Studies have shown that tympanometry in infants 0–7 months of age is inaccurate due to the high compliance of the ear canal in these patients.
- Recent ear surgery, such as stapedectomy, myringoplasty, or tympanoplasty.

Relative

- Blocked ear canal.
- Ear canal with copious drainage.
- Uncooperative or screaming patient.

EQUIPMENT

- Otoscope.
- Ear curettes.
- Tympanometer with probe tips.
  - All instruments use acoustic energy to measure the combined admittance (compliance) of the ear canal and middle ear.
  - The most commonly used instruments deliver a probe tone of 225 Hz.

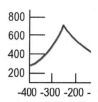

• High-frequency instruments, sometimes used in infants, deliver a tone of 678 Hz.

PEARLS AND TIPS

- Before beginning the procedure, make sure that the probe assembly is securely fastened together; leaks will obscure the test results.
- Also, ensure that the probe tube and tips are dry; wet equipment may clog, making it impossible to continue the test.

PATIENT PREPARATION

- Describe the procedure to the parents and patient and answer any questions.
- Be sure to inform the patient that he or she will be hearing some brief, but potentially loud, sounds.

PATIENT POSITIONING

- The child needs to sit still during the procedure; if necessary, have the child sit on a parent's lap for reassurance.

ANATOMY

- Hearing results from the conduction of sound into the ear canal. Sound stimulates the tympanic membrane, which then vibrates.
- The malleus (the first bone of the ossicular chain, attached to the eardrum) also starts vibrating, which sets the incus and stapes into motion (Figure 44–1).
- The stapes is set in the oval window, the opening of the inner ear. The sound is conducted into the inner ear, which translates sound energy into nerve impulses to the brain.
- The eustachian tube, an extension of the nasopharynx, equalizes middle ear pressure with atmospheric pressure (the pressure within the ear canal).

PROCEDURE

- Using an otoscope, examine the ear canal and remove any occluding cerumen.
- Choose the appropriate sized ear tip for the patient's ear canal and affix it to the probe.
- Grasp the helix and pull back and up gently to straighten the ear canal.
- Insert the probe into the entrance of the ear canal, obtaining an airtight seal. When the probe is positioned properly, the recording device will be triggered.
- The tympanometer then introduces a known amount of sound energy into the ear and measures the amount of energy that returns to the probe. The difference of these 2 values indicates the compliance of the ear.

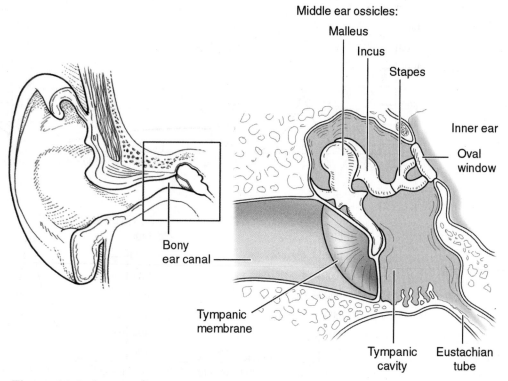

Middle ear ossicles:
Malleus
Incus
Stapes
Inner ear
Oval window
Bony ear canal
Tympanic membrane
Tympanic cavity
Eustachian tube

Figure 44–1. *Anatomy of ear.*

- The tympanometer varies the amount of pressure introduced into the ear gradually and records the compliance of the ear at each pressure point.
- Leave the probe in position until the tympanometer signals the conclusion of the test.
- Repeat in the contralateral ear.

INTERPRETATION AND MONITORING

- The tympanometer reports the ear canal volume, compliance and pressure peaks, and the pressure gradient.
- A tympanogram, a graph that reflects the change in compliance of the middle ear system as pressure varies, is also generated.
- In general, stiffening of the middle ear system (effusion, sclerosis) reduces compliance and produces tympanograms with low peaks; loosening of the middle ear system (flaccidity of the membrane, ossicular disruption) increases compliance and produces tympanograms with high peaks.
- Five typical tympanogram classifications exist (Figure 44–2).
  - Type A shows normal pressure-compliance functions.
  - Type As curves are shaped like type A curves but are shallower and are associated with decreased compliance.
  - Type Ad curves are also shaped like type A curves but are deeper and associated with increased compliance.

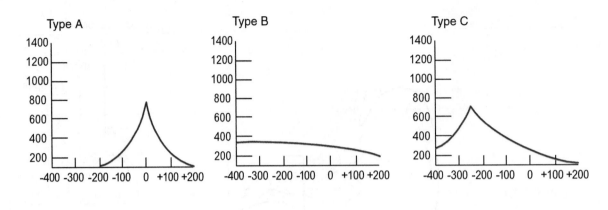

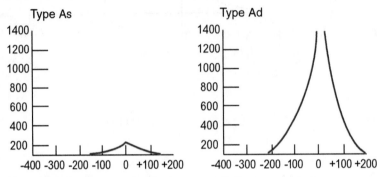

Figure 44–2. *Five typical tympanogram classifications.*

- Type B curves are flat, showing no pressure at which the membrane becomes compliant, and suggest fluid in the middle ear, ear canal blockage, or tympanic membrane perforation.
- Type C shows the peak of compliance when the pressure in the ear canal is negative, such as in eustachian tube dysfunction or other conditions that cause difficulties with pressure equalization in the middle ear.

■ In the diagnosis of effusion, the shape of the tympanogram is the measure with the highest degree of sensitivity and specificity.

■ The more rounded the peak and the wider the tympanogram, the higher the probability of effusion.

■ Ear canal volume estimates can be useful in diagnosing other types of ear pathologies.

- An abnormally high ear canal volume can indicate a tympanic membrane perforation, especially when it is associated with a flat tympanogram.
- An abnormally small ear canal volume can be evidence of poor probe fit, obstructed probe, or ear canal occlusion with cerumen or debris.

CAVEATS

■ Tympanometry cannot distinguish between middle ear effusion due to otitis media with effusion and acute otitis media.

- Tympanometry can only document the presence of an effusion.

- Further history and physical signs must be used to diagnose acute otitis.

- Guidelines established by the American Academy of Pediatricians, American Academy of Family Physicians, and Agency for Healthcare Research Quality on otitis media with effusion recommends optional use of tympanometry in confirming suspected otitis media with effusion.

- Tympanometry is as effective as pneumatic otoscopy in diagnosing middle ear fluid when the examiner is an experienced otoscopist; in those cases, tympanometry will have little additional benefit.

- However, in practical application or uncertain diagnoses, tympanometry can add useful information; 1 study of diagnostic methods reported a 30% decrease in diagnosis of otitis media.

- Among cooperative children, sensitivity and specificity of tympanometry have been shown to be 79–94% and 86–93%, respectively, for diagnosis of middle ear effusion.

- Among uncooperative children, sensitivity and specificity are 71% and 38%, respectively.

- Sensitivity and specificity increase when tympanometry is coupled with pneumatic otoscopy.

- One recent study showed that while pediatricians were able to accurately perform tympanometry, they did not incorporate the results in their diagnosis.

- Thus, otitis media is overdiagnosed in 14–40% of cases, suggesting that further education and familiarity with tympanometry is needed.

- Research to develop accurate tympanometry in infants younger than 7 months is ongoing. Some promise is shown with different probe frequencies, but no method has been validated at this time.

REFERENCES

American Academy of Family Physicians; American Academy of Otolaryngology-Head and Neck Surgery; American Academy of Pediatrics Subcommittee on Otitis Media With Effusion. Otitis media with effusion. *Pediatrics.* 2004;113:1412–1429.

Behrman RE, Kliegman RM, Jenson HB, eds. *Nelson Textbook of Pediatrics.* 17th ed. Philadelphia: WB Saunders Company; 2004.

Blomgren K, Pitkaranta A. Current challenges in diagnosis of acute otitis media. *Int J Pediatr Otorhinolaryngol.* 2005;69:295–299.

Finitzo T, Friel-Patti S et al. Tympanometry and otoscopy prior to myringotomy: issues in diagnosis of otitis media. *Int J Pediatr Otorhinolaryngol.* 1992;24:101–110.

Hoekelman RA. *Primary Pediatric Care.* St. Louis: Mosby; 2001.

Johansen EC, Lildholdt T, Damsbo N, Eriksen EW. Tympanometry for diagnosis and treatment of otitis media in general practice. *Fam Pract.* 2000;17:317–322.

Koivunen P, Alho OP, Uhari M, Niemela M, Luotonen J. Mini-tympanometry in detecting middle ear fluid. *J Pediatr.* 1997;131:419–422.

Onusko E. Tympanometry. *Am Fam Physician.* 2004;70:1713–1720.

Shanks J, Shelton C. Basic principles and clinical applications of tympanometry. *Otolaryngol Clin North Am.* 1991;24:299–328.

Spiro DM, King WD, Arnold DH, Johnston C, Baldwin S. A randomized clinical trial to assess the effects of tympanometry on the diagnosis and treatment of acute otitis media. *Pediatrics.* 2004;114:177–181.

Takata GS, Chan LS, Morphew T, Mangione-Smith R, Morton SC, Shekelle P. Evidence assessment of the accuracy of methods of diagnosing middle ear effusion in children with otitis media with effusion. *Pediatrics.* 2003;112(6 Pt 1):1379–1387.

CHAPTER 45

Myringotomy and Tympanostomy Tube Insertion

Lauren Holinger, MD and Sue Kim, MD

INDICATIONS

- Otitis media with effusion (OME) persisting longer than 3 months.
- Hearing loss > 30 dB in patients with OME.
- Recurrent episodes of acute otitis media.
  - More than 3 episodes in 6 months.
  - More than 4 episodes in 12 months.
- Barotrauma and patients undergoing hyperbaric oxygen therapy.

CONTRAINDICATIONS

Absolute

- Aural atresia.
- Ectopic or aberrant carotid artery into the middle ear space.

Relative

- Otitis externa causing stenosis of the external auditory meatus.
- High-riding jugular bulb into the middle ear space.
- Mass behind the tympanic membrane.

EQUIPMENT

- Microscope.
- Ear speculum.
- Cerumen curette.
- Myringotomy knife.
- Suction cannula (3F, 5F, and 7F) with suction canister and apparatus for cultures.
- Tympanostomy tube.
  - For children aged 6 months to 2 years, use short-term ventilation tubes (eg, straight tube, grommet tube, Reuter collar button tube).
  - For children aged 3–5 years with chronic eustachian dysfunction (such as children with cleft palates), use long-term ventilation tubes (eg, T-tubes or large inner-flanged tubes).

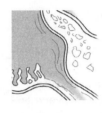
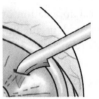

- Alligator forceps.
- Ear pick.

RISKS

- Risks of anesthesia.
- Bleeding.
  - Temporary; usually resolves spontaneously within 24 hours.
  - Due to outer ear or ear canal laceration.
  - Due to myringotomy incision.
  - Due to inflamed middle ear mucosa.
- Otorrhea occurs in approximately 20–30% of patients with tympanostomy tubes.
  - Postoperative otorrhea (16%): Most likely related to the presence of purulent fluid or inflamed middle ear mucosa.
  - Recurrent otorrhea (7–26%): Usually occurs due to another episode of acute otitis media.
  - Persistent or chronic otorrhea (3.8%): Can occur from reactive inflammation to the tube itself and may require tube removal.
- Tympanic membrane perforation occurs in 5–15% of patients.
  - Short-term ventilation tubes: Less than 5%.
  - Long-term ventilation tubes: Higher rate of perforation at approximately 15%.
  - Less than 3% require surgical closure of the perforation.
- Tube that is retained for longer than 5 years, with or without granuloma formation, can act as a foreign body.
  - If the patient has chronic unresolving otorrhea or granulation tissue around the tympanostomy tube, it should be removed.
  - Granulation tissue formation occurs in approximately 5% of patients.
- Medial displacement of the tympanostomy tube (0.5%); not a problem.
- Myringosclerosis is the submucosal hyaline degeneration in the fibrous layer of the tympanic membrane, resulting in a whitish "plaque."
  - Can occur in as many as 30–40% of patients with tympanostomy tubes.
  - In most cases, there is no clinical significance.
- Other structural changes of the tympanic membrane.
  - Flaccid tympanic membrane (25%).
  - Retracted tympanic membrane (3.1%).
- Cholesteatoma.
  - Occurs in less than 1% of patients.
  - May result from squamous debris being trapped in the middle ear around the tympanostomy tube.

PEARLS AND TIPS

- Clinicians should use pneumatic otoscopy as the primary method to diagnose OME.
- During the myringotomy and tube insertion, be careful not to traumatize the anterior bony canal wall. Should trauma occur, place a cotton wick impregnated with oxymetazoline in the ear canal for 5 minutes.
- Use the largest ear speculum that fits into the ear canal to maximize exposure of the tympanic membrane.
- Place incision in the anterior-inferior quadrant; avoid the posterior-superior quadrant since this is where the ossicles are located.
- If the ear tube falls past the incision into the middle ear space, there are 2 options:
  - Try to retrieve it with an empty alligator if the tube is sitting just past the myringotomy incision, away from the ossicles and in plain sight.
  - Leave the tube in the middle ear space and insert another tympanostomy tube if the tube is not easily retrievable or is not visible.
- Ototopical antibiotic drops are used to treat otorrhea after tube placement.

PATIENT PREPARATION

- Preoperative audiogram and tympanogram.
- Routine preparation for general anesthesia.
- Certain cooperative children may tolerate procedure with local anesthesia only.
  - Eutectic mixture of local anesthetic (EMLA) cream.
  - Phenol applied to tympanic membrane.
  - 4-point external auditory canal injection with 1% lidocaine with 1:100,000 epinephrine.

PATIENT POSITIONING

- Supine with head turned away from the clinician.

ANATOMY REVIEW

- Figure 45–1 shows the anatomy of the ear.

PROCEDURE

- Administer general anesthesia by mask ventilation or apply local anesthesia.
- Place the operating microscope at the head of the bed.
- Position an ear speculum into the external auditory meatus.
- Gently clear cerumen from the ear canal with a wax curette or suction cannula under direct microscopic visualization.

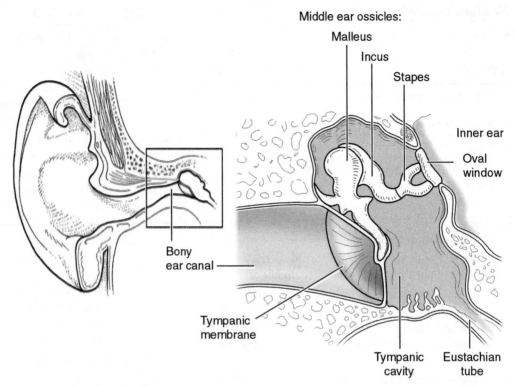

Figure 45–1. *Anatomy of ear.*

- Inspect the external auditory meatus and tympanic membrane.
- Identify the ossicles (specifically, the short process of the malleus, manubrium, and umbo).
- Determine site for the myringotomy incision; possibilities include the following:
  - Anterior-inferior quadrant (preferred).
  - Anterior-superior quadrant.
  - Posterior-inferior quadrant.
- Use a myringotomy knife to make a radial incision in the tympanic membrane (Figure 45–2).
- Aspirate fluid from the middle ear with a 3F suction cannula, preferably without touching the tympanic membrane.
- Use larger suction cannulas (5F or 7F) for thick mucoid.
- Enlarge the myringotomy if necessary once the fluid is evacuated. The incision should be slightly larger than the medial flange of the tympanostomy.
- Load the alligator with a tympanostomy tube, and insert the medial flange into the myringotomy incision.
- Use an ear pick to manipulate the tube so that the entire medial flange of the tympanostomy tube is fully inserted.
- Confirm the position of the tube.
- Insert ear drops in the external auditory canal.

MONITORING

- If the child undergoes general anesthesia, monitor the patient in a recovery room setting.
- Patient can be discharged when ambulatory center guidelines are met.

CAVEATS

- Antihistamines and decongestants are not effective treatment for OME.
- Antibiotics and corticosteroids are not recommended for routine management of OME.
- As many as 30% of children undergoing myringotomy with insertion of ear tubes require another tube within 5 years.
- Adenoidectomy is recommended for children with OME who require a second set of tubes.

FOLLOW-UP

- Postoperative visit in 1–2 weeks to document healing and patency of tubes.
- Postoperative audiogram to document hearing and tube patency.
- Follow-up visits every 6 months to assess tubes and symptoms.

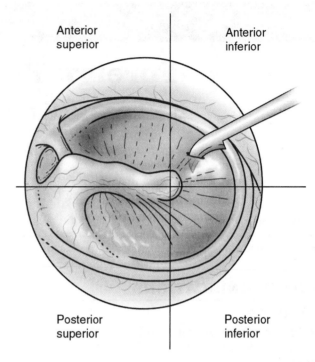

Figure 45–2. *Incision of tympanic membrane.*

REFERENCES

Rosenfeld RM, Culpepper L, Doyle KJ et al; American Academy of Pediatrics Subcommittee on Otitis Media with Effusion; American Academy of Family Physicians; American Academy of Otolaryngology–Head and Neck Surgery. Clinical practice guideline: Otitis media with effusion. *Otolaryngol Head Neck Surg.* 2004;130(5 Suppl):S95–S118.

Paradise JL, Feldman HM, Campbell TF et al. Effect of early or delayed insertion of tympanostomy tubes for persistent otitis media on developmental outcomes at the age of three years. *N Engl J Med.* 2001;344:1179–1187.

Kay DJ, Nelson M, Rosenfeld RM. Meta-analysis of tympanostomy sequelae. *Otolaryngol Head Neck Surg.* 2001;124:374–380.

Brackmann DE, ed. *Otologic Surgery.* Philadelphia: WB Saunders Company; 2001:68–81.

Becker W, ed. *Atlas of Ear, Nose and Throat Diseases.* 2nd ed. New York: Thieme; 1984:20.

CHAPTER 46

Foreign Body Removal: External Auditory Canal

Jennifer Trainor, MD

INDICATIONS

- Foreign body lodged in the external auditory canal.

CONTRAINDICATIONS

Absolute

- Perforated tympanic membrane.

Relative

- Inability to visualize the tympanic membrane.

EQUIPMENT

- Alligator forceps.
- Simple forceps.
- Ear curette (metal or plastic).
- Right-angle hook.
- Irrigation setup (water pik device or 20–60-mL syringe attached to cut-off butterfly tubing or angiocatheter).
- Otoscope with operating head.
- Lidocaine spray or viscous lidocaine suspension.
- Frazier tip or Schuknecht suction.
- Cyanoacrylate glue adhesive.

RISKS

- Failed removal (20–30%).
- Canal laceration or bleeding (10–50%).
- Psychological stress (common; child is restrained for procedure).
- Perforation of the tympanic membrane (1–2%).
- Damage to the ossicles (< 1%).

PEARLS AND TIPS

- If the child cannot be adequately restrained, do not attempt removal.

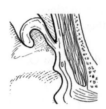
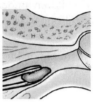

- Most foreign bodies do not require urgent removal, and the child can be referred to an otolaryngologist if efforts fail.
- Never use irrigation to remove disc batteries, vegetable matter, or expansible objects (eg, sponge).
- Hard spherical objects can be difficult to remove. Do not use forceps because they may push the object further into the canal.
- Sharp objects pose a higher risk of tympanic membrane perforation. Proceed with caution or refer to an otolaryngologist for removal with an operating microscope.
- The first attempt is the best attempt. Repeated attempts with a struggling child are not likely to be successful.
- Test for and document any dizziness or hearing loss before removal attempts. Document an additional examination after the foreign body has been removed.

PATIENT PREPARATION

- Reassure the child that no needles will be used.
- Show the child the instrument that you are going to use and let him or her feel that it is not sharp.
- Explain that holding still is extremely important in order to minimize the likelihood of pain.

PATIENT POSITIONING

- A toddler may be restrained in the parent's lap, facing the parent, with the head turned to 1 side and pressed up against the parent's chest.
- The parent then gives the child a bear hug, wrapping 1 arm around the patient's body and arms and the other arm restraining the head.
- It is important that the head be fully turned because the child has less strength in this position to break free from the parent's grasp.
- An older child should be placed supine on the examining table, with the head turned so that the affected ear is facing up.
- Immobilization of the head by an assistant is recommended, even if the child appears cooperative.
- The inner two-thirds of the external auditory canal is exquisitely sensitive to pain. With even minor manipulation, the child may suddenly jerk his or her head, causing trauma to the external auditory canal.
- If the child is uncooperative, the shoulders and torso need to be restrained as well.
- A parent or assistant may assume a position at the foot of the bed, leaning over the patient, and holding the child's arms at his or her sides.

ANATOMY REVIEW

- Figure 46–1 shows the anatomy of the ear.

PROCEDURE

- In order to optimize visualization, the examiner should retract the pinna to straighten the ear canal.
- The foreign body should then be visualized with an otoscope, preferably with an operating head.
- Size, shape, and location of the foreign body should be noted.
- Based on the visualized foreign body type and the operator's prior experience, use either the direct instrumentation method, irrigation method, or cyanoacrylate method to remove the foreign body.

Direct Instrumentation Method

- This approach uses forceps and is most successful for irregularly shaped, graspable objects.
- If an otoscope with an operating head is not available, but the foreign body can be visualized by simple visual inspection, grasp the object with forceps and pull it from the canal.
- Alligator forceps are most useful when the foreign body is narrow or has a small leading edge (Figure 46–2).
- An object not easily grasped with forceps that does not completely occlude the canal can be removed by sliding an ear curette beyond the foreign body, then pulling forward.
- A right-angle hook can be used in the same manner by sliding the instrument past the foreign body, then turning it 90 degrees so the angle captures the foreign body, pulling it forward and out of the canal.
- Suction may be used for smooth-surfaced foreign bodies that occlude the canal.
- Proceed cautiously, however, to prevent pushing the foreign body deeper into the canal, injuring the tympanic membrane.

Irrigation Method

- Irrigation is best used for hard, nongraspable objects that do not completely occlude the canal.
- Use warmed saline or water to minimize discomfort.
- Insert butterfly tubing or angiocatheter beyond the foreign body and flush with approximately 20–60 mL of liquid.
- Aim the stream at the posterior, superior canal wall and not at the tympanic membrane.
- To remove live insects, precede irrigation attempts with instillation of viscous lidocaine.
- Lidocaine has been reported to cause live cockroaches to spontaneously exit the canal, obviating the need for either instrumentation or irrigation.

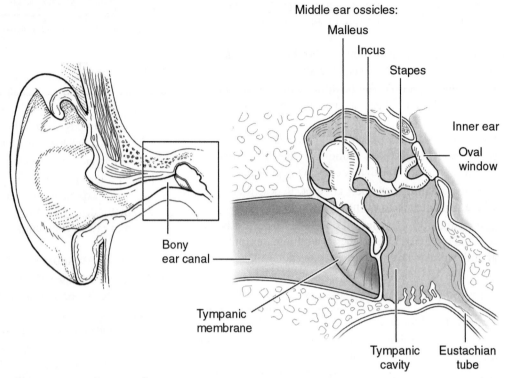

Figure 46–1. *Anatomy of ear.*

■ If lidocaine is not available, the insect can be killed with mineral oil before extraction attempts.

Cyanoacrylate Method

■ Apply cyanoacrylate (tissue adhesive) glue to the blunt end of a wooden cotton swab tip.

■ Introduce the tip into the ear canal to make contact with the foreign body, taking care not to touch the ear canal.

■ Allow the glue to remain in contact with the foreign body for approximately 1 minute before retracting the stick.

■ If the stick becomes adherent to the canal wall inadvertently, mineral oil may be used to detach it.

MONITORING

■ Examine the ear canal after object removal for signs of trauma, bleeding, or perforated tympanic membrane.

■ Verify the tympanic membrane is intact with pneumatic otoscopy.

■ If there are lacerations or abrasions present, consider discharging the patient on short course of topical antibiotic and anti-inflammatory suspension.

■ Describe the procedure and document findings in the medical record.

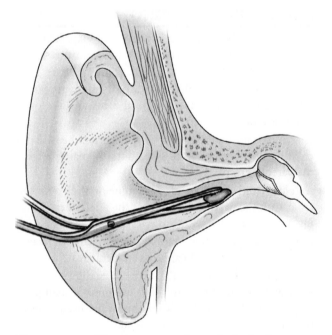

Figure 46–2. *Direct instrumentation method using forceps.*

COMPLICATIONS

- Retained foreign body.
- External auditory canal laceration or abrasion.
- Perforation of the tympanic membrane.
- Damage to the ossicles.
- Hearing loss.

CAVEATS

- Techniques for removal of ear foreign bodies are similar to cerumen removal, a procedure commonly performed by pediatric practitioners.
- Limited data suggest that hard, round, smooth objects are more difficult to remove and result in higher rates of complications and retained foreign bodies than other foreign body types.
- Objects that completely occlude the external auditory canal do not allow passage of an instrument beyond the foreign body and may make removal more difficult.
- Removal attempts may result in the object being pushed further into the canal, perforating the tympanic membrane, or causing ossicular damage, a rare but reported complication that has the potential to cause hearing loss.
- Live insects are best removed with either lidocaine instillation or irrigation. Use of forceps may result in fragmentation of the insect, and retained fragments have the potential to cause infection.

- In contrast to most other foreign bodies, disc batteries need to be urgently removed because leakage of chemicals can cause liquefaction necrosis of the ear canal.

FOLLOW-UP

- If trauma to the canal occurs, a follow-up visit is warranted.
- Patients should be referred to an otolaryngologist if they complain of dizziness or if there is any damage to the tympanic membrane.

REFERENCES

Ansley J, Cunningham M. Treatment of aural foreign bodies in children. *Pediatrics.* 1998;101:638–641.

Bressler K, Shelton C. Ear foreign-body removal: a review of 98 consecutive cases. *Laryngoscope.* 1993;103:367–370.

Brown L, Denmark TK, Wittlake W, Vargas EJ, Watson T, Crabb JW. Procedural sedation use in the ED: management of pediatric ear and nose foreign bodies. *Am J Emerg Med.* 2004;22:310–314.

DiMuzio J, Deschler D. Emergency department management of foreign bodies of the external auditory canal in children. *Otol Neurotol.* 2002;23:473–475.

Henretig FM, King C. *Textbook of Pediatric Emergency Procedures.* Baltimore: Williams & Wilkins; 1996.

Walsh-Sukys MC, Krug SK. *Procedures in Infants and Children.* Philadelphia: WB Saunders Company; 1997.

Marin J, Trainor J. Foreign body removal from the external auditory canal. 2005 Pediatric Academic Societies Annual Meeting. 2005. Abstract 1866.

CHAPTER 47

Foreign Body Removal: Nasal Cavity

Jennifer Trainor, MD

INDICATIONS

- Foreign body lodged in the nasal cavity.

CONTRAINDICATIONS

Absolute

- Respiratory distress.
- Penetrating injury.
- Bleeding diathesis.
- Disc battery impaction.

Relative

- Fractured nasal bone.
- Inability to visualize the foreign body.

EQUIPMENT

- Vasoconstrictor nasal spray or drops (.25% phenylephrine hydrochloride).
- Topical anesthetic (1–4% lidocaine).
- Alligator forceps.
- Right-angle hook.
- Ear curette (metal or plastic).
- Nasal speculum.
- Suction apparatus.
- Self-inflating ventilation bag (ie, Ambu) and mask.

RISKS

- Failed or incomplete removal (10–30%).
- Epistaxis (10–30%).
- Psychological stress (minimal if parent kiss technique is used).
- Septal hematoma or perforation (rare).
- Aspiration (rare).

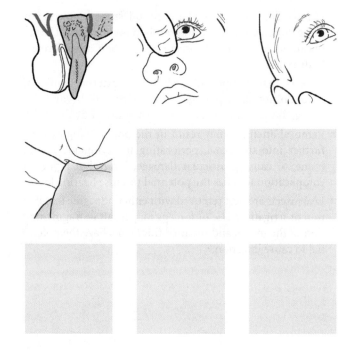

- The equipment needed depends on the method of removal.

- Risks depend on the method of removal.

PEARLS AND TIPS

- The parent kiss technique is the least invasive method and should be attempted first for smooth objects lodged high in the nasal passage.
- Precede all attempts with vasoconstrictive nose drops to minimize bleeding and reduce edema.
- If the child cannot be adequately restrained, do not attempt instrument removal.
- Never use irrigation to remove disc batteries, vegetable matter, or expansible objects (eg, sponge).
- The first attempt is the best attempt.

PATIENT PREPARATION

Parent Kiss Technique

- Explain to the child that his or her parent will give him or her a special kiss on the mouth to remove the object.
- The child will need to keep his or her mouth open for the kiss.
- This is the only cooperation required, and there will be no instruments used.
- Explain to the parent, out of earshot of the child, that the parent must blow with 1 forceful puff into the child's mouth while simultaneously occluding the uninvolved nostril.
- If successful, the object will be expelled from the nasal cavity, obviating the need for instrument removal.
- The technique is less frightening to the child and less likely to result in local trauma.

Instrument Removal Technique

- Reassure the child that no needles will be used.
- Show the child the instrument that you are going to use and let him or her feel that it is not sharp.
- Explain that holding still is extremely important in order to minimize the likelihood of pain.
- Warn the parent that small amounts of bleeding are common.

PATIENT POSITIONING

Positive Pressure Techniques

- Can be performed in several positions:
  - Child sits upright on the examining table or reclines back against a parent who is sitting on the examining table.
  - Child stands with back and head against a wall.
  - Child lies supine on the examining table.
- For the parent kiss and self-expel techniques, no restraint is required.
- For the self-inflating ventilation bag technique, an assistant needs to hold the head and mask in place during the procedure.

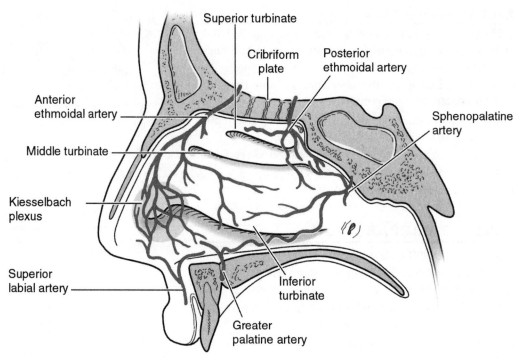

Figure 47–1. *Sagittal view of nasal cavity.*

Instrument Removal Technique

- Child should be supine on the examining table.
- Immobilization of the head by an assistant is recommended, even if the child appears cooperative.
- If the child is uncooperative, the shoulders and torso need to be restrained as well.
- A parent or assistant may assume a position at the foot of the bed, leaning over the patient, and holding the child's arms at the sides.
- Alternatively, a papoose board may be used for restraint.

ANATOMY REVIEW

- The floor of the nasal cavity is oriented perpendicular to the plane of the face.
- Figure 47–1 shows the position of the inferior, middle, and superior turbinates.
- The cribriform plate lies just above the superior turbinate.

PROCEDURE

- Before any removal attempts are made, visualize the foreign body, and determine its location, size, and composition.
- Relatively anteriorly placed foreign bodies may be seen by simply tipping up the nose in a cephalad direction to open the nares and allow visualization of the floor of the nasal cavity (Figure 47–2).

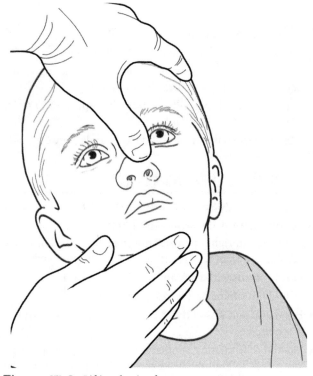

Figure 47–2. *Lifting the tip of nose.*

- For objects not visualized in this manner, a nasal speculum should be used (Figure 47–3).
- Orient the speculum in the superior-inferior position, so it does not exert pressure against the nasal septum.
- Apply vasoconstrictive nose drops (or spray) to the affected nasal cavity before attempting removal.
- Lidocaine may also be used topically as a local anesthetic.

Positive Pressure Techniques

A. PARENT KISS

- Have the parent lean over the child, occluding the uninvolved nostril with 1 finger, and placing his or her lips around the patient's lips (as if to give a mouth-to-mouth breath).
- The parent then quickly and forcefully exhales once into the child's mouth (Figure 47–4).
- If successful, the foreign body will be expelled.
- Occasionally, this just moves the object into the anterior portion of the nasal cavity.
- The object can then be coaxed out of the nostril before the child sniffs it back up into the nasal cavity.

B. SELF-EXPEL

- An older, cooperative child may perform the technique himself or herself.
- Instruct the child to occlude the unaffected nostril, inhale deeply by mouth, then forcefully exhale through the nose, expelling the lodged object.

C. SELF-INFLATING VENTILATION BAG

- A self-inflating ventilation bag connected to appropriately sized mask is applied to the patient's mouth.
- The uninvolved nostril is occluded, and 1 compression of the bag is delivered.

D. HIGH-FLOW OXYGEN

- If an oxygen or high-flow air source is available in the office, place oxygen tubing delivering 10–15 L/min of flow into the uninvolved nostril while the child maintains a closed mouth.
- The object is then expelled.

Instrument Removal Technique

- The nasal turbinates are perpendicular to the face not parallel to the nasal bone.
- Attempt direct removal by advancing the forceps straight back to grasp the foreign body and remove.
- To remove a nongraspable object that does not completely occlude the nasal cavity, slide an instrument (eg, right-angle hook, cerumen loop) along the nasal septum beyond the foreign body, and turn it 90 degrees to catch and pull the object forward.

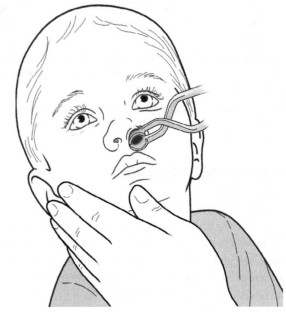

Figure 47–3. *Using nasal speculum.*

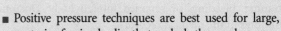

- Positive pressure techniques are best used for large, posterior foreign bodies that occlude the nasal passage.
- The parent kiss technique is least traumatic to the child but requires a cooperative parent.
- Other positive pressure techniques require more restraint and patient cooperation as well as a self-inflating ventilation bag and mask or oxygen source.

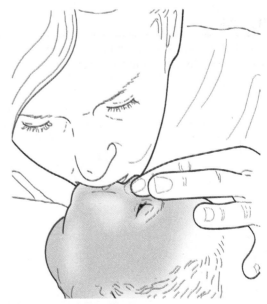

Figure 47–4. *Parent kiss technique.*

- A right-angle hook can also be used to pierce a foreign body composed of vegetable material (eg, bean) to facilitate removal.
- Alternatively, use a Frazier tip or Schukneckt foreign body extractor to remove an anteriorly lodged, smooth-surfaced foreign body.
- Foreign bodies lodged posteriorly may be pushed further back with this method, risking drop into the oropharynx and aspiration.

Cyanoacrylate Method

- Apply cyanoacrylate (tissue adhesive) glue to the blunt end of a wooden cotton swab tip.
- Introduce the tip into the nasal cavity to make contact with the foreign body, taking care not to touch the nasal mucosa.
- Allow the glue to remain in contact with the foreign body for about 30–60 seconds before retracting the stick.
- If the stick inadvertently adheres to the mucosa, use mineral oil to detach it.

MONITORING

- Examine the nasal cavity after object removal for signs of trauma, bleeding, or retained foreign body. Document findings in the medical record.

COMPLICATIONS

- Epistaxis.
- Retained foreign body.
- Aspiration.
- Perforation of the cribriform plate.

CAVEATS

- Objects that are located superior and medial to the middle turbinate are in close proximity to the cribriform plate.

- Use caution in this area because aggressive instrumentation may lead to fractures of the cribriform plate, resulting in leak of cerebrospinal fluid and risk of meningitis.
- Avoid the nasal septum because it is richly vascularized.
- If bleeding occurs, pinch the cartilaginous portion of the nose for 5–10 minutes.
- Crushed ice may also be applied to increase vasoconstriction.
- Although the risk of barotrauma is low with any of the positive pressure techniques, the ears, nose, and oral pharynx should still be examined for evidence of trauma.

FOLLOW-UP

- No specific follow-up is indicated.
- Instruct parents that the child needs to return for reexamination if he or she has persistent unilateral nasal discharge.
- After retained foreign body has been ruled out, a short course of antibiotics would be indicated for rhinosinusitis.

REFERENCES

Backlin SA. Positive-pressure technique for nasal foreign body removal in children. *Ann Emerg Med.* 1995;25:554–555.

Brown L, Denmark TK, Wittlake W, Vargas EJ, Watson T, Crabb JW. Procedural sedation use in the ED: management of pediatric ear and nose foreign bodies. *Am J Emerg Med.* 2004; 22:310–314.

Chan TC, Ufber J, Harrigan RA, Vilke GM. Nasal foreign body removal. *J Emerg Med.* 2003;12:441–445.

Davies PH, Benger JR. Foreign bodies in the nose and ear: a review of techniques for removal in the emergency department. *J Accid Emerg Med.* 2000;17:91–94.

Henretig FM, King C. *Textbook of Pediatric Emergency Procedures.* Baltimore: Williams & Wilkins; 1996.

Navitsky RC, Beamsley A, McLaughlin S. Nasal positive-pressure technique for nasal foreign body removal in children. *Am J Emerg Med.* 2002;20:103–104.

Walsh-Sukys MC, Krug SK. *Procedures in Infants and Children.* Philadelphia: WB Saunders Company; 1997.

CHAPTER 48

Anterior Nasal Packing

Lauren Holinger, MD and Sue Kim, MD

INDICATIONS

- Persistent epistaxis localized anteriorly on the nasal septum that does not respond to digital pressure, topical vasoconstrictive agents, or cautery.

EQUIPMENT

- Headlight.
- Nasal speculum.
- Frazier suction, 8F and 10F.
- Bayonet forceps.
- Yankauer suction.
- Tongue retractor/tongue blade.
- Absorbable topical vasoconstrictor (oxymetazoline).
- Expandable cellulose intranasal tampons.
- Antibiotic ointment (eg, bacitracin).
- Layered quarter-inch gauze with petroleum.
- Silver nitrate sticks.
- Hemostatic material.
- Cottonoid pledgets.
- 4% topical lidocaine or tetracaine hydrochloride.

RISKS

- Mucosal abrasion.
- Septal perforation if excessively tight packing or bilateral cauterization.
- Neurogenic syncope during packing.

PEARLS AND TIPS

- As in any patient who is hemorrhaging, assess airway, breathing, and circulation first.
- Wear protective eyewear, gown, and gloves; maintain universal precautions.
- Once hemorrhage is controlled, instruct the patient against sneezing or coughing with his or her mouth closed, bending over, straining, or nose picking or blowing.

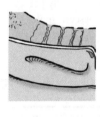

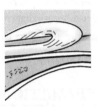

- Do not discharge a patient as soon as the bleeding stops; rather, observe him or her for at least 30 minutes to ensure that the patient is stable and the bleeding does not recur.
- Always look in the posterior oropharynx, behind the uvula, to ensure that blood is not dripping down and being swallowed.
- Do not cauterize both sides of the septum. Loss of the perichondrial layers on both sides of the septum can result in cartilage necrosis and septal perforation.
- If a patient has recurrent epistaxis, consider a neoplastic process, especially if bleeding always occurs on the same side.
  - Juvenile nasopharyngeal angiofibromas are highly vascular tumors arising in the nasopharynx that usually present as recurrent unilateral hemorrhage in pubescent males.
- Always provide systemic antibiotic coverage against *Staphylococcus* species.

PATIENT PREPARATION

- Severe epistaxis may require endotracheal intubation (for airway obstruction), cardiac monitoring and pulse oximetry, and vascular access (to administer intravenous crystalloid solution).
- Obtain a history, if possible, about digital nasal trauma, foreign bodies, hematologic disorders, medications, and nasal fracture.
- Obtain a blood count, clotting screen, and a sample for a cross-match.
- Inform the patient and parents that bleeding will be controlled in a stepwise fashion.
- If the patient is stable, have patient or assistant maintain firm digital pressure by pinching the nose closed with a gauze sponge.
- Consider sedation.

PATIENT POSITIONING

- Have the patient sit upright (unless hypotensive) and tilt head forward to prevent blood from pooling in the posterior pharynx.

ANATOMY REVIEW

- The nasal mucosa is richly supplied with an arborizing network of submucosal vessels (Figure 48–1, see Figure 47–1).
- Kiesselbach area (also called Little's area) is an area on the anteroinferior septum; it is the most common site for anterior epistaxis.
- The anterior end of the inferior turbinate is another site where bleeding can be seen.
- Posterior epistaxis is predominantly from the sphenopalatine artery and anterior ethmoid artery.

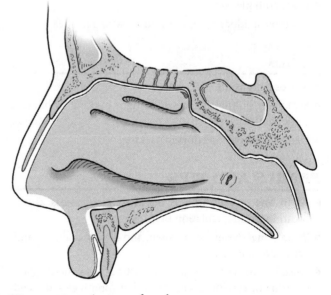

Figure 48–1. *Anatomy of nasal mucosa.*

PROCEDURE

- Manage anterior nasal hemorrhage systematically.
- Reassess the patient after digital pressure is maintained for 10 minutes to see if the epistaxis has resolved.
- Use a bright headlight because it provides good visualization and keeps both hands free.
- If the patient is still bleeding, have the patient blow the clots from his nose and quickly inspect for a bleeding site using a nasal speculum and Frazier suction tip.
- Try to identify whether bleeding is anterior or posterior.
- Use a tongue blade to see if blood is in the oropharynx.
- Insert oxymetazoline-soaked cotton pledgets into both nostrils with bayonet forceps for 5–10 minutes.
- If the bleeding continues, and an anterior site is localized, silver nitrate sticks can be used to cauterize the area.
- Avoid cauterizing both sides because loss of both perichondrial layers on the septum can lead to cartilage necrosis and septal perforation.
- If bleeding persists or a bleeding site cannot be identified, proceed to anterior nasal packing.

Anterior Nasal Packing Using Intranasal Tampon

- Intranasal tampon is coated with antibiotic ointment and placed into the nasal cavity using a bayonet and nasal speculum.
- Saline is then instilled onto the cellulose tampon to allow it to expand and tamponade the area of bleeding.
- Determine whether bleeding has been controlled, and evaluate the opposite side.
- If bleeding is identified on the opposite side, repeat insertion with an additional intranasal tampon.
- Administer and prescribe antistaphylococcal antibiotics for 7–10 days to minimize risk of toxic shock syndrome.

Anterior Nasal Packing Using Layered Quarter-Inch Gauze

- Topical anesthetic (4% lidocaine or tetracaine) is placed on cotton pledgets and inserted into the nasal cavity.
- A quarter-inch × 72-inch petroleum gauze strip is impregnated with antibiotic ointment by rubbing the ointment into the gauze.
- Use a nasal speculum and begin packing the nasal cavity by grasping the gauze ribbon, about 6 inches from its end, with a bayonet forceps and placing the packing as far back as possible (Figure 48–2).
- Ensure that the free end protrudes from the nose.
- Push down the packing against the floor of the nose.

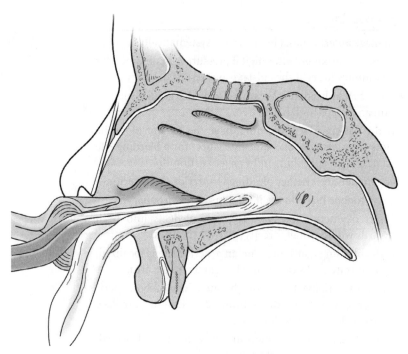

Figure 48–2. *Nasal packing using nasal speculum and gauze.*

- The gauze ribbon is grasped about 4–5 inches from the nasal alae and repositioned in the nasal speculum so that the lower blade holds the ribbon against the lower border of the nasal alae while another layer is inserted into the nasal cavity.
- Continue layering the gauze from the floor of the nose toward the top of the nasal cavity until the affected side is tightly filled.
- Both ends of the ribbon must protrude from the naris and be secured in place by taping to the nose.
- Assess to see if the bleeding has stopped.
- If unilateral anterior nasal packing does not provide enough pressure, packing the opposite side of the nose anteriorly can sometimes increase the pressure by preventing the septum from bowing to the opposite side of the nose.
- The packing is maintained in place for 72 hours.
- Administer and prescribe antistaphylococcal antibiotics for 7–10 days to minimize risk of toxic shock syndrome.

MONITORING

- Observe patient for 15–30 minutes after any intervention to ensure that the bleeding is controlled.
- Assess vital signs and hematocrit to determine whether the patient needs admission for observation.

- Most patients can be discharged home with outpatient follow-up.

COMPLICATIONS

- Toxic shock syndrome (1 in 100,000).
- Septal hematomas or abscesses from traumatic packing.
- Sinusitis.

FOLLOW-UP

- Remove packing in 3–5 days.
- In most cases, the problem is resolved.
- If bleeding persists, packing should be replaced and the patient referred to an otolaryngologist for further management.

REFERENCES

Alvi A, Joyner-Triplett N. Acute epistaxis. *Postgrad Med.* 1998; 99:83–96.

Fairbanks DNF. Complications of nasal packing. *Otolarynol Head Neck Surg.* 1986;94:412–415.

Josephson GD, Godley FA, Stierna P. Practical management of epistaxis. *Med Clin North Am.* 1991;75:1311–1320.

Tan LK, Calhoun KH. Epistaxis. *Med Clin North Am.* 1999;83: 43–56.

CHAPTER 49

Foreign Bodies: Eyelid Eversion and Retraction

Yiannis L. Katsogridakis, MD, MPH

INDICATIONS

- Suspected foreign body or corneal abrasion.
- History of eye trauma or irritability in a nonverbal patient.
- Abnormal sensation or eye pain, foreign body sensation, photophobia.

CONTRAINDICATIONS

Absolute

- Penetrating trauma and globe rupture.

EQUIPMENT

- Examination gloves.
- Sterile isotonic irrigation solution (0.9% saline or lactated Ringer's). Tap water at room temperature is an acceptable alternative to prevent treatment delay.
- Topical ophthalmic anesthetic solution (proparacaine 0.5% or tetracaine 0.5%).
- Cotton-tipped swab.
- Eyelid retractor.

RISKS

- Pain or discomfort.
- Eyelid laceration.
- Contusion of the lid or globe.
- Corneal abrasion.

PEARLS AND TIPS

- Suspect an embedded eyelid foreign body when no object can be visualized and symptoms are persistent.
- If possible, do not apply a topical ophthalmic anesthetic until a foreign body is visualized or you are confident that none is present.
  - Patients can help localize a foreign body but sensation will be eliminated by the topical anesthetic.

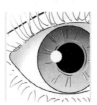
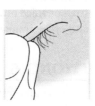

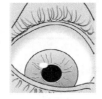
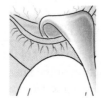

- Patient's inability to feel increases the potential for abrasions since there is no further pain or apprehension with blinking, eye movement, or rubbing.
- A smooth, uncoated metal clip can be bent to into an appropriate shape to be used as a retractor after sterilization with alcohol.
- Copious irrigation and mechanical removal of a foreign body is necessary to prevent corneal abrasions, infections, ulcerations, perforations, and metallic rust rings.

PATIENT PREPARATION

- Apply topical ophthalmic anesthetic solution after foreign body has been visualized or ruled out to decrease pain and facilitate procedure and eye examination.

PATIENT POSITIONING

- Age-appropriate positioning and restraint as necessary to complete procedure and eye examination.

ANATOMY REVIEW

- Figure 49–1 shows the anatomy of the eye.
- Eyelid margin: Junction of the internal and external portions of the eyelid where the eyelashes are located.
- Palpebral fissure: Space between the upper and lower eyelid margins when the eyelids are open.
- Medial commissure: Medial junction of upper and lower eyelids.
- Lateral commissure: Lateral junction of upper and lower eyelids.

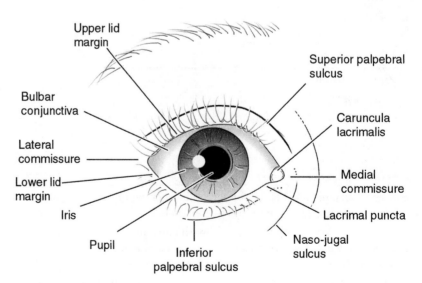

Figure 49–1. *Anatomy of eye.*

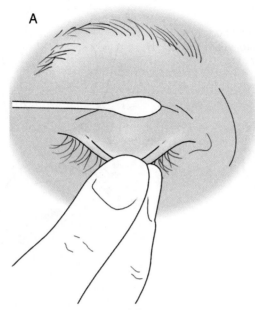
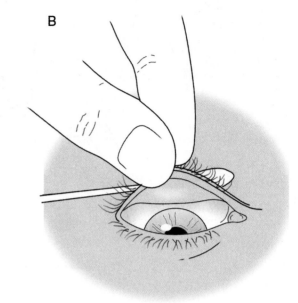

Figure 49–2. *Upper eyelid eversion.*

- Lacrimal puncta: Located on the eyelid margin before the medial commissure.
- Conjunctiva: Thin transparent membrane.
  - Palpebral conjunctiva: Covers the inner surface of the eyelid.
  - Bulbar conjunctiva: Covers the anterior portion of the eye except for the central cornea.
  - Fornix: Transition between the palpebral and bulbar conjunctiva.
- Muscles of the eyelid.
  - Orbicularis muscle: Closes the eyelids.
  - Levator muscle: Opens the eyelids.

PROCEDURE

Upper Eyelid Eversion

- Ask the patient to direct gaze downward.
- Grasp the eyelashes and distal upper eyelid between the index finger and thumb and pull downward.
- Place a cotton-tipped swab across the mid-body of the upper eyelid.
- In a single maneuver, move the swab downward and pull the eyelid upward (Figure 49–2), bending the eyelid over the swab and exposing the palpebral conjunctiva.
- After the examination is complete, instruct patient to gaze downward and gently fold the lid over the eye.

Lower Eyelid Eversion

- A single digit is used to pull the lower lid downward and back (Figure 49–3).
- Instruct the patient to gaze upward during the procedure.

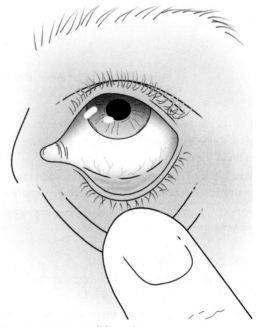

Figure 49–3. *Lower eyelid eversion.*

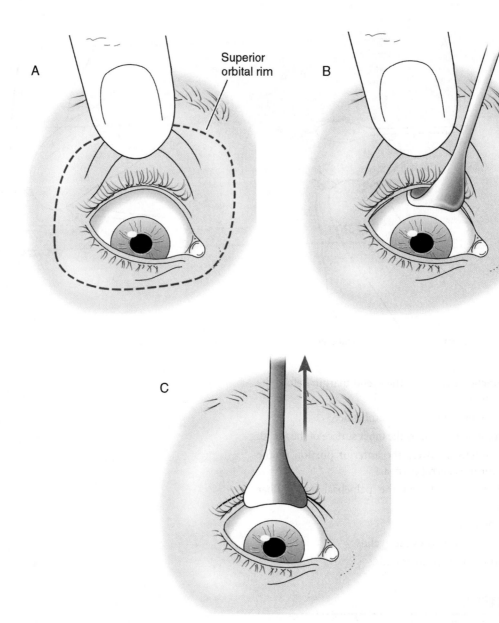

Figure 49–4. *Upper eyelid retraction.*

Upper Eyelid Retraction

- Place a single digit on the superior orbital rim and pull the skin at the eyelid upward.
- Slip the blade of the retractor under the eyelid margin and exert upward traction away from the globe (Figure 49–4).
- Downward gaze by the patient during the procedure improves success.

Lower Eyelid Retraction

- Place a single digit on the inferior orbital rim and firmly pull the skin at the eyelid downward.
- Slip the blade of the retractor under the eyelid margin and exert downward traction away from the globe (Figure 49–5).

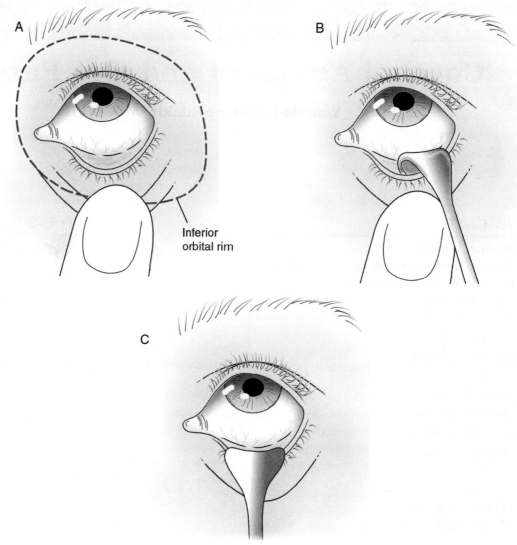

Figure 49–5. *Lower eyelid retraction.*

- Upward gaze by the patient during the procedure improves success.

FOLLOW-UP

- Immediate referral to an ophthalmologist for any penetrating foreign body or metallic foreign body with rust ring.
- Topical ophthalmic antibiotic ointment or drops for 3 days.
- If patient is asymptomatic in 24 hours, no follow-up is necessary.
- If patient is symptomatic after 24 hours, reevaluation is necessary.
- If patient is symptomatic after 48 hours, reevaluation by an ophthalmologist is needed.
- Patients who wear contact lenses should refrain from using them for 1 week.

REFERENCES

Bachur R. Minor Trauma. In: Green-Hernandez C, Singleton JK, Aronzon DZ, eds. *Primary Care Pediatrics.* Philadelphia: Lippincott Williams & Wilkins; 2001:520–521.

Carlson DW, Digiulio GA, Gewitz MH et al. Illustrated Techniques of Pediatric Emergency Procedures. In: Fleisher GR, Ludwig S, Henretig FM, Ruddy RM, Silverman BK, eds. *Textbook of Pediatric Emergency Medicine.* 4th ed. Philadelphia: Lippincott Williams & Wilkins; 2000:1822–1823.

Levin AV. Eye Trauma. In: Fleisher GR, Ludwig S, Henretig FM, Ruddy RM, Silverman BK, eds. *Textbook of Pediatric Emergency Medicine.* 4th ed. Philadelphia: Lippincott Williams & Wilkins; 2000:1397–1406.

Levin AV. General Pediatric Ophthalmologic Procedures. In: Henretig FM, King C, Joffe MD, King BR, Loiselle J, Ruddy RM, Wiley JF, eds. *Textbook of Pediatric Emergency Procedures.* Baltimore: Williams & Wilkins; 1997:579–592.

McLeod M. Eye Problems. In: Green-Hernandez C, Singleton JK, Aronzon DZ, eds. *Primary Care Pediatrics.* Philadelphia: Lippincott Williams & Wilkins; 2001:359–372.

CHAPTER 50

Corneal Abrasion and Eye Patching

Yiannis L. Katsogridakis, MD, MPH

INDICATIONS

- Suspected corneal abrasion.
- History of eye trauma, prolonged use of contact lenses, or irritability in a nonverbal patient.
- Abnormal vision.
  - Decreased visual acuity.
  - Diplopia.
- Abnormal sensation.
  - Eye pain.
  - Photophobia.
  - Foreign body sensation.
- Abnormal appearance.
  - Blepharospasm.
  - Tearing.
  - Conjunctival erythema.
  - Visible corneal defect.
  - Visible corneal foreign body.

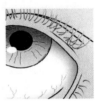

CONTRAINDICATIONS

Absolute

- Penetrating trauma with suspected globe rupture.
- Chemical burn.
- Retained contact lens.
- Hypersensitivity to fluorescein.
- Eye patching of an abrasion caused by a contact lens or a contaminated surface is contraindicated due to increased risk of infection.

Relative

- Suspected minor chemical burn.

EQUIPMENT

- Examination gloves.

- Sterile isotonic irrigation solution (0.9% saline or lactated Ringer's). Copious tap water at room temperature is an acceptable alternative to prevent treatment delay.
- Topical ophthalmic anesthetic solution (proparacaine 0.5% or tetracaine 0.5%).
- Fluorescein dye (single-dose dropper or dye-impregnated ophthalmic paper strip).
- Cobalt blue light (handheld direct ophthalmoscope or slit lamp) or ultraviolet light (Wood's lamp).
- Eye patch (occlusive or standard).

RISKS

- Hypersensitivity reaction to fluorescein.
- Permanent fluorescein staining of a contact lens.
- Iatrogenic corneal abrasion if fluorescein strip touches the eye.
- Eye patching may increase discomfort and risk of infection.

PEARLS AND TIPS

- A corneal abrasion is a simple scratch limited to the corneal epithelial surface.
- A corneal or conjunctival foreign body is irritating, and rubbing may lead to further abrasions.
- Suspect an embedded eyelid foreign body when no object can be visualized and symptoms are persistent.
- Copious irrigation and mechanical removal of a persistent foreign body is necessary to prevent further abrasions.
- If possible, do not apply a topical ophthalmic anesthetic until a foreign body is visualized or you are confident that none is present.
  - Patients can help localize a foreign body but sensation will be eliminated by the topical anesthetic.
  - Patient's inability to feel increases the potential for abrasions since there is no further pain or apprehension with blinking, eye movement, or rubbing.

PATIENT PREPARATION

- Apply topical ophthalmic anesthetic solution after foreign body has been visualized or ruled out to decrease pain and facilitate procedure and eye examination.

PATIENT POSITIONING

- Age-appropriate positioning and restraint as necessary to complete eye examination.

ANATOMY REVIEW

- Figure 50–1 shows the anatomy of the eye.

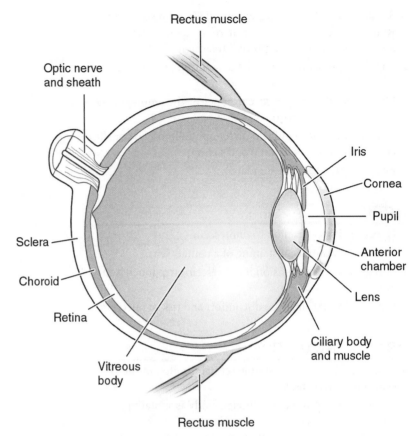

Figure 50–1. *Anatomy of eye.*

- The cornea is the transparent outermost layer that covers the iris and pupil of the eye. Cornea must remain transparent to refract light properly.
- The corneal tissue is arranged in 5 layers:
  - Epithelium: The outermost layer that contains sensory nerves and comprises about 10% of the cornea.
  - Bowman's layer: The basement membrane for epithelial cells.
  - Stroma: Provides support and is primarily composed of water and collagen and comprises about 90% of the cornea.
  - Descemet's membrane: Provides elasticity and is composed of collagen.
  - Endothelium: The thin innermost layer of the cornea.

PROCEDURE

- Moisten a fluorescein paper strip with the patient's tears (Figure 50–2), sterile isotonic solution, or topical ophthalmic anesthetic solution.
- Pull down the lower eyelid to expose the palpebral conjunctiva that lines the inner surface of the eyelid.
- Gently place a drop of fluorescein dye or a moistened strip on the palpebral conjunctiva.
- Ask the patient to close and open the eye.

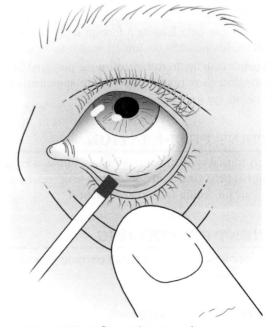

Figure 50–2. *Moisten fluorescein paper strip.*

- The solution disperses across the ocular surface with each subsequent blink.
- Evaluate the eyes for corneal or conjunctival fluorescein uptake with a cobalt blue light or an ultraviolet light.
- Secure an eye patch to the patient's face by an adhesive border or 1-inch wide medical tape.

INTERPRETATION AND MONITORING

- A corneal epithelial defect is revealed by yellow-green fluorescence of the exposed basement membrane underlying the epithelium.
- A foreign body will be surrounded by a yellow-green ring.
- Patients with a foreign body sensation or multiple abrasions require examination of the conjunctival surface of the upper and lower lids to exclude a foreign body.
- The lower lid should be pulled down and the upper lid everted.
- A teardrop or irregular pupil indicates penetration into the deeper corneal tissues.
- A positive Seidel test.
  - Rapid flow of fluorescein away from a defect indicates globe perforation with extravasation of vitreous humor.

CAVEATS

- Topical anesthetics should not be prescribed for home use.
  - Anesthetics are toxic to the corneal epithelium.
  - Repeated use impedes healing, which may result in corneal infection and ulceration.
- The efficacy of eye patching in treatment of corneal abrasions is controversial.
- Children resist eye patching.
- Possible advantages of eye patching include decreased pain in the affected eye and production of a stable corneal environment that promotes migration and proliferation of epithelial cells.
- Possible disadvantages of eye patching include decreased corneal oxygenation and increased local temperature, which may delay healing and increase risk of infection.
- Current studies suggest that eye patching is not beneficial in the treatment of corneal abrasions compared with topical antibiotic alone.
  - There is no reported difference in rate of healing, degree of discomfort, interference in activities of daily living, or complications.

- Eye patching impairs binocular vision and reduces the visual field.

FOLLOW-UP

- Corneal abrasions usually heal in 24–48 hours.
- Topical ophthalmic antibiotic ointment or drops for 3 days.
- If patient is asymptomatic in 24 hours, no follow-up is necessary.
- If patient is symptomatic after 24 hours or if the abrasion was large or centrally located, reevaluate the patient for improvement.
- If patient shows no improvement after 48 hours, an ophthalmologist should reevaluate the patient.
- Patients who wear contact lenses should refrain from using them for 1 week and be evaluated by an ophthalmologist.

REFERENCES

Arbour JD, Brunette I, Boisjoly HM, Shi ZH, Dumas J, Guertin MC. Should we patch corneal erosions? *Arch Ophthalmol.* 1997;115:313–317.

Bachur R. Minor Trauma. In: Green-Hernandez C, Singleton JK, Aronzon DZ, eds. *Primary Care Pediatrics.* Philadelphia: Lippincott Williams & Wilkins; 2001:520–521.

Eye Disorders. In: *Diseases.* 3rd ed. Springhouse, PA: Lippincott Williams & Wilkins; 2001:1135–1150.

Flynn CA, D'Amico F, Smith G. Should we patch corneal abrasions? A meta-analysis. *J Fam Pract.* 1998;47:264–270.

Horton JC. Disorders of the Eye. In: Kasper DL, Fauci AS, Longo DL et al, eds. *Harrison's Principles of Internal Medicine.* 16th ed. New York: McGraw-Hill; 2005:165.

Le Sage N, Verreault R, Rochette L. Efficacy of eye patching for traumatic corneal abrasions: a controlled clinical trial. *Ann Emerg Med.* 2001;38:129–134.

Levin AV. Eye Trauma. In: Fleisher GR, Ludwig S, Henretig FM, Ruddy RM, Silverman BK, eds. *Textbook of Pediatric Emergency Medicine.* 4th ed. Philadelphia: Lippincott Williams & Wilkins; 2000:1397–1406.

McLeod M. Eye Problems. In: Green-Hernandez C, Singleton JK, Aronzon DZ, eds. *Primary Care Pediatrics.* Philadelphia: Lippincott Williams & Wilkins; 2001:359–372.

Michael JG, Hug D, Dowd MD. Management of corneal abrasion in children: a randomized clinical trial. *Ann Emerg Med.* 2002;40:67–72.

Rittichier KK, Roback MG, Bassett KE. Are signs and symptoms associated with persistent corneal abrasions in children? *Arch Pediatr Adolesc Med.* 2000;154:370–374.

CHAPTER 51

Vision Screening

Sharon M. Unti, MD

INDICATIONS

- All newborn infants and all children at subsequent well-child health supervision visits.
- All premature infants.
- Children with significant developmental delay or neurologic disorders.
- Children with systemic disease associated with eye abnormalities.
- All children with a family history of congenital cataracts, retinoblastoma, and metabolic or genetic diseases.

CONTRAINDICATIONS

Relative
- Costs associated with the further evaluation of children with false-positive screening results.

EQUIPMENT

Vision Assessment (Newborn to age 3 years)
- Any object to assess ability to fix and follow.

Visual Acuity (Age 3 years and older)
- Picture tests, such as Allen cards or LEA symbols (flash cards with figures or symbols), are suggested for children 3–4 years of age.
- Tumbling E test (which involves matching the orientation of the legs of the letter E with the child's fingers) or HOTV test (which involves matching the letters H, O, T, V on a wall chart with the correct letter on a testing board) is suggested for children ages 3–5 years.
- Snellen acuity chart (using Snellen letters or numbers) is suggested for children 6 years of age and older.
- Occluders are used to obtain complete coverage of the untested eye.

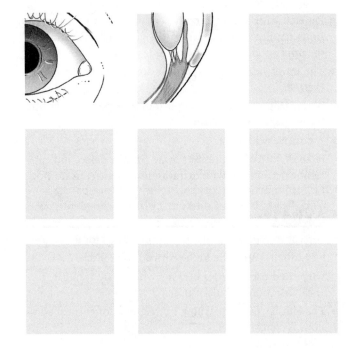

- Depends on age and what is being assessed.

External Inspection of the Eyes and Lids

- Penlight.

Ocular Alignment

- Cross cover test uses any object to focus on and an occluder.
- Random dot E stereo test uses raised and recessed E cards.
- Titmus test uses objects printed on material polarized at 90 degrees and polarized filter spectacles.
- Simultaneous red reflex test (Bruckner test) uses direct ophthalmoscope.

Ocular Media Clarity

- Red reflex uses direct ophthalmoscope.

PEARLS AND TIPS

- When testing visual acuity, the test requiring the highest level of cognitive function that the child is capable of performing should be used.
- Children who wear eyeglasses should have their visual acuity tested while wearing the eyeglasses.
- It is recommended that visual acuity be tested using commercially available occluders that provide complete occlusion rather than cardboard or paddle occluders, which can allow for peeking.
- When testing visual acuity, tests that use a line of figures are preferred over tests using single figures.

PATIENT PREPARATION

- The child should be examined while in good health.
- The child should be comfortable; for younger children this may require that the child be sitting on a parent's or guardian's lap.
- Keep distractions to a minimum.

PATIENT POSITIONING

- The child should be visually fixing on an object, particularly when assessing ocular alignment.
- When measuring visual acuity, it is imperative that the child be 10 feet away from the testing equipment.

ANATOMY REVIEW

- Figure 51–1 shows the anatomy of the eye.
- Adnexa: Examine tissues surrounding the eyes and orbit.
- Orbit: Check for proptosis, orbital position, and bony abnormalities.

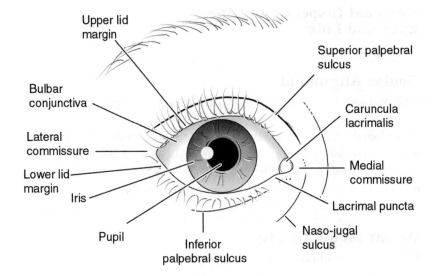

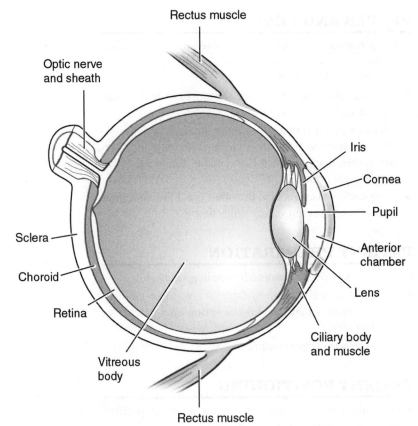

Figure 51–1. *Anatomy of the eye.*

- Lids: Examine contour, position, ptosis, retractor, epicanthus, and possible inflammation.
- Lashes: Examine for missing lashes.
- Lacrimal duct and tears: Examine for inflammation or deficient tearing.
- Conjunctiva: Examine for inflammation, discharge, foreign bodies, or masses.

- Cornea: Examine for clarity.
- Anterior chamber: Examine for clarity.
- Iris: Examine papillary margins and check for masses.

PROCEDURE

Ocular History

- Do you have any concerns about your child's ability to see?
- Does your child seem to hold objects too close to his or her face?
- Do your child's eyes always appear to be straight?
- Do your child's eyelids droop?
- Do your child's eyelids appear to be symmetric?
- Have your child's eyes ever been injured?
- Do you have any concerns about your child's eyes?
- Obtain family history regarding eye disorders.

Vision Assessment (Newborn to age 3 years)

- Determine whether each eye can fix on an object, maintain fixation, and then follow the object in different gaze directions.
- Assess each eye independently and both eyes together.

Visual Acuity Measurement (3 years of age and older)

- *For acuity charts,* such as the Snellen, tumbling E, or HOTV test, the child should be standing 10 feet from the chart.
- Test 1 eye at a time using an occluder, and instruct the child to keep both eyes open during testing. If the child wears eyeglasses, the child should be tested with them on.
- Ask the child to read the practice line. If the child fails, move up to the next larger line. Continue moving up the chart until a line is identified that the child can read.
- Then move down the chart until the child fails to read a line.
- To pass a line, the child must identify at least 4 of the 6 symbols on the line correctly.
- *For card tests,* such as the Allen cards, it is important that the child is able to identify verbally or correctly match all the figures on the cards. Testing is done with both of the child's eyes open.
- Present cards and ask the child to identify the figures.
- Continue to walk backward 2 feet at a time while presenting different cards.
- When the child cannot correctly identify the figures, move forward to confirm the farthest distance at which the child is able to identify figures accurately.

External Examination

- Using a penlight, directly examine the eyelids, conjunctiva, sclera, cornea, and iris.

Ocular Motility Assessment

- *For the cross cover test,* ask the child to look straight ahead and focus on an object 10 feet away.
- Cover 1 eye with an occluder and immediately look for movement of the uncovered eye.
- Now cover the other eye, checking for movement of the uncovered eye.
- If there is no apparent movement of either eye, move the occluder back and forth between the 2 eyes, waiting about 1–2 seconds between movements.
- *For the tests measuring stereopsis* (random dot E or Titmus), hold the cards or booklet 16 inches from the child's eyes and explain the test to the child.
- Place the stereo glasses on the child and be certain that the child is looking straight ahead. If the child wears eyeglasses, place the stereo glasses over the child's eyeglasses.
- In the case of the random E test, hold both cards (the blank card and the raised or recessed E card) straight in order to avoid darkness and glare.
  - Ask the child to look at both cards and point to the card with the E.
  - Repeat 6 times, switching the E card randomly from side to side.
  - To pass the test, the child must correctly identify the E card at least 4 out of 6 times.

Pupil Examination

- Using a penlight, examine each pupil looking for any asymmetry of pupil size, shape, or color.
- Assess each pupil for reactivity to light.

Red Reflex Examination

- The examination room should be darkened to maximize dilation of the pupils.
- Using a direct ophthalmoscope, focus on 1 pupil at a distance 12–18 inches away from the eye and assess the color of the reflex.
- Repeat the examination on the other pupil.
- Now view the red reflex in both eyes simultaneously (Bruckner test) from a distance of 3 feet away. The red reflexes should be equal in size, color, and brightness.

Ophthalmoscopy

- Ask the child to fixate on an object.
- Use the ophthalmoscope to examine the optic disc, retinal vasculature, and macula.

INTERPRETATION

Vision Assessment

- In a cooperating child, failure to fix and follow objects indicates significant visual impairment.
- If failure is found in 1 eye or in both eyes, referral for a more formal vision assessment is advised.

Visual Acuity Measurement

- *For acuity charts,* the child's vision is determined based on the chart line that they passed (correctly identified at least 4 out of 6 symbols). For example, if a child correctly reads the 10/20 line, then the child's vision is 10/20 or 20/40.
- *For card tests,* the furthest distance where the child can correctly identify figures is the numerator; the denominator is 30. For example, if the child correctly identified figures on the cards at 15 feet, then the child's vision is 15/30 or 30/60 or 20/40.

External Examination

- Increased discharge or persistent tearing may be secondary to infection, allergy, blocked lacrimal duct, or glaucoma.
- The presence of cloudy or asymmetrically enlarged corneas may be secondary to congenital glaucoma.
- Findings of ptosis require further evaluation and referral. Unilateral ptosis can lead to amblyopia, and bilateral ptosis may be associated with other disease processes, such as myasthenia.

Ocular Motility Assessment

- Abnormalities that may be noted include strabismus and nystagmus. These can represent significant eye or neurologic disorders and require referral.

Pupil Examination

- Slow or poorly reactive pupils can suggest retinal or optic nerve dysfunction.
- Asymmetric pupil size (usually > 1 mm) can indicate a sympathetic (eg, Horner syndrome) or parasympathetic (eg, third nerve palsy) disorder.

Red Reflex Examination

- Opacity noted in 1 eye can suggest a cataract, corneal abnormality, retinoblastoma, or retinal detachment, depending on the location of the opacity.
- When viewing both eyes, any asymmetry in color, brightness, or size may indicate an amblyogenic condition, such as strabismus.
- The child with an abnormal red reflex examination should be referred to an ophthalmologist.

FOLLOW-UP

- Parents or caretakers should be notified of all examination and testing results, including clear instructions for follow-up care and referrals.
- Any child who fails a vision screening or is found to have an abnormality should be referred to an ophthalmologist experienced in the care of children.
- Any child who is unable to be tested after 2 attempts should be referred to an ophthalmologist experienced in the care of children.

REFERENCES

Committee on Practice and Ambulatory Medicine, and Section on Ophthalmology. Eye examination in infants, children, and young adults by pediatricians. *Pediatrics.* 2003; 111(4Pt1):902–907.

Curnyn KM, Kaufman LM. The eye examination in the pediatrician's office. *Pediatr Clin North Am.* 2003;50:25–40.

Friedman LS, Kaufman LM. Guidelines for pediatrician referrals to the ophthalmologist. *Pediatr Clin North Am.* 2003;50:41–53.

Robbins SL, Christian WK, Hertle RW, Granet DB. Vision testing in the pediatric population. *Ophthalmol Clin North Am.* 2003;16:253–267.

CHAPTER 52

Hearing Screening

Thomas Valvano, MD and Kimberley Dilley, MD, MPH

INDICATIONS

- Conductive hearing loss results from an obstruction of the air conduction pathway in the outer or middle ear.

- Sensorineural hearing loss results from a defect in the cochlea or auditory nerve.

- Both forms of hearing loss may be congenital or acquired.

- The American Academy of Pediatrics recommends universal newborn hearing screening (UNHS) for all infants for the following reasons:

  - Hearing loss in infants is not readily detectable by routine clinical observation.

  - Screening programs based on the presence of risk factors or family history will miss up to 50% of children with hearing loss because these children lack identifiable risk factors.

  - Infants identified before age 6 months demonstrate better language development than those identified later.

- Screening should be completed during the hospital birth admission; before discharge from the neonatal intensive care unit; or for alternative birth locations, such as home births before 1 month of age.

- When UNHS is not available, infants with the following risk factors should be screened before 1 month of age:

  - Stay in neonatal intensive care unit of 48 hours or more.

  - Stigmata or other findings associated with syndrome known to include hearing loss.

  - Family history of permanent childhood hearing loss.

  - Craniofacial anomalies, including abnormalities of the pinna and ear canal.

  - In utero infections associated with hearing loss, including cytomegalovirus (CMV), herpes, toxoplasmosis, or rubella.

- Children with the following risk factors for progressive or delayed-onset hearing loss should be tested every 6 months until at least 3 years of age, even if they passed the newborn screening:

  - Parental or caregiver concern regarding hearing, speech, language, or developmental delay.

  - Family history of permanent childhood hearing loss.

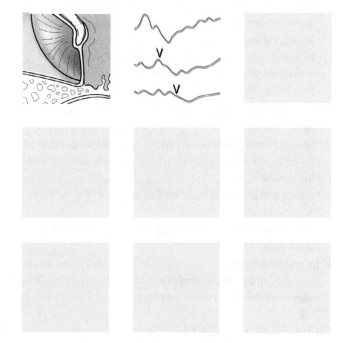

- Stigmata or other findings associated with a syndrome known to include hearing loss or eustachian tube dysfunction.
- Postnatal infections associated with hearing loss, including bacterial meningitis.
- In utero infections, such as CMV, herpes, toxoplasmosis, rubella, and syphilis.
- Neonatal indicators including hyperbilirubinemia requiring exchange transfusion, persistent pulmonary hypertension of the newborn associated with mechanical ventilation, and conditions requiring extracorporeal membrane oxygenation (ECMO).
- Syndromes associated with progressive hearing loss, such as neurofibromatosis, osteopetrosis, and Usher syndrome.
- Neurodegenerative disorders, such as Hunter syndrome, or sensorimotor neuropathies, such as Friedreich ataxia and Charcot-Marie-Tooth disease.
- Head trauma.
- Recurrent or persistent otitis media with effusion for at least 3 months.

■ The American Academy of Pediatrics recommends that all children receive hearing screening at their annual well-child visits:
- Age-appropriate objective testing at ages 4, 5, 6, 8, 10, 12, 15, and 18 years of age.
- Subjective evaluation by history at all other annual well-child visits.

■ In addition to otoacoustic emissions, auditory brainstem response, and conventional pure tone audiometry, audiologists may use behavioral assessments.

CONTRAINDICATIONS

Relative

■ Wax in the ear canal may interfere with otoacoustic emissions.

ANATOMY REVIEW

■ The external ear includes the external acoustic meatus to the tympanic membrane.
■ The middle ear includes the tympanic cavity and ossicles (Figure 52–1).
■ The inner ear includes the semicircular canals, vestibule, and cochlea.
■ The hair cells are located in the spiral organ within the cochlea and connect to nerve fibers of the cochlear nerve.

OTOACOUSTIC EMISSIONS (OAE)

PEARLS AND TIPS

■ Indirectly measures hearing by measuring hair cell function of cochlea.

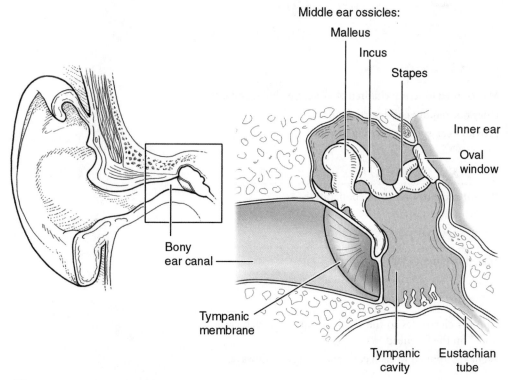

Figure 52-1. *Anatomy of the ear.*

- May be used to screen children of all ages, including infants.
- Does not require child participation.
- Can isolate hearing loss to specific ear.

PATIENT PREPARATION

- Patient must be quiet and cooperative because noise from the surroundings or from the child will affect reliability.

PATIENT POSITIONING

- Seated in parent's lap.

PROCEDURE

- Place probe containing a microphone in the ear.
- Tone from probe stimulates hair cells in cochlea to emit sound that is picked up by microphone.

INTERPRETATION

- Presence of sound indicates normally functioning cochlea and middle ear.

CAVEATS

- Presence of middle ear fluid may interfere with test.
- Does not measure degree of hearing loss.

AUDITORY BRAINSTEM RESPONSE (ABR)

PEARLS AND TIPS

- May be used to screen children of all ages, including infants.
- Does not require child participation.
- Provides ear-specific hearing thresholds.

PATIENT PREPARATION

- Patient must be quiet and cooperative.

PATIENT POSITIONING

- Seated in parent's lap.

PROCEDURE

- Apply 4 electrodes to the child's scalp: 1 on each earlobe and 2 on the forehead.
- A click is applied to each ear, generating a brainwave.

INTERPRETATION

- Brainwave has 7 identifiable and reproducible waveforms. Wave V is the largest and most identifiable.
- Wave V diminishes as the intensity of the click is decreased (Figure 52–2).
- The hearing threshold is reached at the level when Wave V is no longer identifiable.

CAVEATS

- Child must lie quietly to avoid muscle movements, which interfere with test.
- Sedation is often required.

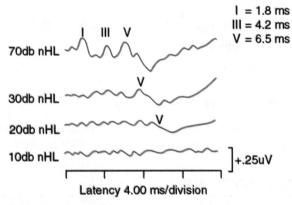

Figure 52–2. *Sample auditory brainstem responses illustrating diminishing waveforms at decreasing decibel levels.*

CONVENTIONAL PURE TONE AUDIOMETRY

PEARLS AND TIPS

- Child must be 5 years of age or older.
- Ear-specific results can be obtained.
- Speech recognition threshold (the lowest intensity at which a 2-syllable word can be repeated) can be tested.

PATIENT POSITIONING

- Seated in a quiet room with earphones on.

PROCEDURE

- Tone is presented through earphones.
- Child raises hand in response to auditory stimuli.

FOLLOW-UP

- Refer to an audiologist for additional testing when any of the following is present:
  - Failed screen in either ear.
  - Risk factors for progressive or delayed-onset hearing loss (these children should be tested every 3 months until age 3).
  - Parental concern regarding hearing, speech, or language delay.

———————[■■■]———————

BEHAVIORAL ASSESSMENTS

- Behavioral Observation Audiometry
  - May be used in infants younger than 6 months of age.
  - A speaker or noisemaker is placed on each side of infant.
  - Behavioral changes, including eye blinking, startle response, head turning, and cessation of movement, are observed in response to auditory stimulation.
  - Can rule out severe or profound hearing loss but may miss mild or moderate hearing loss.
- Visual Reinforcement Audiometry
  - May be used in children 6 months to 3 years of age.
  - Child is seated between 2 speakers.
  - When child turns toward the sound from 1 of the speakers, an animated or illuminated toy appears on that side to reinforce the child's behavior.
  - The intensity of the stimulus is progressively lowered to determine the child's minimum response level.
  - Cannot determine ear-specific thresholds.
  - May not detect unilateral hearing loss.
- Conditioned Play Audiometry
  - May be used in children ages 3–5 years.
  - Child is taught to perform a fun task in response to an auditory stimulus, such as placing a block in a bucket.
  - Stimuli are presented through earphones so that ear-specific results can be obtained.

REFERENCES

American Academy of Pediatrics. Year 2000 Position Statement: Principles and guidelines for early hearing detection and intervention programs. *Pediatrics.* 2000;106:798–817.

American Academy of Pediatrics Committee on Practice and Ambulatory Medicine and the Section on Otolaryngology and Bronchoesophagology. Hearing assessment in infants and children: recommendations beyond neonatal screening. *Pediatrics.* 2003;111:436–440.

Applebaum EL. Detection of hearing loss in children. *Pediatr Ann.* 1999;28:351–356.

Elden LM, Potsic WP. Screening and prevention of hearing loss in children. *Curr Opin Pediatr.* 2002;14:723–730.

Folsom RC, Diefendorf AO. Physiologic and behavioral approaches to pediatric hearing assessment. *Pediatr Clin North Am.* 1999;46:107–120.

Gregg RB, Wiorek LS, Arvedson JC. Pediatric audiology. *Pediatr Rev.* 2004;25:224–234.

Stockard-Pope JE. Auditory development and hearing evaluation in children. *Adv Pediatr.* 2001;48:273–299.

[CHAPTER 53]

Reduction and Splinting Techniques

Bradley Dunlap, MD and John F. Sarwark, MD

SHOULDER REDUCTION

INDICATIONS

- Any dislocated shoulder (ie, the humeral head is not in concentric relationship within the glenoid fossa).

CONTRAINDICATIONS

- Any associated fracture. Patients with fractures should be evaluated by an orthopedic surgeon before a reduction maneuver is performed.

EQUIPMENT

- Medications for muscle relaxation and an appropriate level of conscious sedation.
- A bed sheet.
- An assistant to perform countertraction.

RISKS

- Inability to reduce the shoulder.
- Additional damage to the humeral head, glenoid, or labrum during the reduction maneuver.
- Traction injury to the brachial plexus and especially the axillary nerve (rare).

PEARLS AND TIPS

- An adequate level of conscious sedation is critical. The patient must have muscle relaxation and should not be "fighting" the reduction maneuver.
- Do not let go once traction is applied to the arm.
- Continuous traction helps relax the muscles that may be holding the humeral head out of the glenoid fossa in a shortened position.
- Perform and document a neurovascular examination both before attempting reduction and after the reduction.

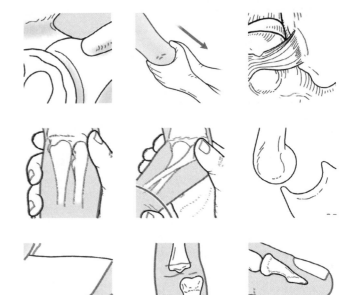

- An anterior shoulder dislocation is most common. The patient holds the arm in abduction and external rotation.
- Obtain radiographs, including an axillary view, to detect possible fracture before any reduction maneuvers.

PATIENT PREPARATION

■ A bed sheet is placed around the patient's chest.

PATIENT POSITIONING

■ Lying supine on the table.

ANATOMY REVIEW

■ The shoulder joint consists of the humeral head, which articulates with the glenoid of the scapula (Figure 53–1).

■ Although a cartilaginous labrum on the glenoid helps provide additional stability, it is an inherently unstable joint.

PROCEDURE

■ After sedation and muscle relaxation, an assistant provides countertraction while the physician holds the arm at the elbow and applies traction by pulling the arm in a longitudinal direction (Figure 53–2).

■ Slight internal and external rotation of the shoulder is used and usually a "clunk" is felt as the humeral head eases into the glenoid and the shoulder reduces.

INTERPRETATION AND MONITORING

■ Obtain radiographs (2 views) to confirm the reduction.

■ The patient is placed in a shoulder immobilizer.

■ If an immobilizer is not available, a sling with an elastic bandage wrap holding the arm to the torso can be substituted.

COMPLICATIONS

■ Recurrent shoulder instability.
  • This is related to the age at which the patient has the dislocation.
  • Recurrence rates of up to 70% have been reported in patients younger than 22 years.

■ Neurologic injury, which often results from traction injuries and generally resolves over weeks to months.

■ Fracture.

FOLLOW-UP

■ Reevaluate the patient in 5–7 days.

REDUCTION OF NURSEMAID'S ELBOW

INDICATIONS

■ Clinical evidence of radial head subluxation.

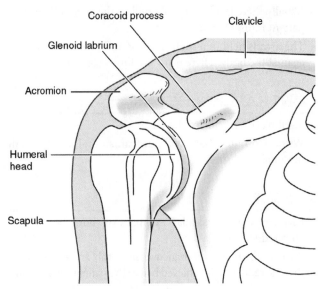

Figure 53–1. *Anatomy of shoulder.*

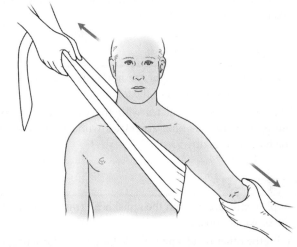

Figure 53–2. *Applying traction to shoulder.*

■ Nursemaid's elbow, or radial head subluxation, usually occurs in children ages 2–5 and results from longitudinal traction on an extended elbow. This allows the radial head to slip through the annular ligament of the elbow.

■ The child holds the forearm in pronation and does not allow any supination because of pain.

■ Usually there is a history of a pull to the arm, followed by patient refusal to use the arm.
■ The arm is held in a slightly flexed and pronated position against the body. There is no swelling or bruising.

CONTRAINDICATIONS

■ Swelling or bruising of the arm.
■ Witnessed injury (fall) with mechanism unlikely to result in radial head subluxation.

PEARLS AND TIPS

■ Perform a neurovascular examination both before and after reduction.
■ Perform the reduction maneuver smoothly and decisively so that the reduction is achieved before the patient senses pain.

PATIENT POSITIONING

■ Sitting on the cart next to the caretaker or in the caretaker's lap.

ANATOMY REVIEW

■ The elbow joint consists of the humerus that articulates with the radius and ulna of the forearm.
■ The radial head articulates with the capitellum of the humerus, while the ulna articulates with the trochlea of the humerus (Figure 53–3).

PROCEDURE

■ Apply gentle pressure on the radial head (the hand cradles the proximal forearm).
■ With the other hand, apply gentle longitudinal traction to the distal forearm, supinate, and flex the arm at the elbow (Figure 53–4A).
■ A click or pop is felt as the radial head becomes repositioned under the annular ligament.
■ Alternate procedure.
  · The affected arm is held at the elbow with 1 hand.
  · The second hand is used to grasp the wrist and hyperpronate (Figure 53–4B).

MONITORING

■ Once the reduction is complete, the child slowly begins to use the arm since it is no longer painful.
■ Full painless pronation and supination of the forearm as well as flexion and extension indicate that reduction has been successful.
■ No immobilization is necessary.

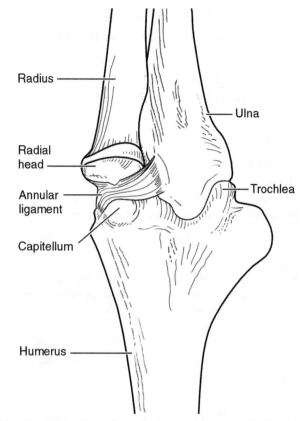

Figure 53–3. *Trapped annular ligament (nursemaid's elbow).*

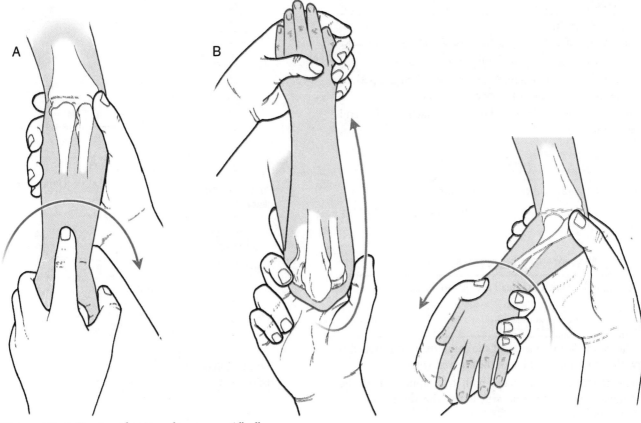

Figure 53–4. *Two procedures to reduce nursemaid's elbow.*

COMPLICATIONS

- Neurovascular injury to the arm resulting from manipulation of an unsuspected fracture.

REDUCTION OF ELBOW DISLOCATION

INDICATIONS

- Elbow dislocation, which is often obvious on radiographs.
- Subtle abnormalities include failure of the radial head to align with the capitellum of the humerus on any radiographic view of the elbow.

CONTRAINDICATIONS

Absolute

- Any associated fracture, which should prompt an evaluation by an orthopedic surgeon before reduction attempt.

EQUIPMENT

- Equipment and medications used for conscious sedation.

- True elbow dislocations involve both the ulna and the radius and are classified according to the position of the forearm relative to the humerus (posterior, medial, lateral, anterior).
- The posterior elbow dislocation is most common.
- Elbow dislocation in children younger than 10 years is rare.

RISKS

- Failed reduction.
  - Rarely, the elbow is unable to be reduced by closed methods because of interposed soft tissue.
  - If closed reduction cannot be achieved, then the patient should have an open operative reduction.
- Injury to the cartilage or bone resulting from forceful manipulation.

PEARLS AND TIPS

- Carefully review radiographs for fractures.
- Perform a neurovascular examination before and after the reduction.

PATIENT POSITIONING

- Sitting in bed with the head at a 30- to 45-degree angle.

ANATOMY REVIEW

- The elbow joint consists of the humerus that articulates with the radius and ulna of the forearm (Figure 53–5).
- The radial head articulates with the capitellum of the humerus, while the ulna articulates with the trochlea of the humerus.

PROCEDURE

- An assistant is needed to hold the humerus steady.
- The joint is first aligned in the medial/lateral plane, then traction is applied for the final reduction (Figure 53–6).
- The reduction is usually felt as it occurs.

MONITORING

- Place the arm in a long-arm posterior mold splint because the elbow can be quite unstable, especially in extension.
- Obtain radiographs to confirm reduction.

COMPLICATIONS

- Neurovascular injury.
- Elbow stiffness. While loss of motion is common after an elbow dislocation, it is generally less of an issue in children (when compared with adults).
- Recurrent elbow instability.

FOLLOW-UP

- Reevaluate the patient in 5–7 days, and the initial examiner should inform the follow-up physician about the degree of instability of the elbow.

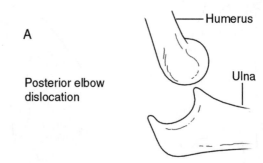

A

Posterior elbow dislocation

Humerus

Ulna

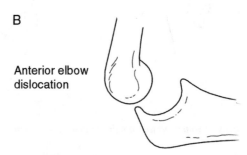

B

Anterior elbow dislocation

Figure 53–5. *Elbow dislocation.*

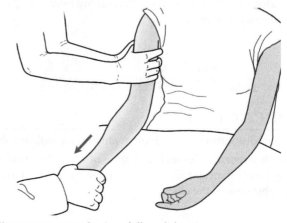

Figure 53–6. *Reduction of elbow dislocation.*

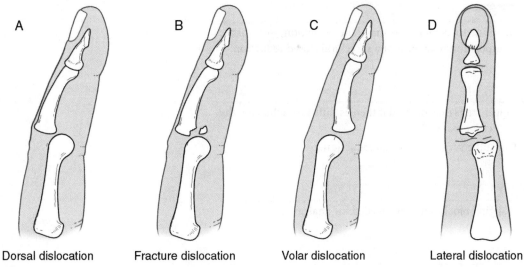

Dorsal dislocation   Fracture dislocation   Volar dislocation   Lateral dislocation

Figure 53–7. *Anatomy of finger.*

REDUCTION OF FINGER DISLOCATIONS

INDICATIONS

■ Dislocation of the PIP or DIP joints.

- Most commonly occur in a dorsal direction (the distal portion is dorsal to the proximal portion) (Figure 53–8).
- PIP or DIP dislocations may have associated intra-articular fractures.

■ Large fragments (> 30%) of the articular surface may result in instability with attempted reduction maneuvers.

CONTRAINDICATIONS

Relative

■ Open dislocations.

- The protrusion of bone through the skin should prompt a surgical evaluation.
- These should be reduced after the joint has been irrigated and gross debris has been removed.

EQUIPMENT

■ Plain lidocaine (no epinephrine) to perform digital block.

■ 10-mL syringe.

■ 18-gauge needle to draw medicine; 25 to 27 gauge to inject.

■ Splinting materials.

■ Common hand injuries usually occur at the proximal interphalangeal joint (PIP) or the distal interphalangeal joint (DIP) (Figure 53–7).

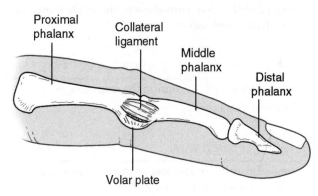

Figure 53–8. *Direction of dislocation.*

RISKS

■ Inability to achieve or maintain reduction; soft tissue interposition may prevent a successful closed reduction.

PEARLS AND TIPS

■ Finger traps may be used if there is difficulty achieving the reduction manually.

■ Consult a surgeon for open reduction.

PATIENT PREPARATION

■ A digital block is usually needed for analgesia.

PATIENT POSITIONING

■ A comfortable position.

ANATOMY REVIEW

■ The finger consists of 3 phalanges: the proximal, middle, and distal.

■ Collateral ligaments limit side-to-side movement, while the volar plate supports the volar joint.

PROCEDURE

■ Apply gentle traction to the distal digit so that the involved phalanx can clear the condyles of the more proximal phalanx and reduce (Figure 53–9).

INTERPRETATION AND MONITORING

■ Obtain radiographs to confirm the reduction.

■ Place finger in a splint.

COMPLICATIONS

■ Long-term stiffness and loss of motion can occur if the finger is immobilized too long.

FOLLOW-UP

■ Orthopedic referral is recommended. This should be arranged within 7–10 days so that early motion, if appropriate, can be instituted.

CAVEATS

■ Reduce simple dislocations promptly so that there is no undue stretch on the surrounding soft tissues and neurovascular structures.

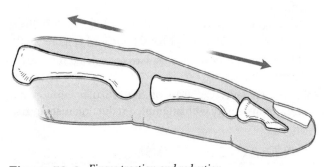

Figure 53–9. *Finger traction and reduction.*

■ Fracture dislocations are more complex but may need to be reduced by a primary care clinician if there is neurovascular compromise.

SPLINTING

INDICATIONS

■ Any fracture or dislocation of an extremity requiring stabilization.

EQUIPMENT

■ Cast padding (cotton bandage or stockinette, or both).
■ Splint material (plaster or fiberglass).
■ Water bucket.
■ Lukewarm water.
■ Elastic wrap.

RISKS

■ Skin necrosis from pressure applied by the splint.

PEARLS AND TIPS

■ Be careful not to cause a burn to a patient by using water that is too hot. In addition, the plaster gives off heat while it sets.
■ Use cast padding liberally. Be sure that all bony prominences are well padded to prevent pressure injury.
■ Do not apply the elastic wrap too tightly because it can have a tourniquet effect.

PATIENT POSITIONING

■ The patient should be comfortable with the affected extremity easily accessible.
■ The extremity should be positioned as appropriate. (For most joints this is a neutral position.)

PROCEDURE

■ Wrap the extremity circumferentially with cast padding (this is cotton and is generally not strong enough to cause a compartment syndrome).
■ Usually 10 strips of plaster are used to make the splint.
  • Measure the length of the plaster needed while it is dry, and then cut appropriately.
  • The width depends on the extremity. Choose a width that allows for coverage of approximately half of the circumference of the affected extremity.

■ Splinting is performed to provide stabilization and reduce further injury to an injured extremity.
■ Because a splint is not circumferential (unlike a cast), it can accommodate swelling with less chance of compartment syndrome developing.
■ Splinting is preferred in acute injuries when there is soft-tissue edema.

■ **Note:** Prefabricated splinting materials are available as an "all-in-one" package, but the principles remain the same.

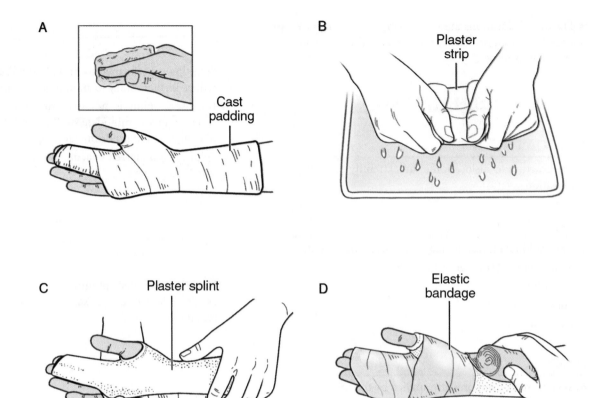

A

Cast padding

B

Plaster strip

C

Plaster splint

D

Elastic bandage

Figure 53–10. *Layers of splint.*

- Dunk the plaster in the water and squeeze out the excess.
- The plaster can also be milked to remove more water so that it is moist but not dripping.
- Place the plaster splint over the padded extremity.
- An additional layer of cast padding is placed to hold the plaster, and to prevent the elastic wrap from sticking to the plaster.
- An elastic wrap is used over the top to hold the splint in place (Figure 53–10).
- Mold the splint into the position desired and allow it to harden.

COMPLICATIONS

- Pressure sores; skin necrosis.
- Reduction of joint function or contractures.

FOLLOW-UP

- Patient should be seen 3–7 days after the splint is placed.
- The primary injury dictates definitive care.

REFERENCES

Beaty JH, Kasser JR, eds. *Rockwood & Wilkins' Fractures in Children.* 5th ed. Philadelphia: Lippincott Williams & Wilkins; 2001.

Cohen MS, Hastings H 2nd. Acute elbow dislocation: evaluation and management. *J Am Acad Orthop Surg.* 1998;6:15–23.

Kang R, Stern PJ. Fracture dislocations of the proximal interphalangeal joint. *J Am Soc Surg Hand.* 2002;2:47–60.

Macias CG, Bothner J, Wiebe R. A comparison of supination/flexion to hyperpronation in the reduction of radial head subluxations. *Pediatrics.* 1998;102:e10.

Walton J, Paxinos A, Tzannes A, Callanan M, Hayes K, Murrell GA. The unstable shoulder in the adolescent athlete. *Am J Sports Med.* 2002;30:758–767.

CHAPTER 54

Arthrocentesis

Bradley Dunlap, MD and John F. Sarwark, MD

INDICATIONS

- Diagnostic: Sampling of fluid for laboratory evaluation (eg, septic joint, inflammatory arthritis).
- Therapeutic.
  - Injection of corticosteroids.
  - Injection of local anesthetic.
  - Removal of hemarthrosis for pain relief following trauma.

CONTRAINDICATIONS

Absolute

- Skin or soft tissue infection (eg, cellulitis, septic bursitis) because there is an increased risk of causing a septic joint.
- Corticosteroid injection into a known or suspected septic joint.

Relative

- Coagulopathy. The procedure may result in hemarthrosis, but one needs to weigh the risk against the need to diagnose a septic joint.
- Bacteremia, because of the increased risk of causing septic joint.

EQUIPMENT

- Syringes (20 mL for knee; 10 mL for ankle).
- 21–25-gauge needles; they must be long enough to enter joint.
- Sterile collection container.
- Povidone-iodine and alcohol for sterile preparation of skin.
- Sterile gloves.
- 4 × 4 gauze.
- Ethyl chloride (optional).
- Lidocaine (optional).

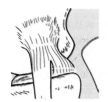
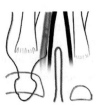

RISKS

- Infection occurs in < 1/10,000 when performed under sterile conditions.
- Bleeding into joint is exceedingly rare, even in patients who are taking anticoagulant medication.
- If corticosteroids are being injected, there is a risk of skin discoloration and fat atrophy following the procedure.

PEARLS AND TIPS

- Do not make an ink mark directly over injection/aspiration site because it will enter the joint when the needle passes through it.
- Instead, use the wood end of a sterile cotton swab or another round object to make an indentation in the skin prior to cleaning with povidone-iodine.
- If infection is a concern, a larger bore needle (18 gauge or 19 gauge) may be needed to aspirate because sometimes purulent fluid will not be drawn into a smaller needle.
- Do not overtighten the needle on to the syringe, and check to make sure the needle easily twists off the syringe before starting the procedure.
- This allows you to empty a full syringe and reattach it without ever pulling the needle out of the joint.
- Lidocaine can be used to numb the skin prior to aspiration/injection, but it can distort anatomic landmarks.
- Alternatively, a topical agent such as ethyl chloride can be used.

ARTHROCENTESIS OF THE KNEE

PATIENT POSITIONING

- Have the patient lie supine on the examination table.
- Place the table at a comfortable height for you and sit or stand at the affected side of the patient.

ANATOMY REVIEW

- The distal femur articulates with the proximal tibia to make up the knee joint.
- The patella sits in a groove anterior to the joint.

PROCEDURE

Knee in Extension

- With the knee extended, have the patient relax the quadriceps.
- Palpate the superior and lateral edge of the patella.

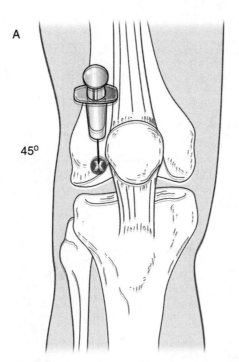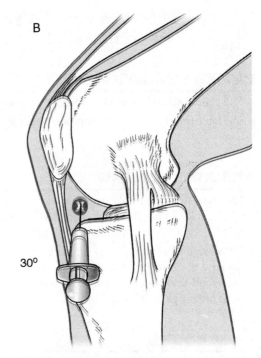

A

45°

B

30°

Figure 54–1. *Anatomy of knee in extension (A) and flexion (B) with needle in aspiration sites.*

- Mark the insertion site just posterior to this edge.
- Prepare the entire area with povidone-iodine.
- Aim the needle at a 45-degree angle posteriorly and a 45-degree angle distally. It should fall under the patella but over the femoral condyle (Figure 54–1A).
- Aspirate as the needle progresses into the joint space.
- If you feel the needle hit bone, pull back slightly and re-direct it.
- Remove as much fluid as possible.
- You may need to move the needle as fibrous septa can create pockets of fluid.

Knee in Flexion
- Have the patient flex the knee to approximately 90 degrees.
- Palpate the inferior edge of the patella. Palpate 2 cm medially or laterally, and 2 cm inferiorly, feel the soft spot, and mark.
- Prepare the area with povidone-iodine.
- Aim the needle at a 30-degree angle superiorly and aspirate as the needle enters the joint (Figure 54–1B).
- Remove as much fluid as possible.
- You may need to move the needle as fibrous septa can create pockets of fluid.

———————[■ ■ ■]———————

- This procedure can be difficult for patients in pain.

ARTHROCENTESIS OF THE ANKLE

PATIENT POSITIONING

■ The patient should be in a comfortable position.

■ The table should be at an appropriate height for the examiner.

ANATOMY REVIEW

■ The distal tibia and fibula articulate with the talus to make up the ankle joint. This joint is crossed by many tendons that function to move the ankle, foot, and toes.

■ Knowledge of location of neurovascular structures, particularly the anterior tibial vessels with the deep peroneal nerve and the superficial peroneal nerve, are essential to prevent iatrogenic injury.

PROCEDURE

■ The ankle joint can be accessed medially or laterally.

■ Medial entry is medial to the anterior tibialis tendon (Figure 54–2).

■ Prepare the area with povidone-iodine.

■ Aspirate as the needle progresses into the joint space.

■ If infection prevents medial access, the lateral entry site is at the lateral one-third of the joint.

■ Avoid the superficial peroneal nerve, which can sometimes be seen through the skin.

INTERPRETATION AND MONITORING

■ Visually inspect joint fluid.

■ Fluid should be sent to the laboratory for analysis of cell count with differential and glucose, and Gram stain and culture (Table 54–1).

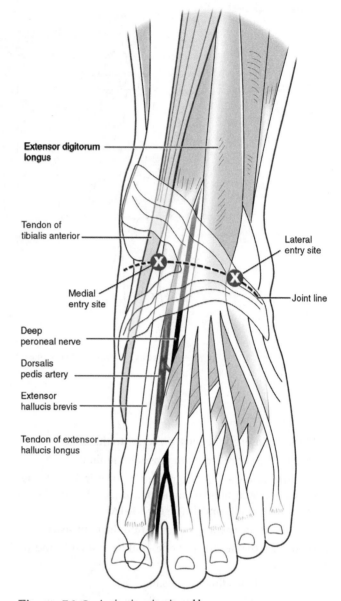

Figure 54–2. *Aspiration sites in ankle.*

Table 54–1. Characteristics of synovial fluid.

Type	White Blood Count	Appearance of Fluid	Culture	Glucose
Normal	Correlates with red blood count	Clear	Negative	Similar to blood glucose
Inflammatory arthritis	> 2000/µL	Turbid	Negative	May be slightly decreased
Septic arthritis	> 50,000/ µL with > 75% polymorphonuclear leukocytes	Purulent	Positive	Decreased to 50% of blood glucose

COMPLICATIONS

- Infection.
- Hemarthrosis.
- Reaccumulation of fluid.

FOLLOW-UP

- Instruct the patient to look for redness and swelling that could be indicative of infection.

REFERENCES

Cole BJ, Schumacher Jr HR. Injectable corticosteroids in modern practice. *J Am Acad Orthop Surg.* 2005;13:37–46.

Luhmann SJ. Acute traumatic knee effusions in children and adolescents. *J Ped Orthop.* 2003;23:199–202.

Nade S. Acute septic arthritis in infancy and childhood. *J Bone Joint Surg Br.* 1983;65:234–241.

Shmerling RH, Delbanco TL, Tosteson AN, Trentham DE. Synovial fluid tests. What should be ordered? *JAMA.* 1990;264:1009–1014.

CHAPTER 55

Regional Nerve Blocks for Bone Fractures

Bradley Dunlap, MD and John F. Sarwark, MD

INDICATIONS

Digital Block

- Provides analgesia in the fingers and toes for treatment of fractures, dislocations, and lacerations.

Hematoma Block

- Analgesia for fracture reduction.
- Most commonly used to reduce distal radius fractures or fractures of the fifth metacarpal (boxer's fractures).

CONTRAINDICATIONS

Absolute

- Skin or soft tissue infection at or near the area to be injected.
- Allergy to lidocaine or other agents used for regional anesthesia.

EQUIPMENT

- 5- or 10-mL syringe.
- 18-gauge needle to draw medicine; 25–27-gauge needle to inject medicine.
- Alcohol swabs to clean skin.
- 1% or 2% plain lidocaine (no epinephrine) or 0.25% bupivacaine (can be combined 1:1).

RISKS

- Inadequate pain relief.
- Allergic reaction.

PEARLS AND TIPS

- Complete and document a neurologic examination before injecting the anesthetic.
- Do not use epinephrine in the digits because it can result in ischemia, necrosis, and potential loss of the digit.

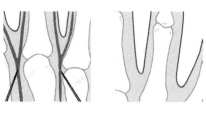

- The maximum lidocaine dose is 5 mg/kg (1% lidocaine has 10 mg/mL; 2% has 20 mg/mL).
- The maximum bupivacaine dose is 2 mg/kg.
- A lidocaine injection provides approximately 2 hours of pain control, while a lidocaine/bupivacaine mixture (1:1) provides approximately 5–7 hours of pain relief.

PATIENT POSITIONING

- For a digital block, pronate the patient's hand and place it on a flat surface.
- For the hematoma block, place the patient's affected extremity on a flat surface.

ANATOMY REVIEW

- There are 2 dorsal nerves and 2 palmar/plantar nerves that innervate each digit; these are the proper digital nerves and they run with the proper digital arteries on the medial/lateral aspect of the digits.

PROCEDURE

Digital Block

- The needle is inserted 1–2 cm proximal to the webspace on 1 side of the digit (Figure 55–1).
- It is advanced palmar/plantar to anesthetize those digital nerves.
- Aspirate to be sure the needle is not intravascular.
- Inject the lidocaine as the needle is slowly pulled out dorsally.
- Repeat the procedure on the other side of the digit.
- This is not a large area; commonly 3–5 mL total of anesthetic is sufficient.
- Massage the area to help spread the agent.

Hematoma Block

- Identify the fracture site and place the needle into the fracture site (dorsal approach for both distal radius and boxer's fractures) (Figure 55–2).
- Continue to aspirate until a flash of blood appears, redirecting the needle as necessary.
- After the flash of blood, slowly inject the lidocaine.

INTERPRETATION AND MONITORING

- Watch for vascular changes; vasospasm can occur but should resolve spontaneously.
- The digit or fracture site is usually fully anesthetized in several minutes.

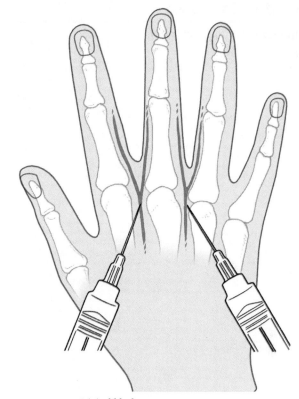

Figure 55–1. *Digital block.*

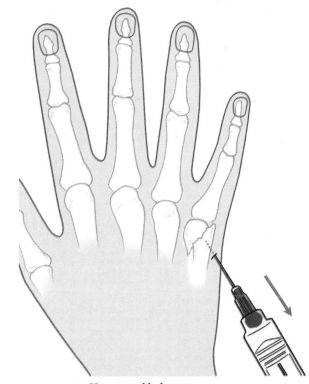

Figure 55–2. *Hematoma block.*

COMPLICATIONS

- Intravascular injection (rare).
- Infection (rare).

REFERENCES

Beaty JH, Kasser JR, eds. *Rockwood & Wilkins' Fractures in Children.* 5th ed. Philadelphia: Lippincott Williams & Wilkins; 2001.

McCarty EC et al. Anesthesia and analgesia for the ambulatory management of fractures in children. *J Am Acad Orthop Surg.* 1999;7:81–91.

New York School of Regional Anesthesia. www.nysora.com

[PART III]

SUBSPECIALTY PROCEDURES

CHAPTER 56

Bronchoscopy

Adrienne Prestridge, MD

INDICATIONS

- Persistent atelectasis.
- Stridor.
- Unexplained or persistent wheeze.
- Suspected foreign body.
- Pneumonia (recurrent, unknown etiology, or in an immunocompromised patient).
- Persistent radiographic infiltrates.
- Hemoptysis (to localize area of bleeding).
- Suspected congenital abnormalities.
- Suspected airway obstruction or compression, including nasal obstruction or associated with sleep disordered breathing.
- Unexplained or persistent cough.
- Excessive bronchial secretions.
- Evaluation of artificial airway (tracheostomy or endotracheal tube).
- Persistent hoarseness.
- Suspected vocal cord dysfunction and paralysis.
- Aspiration.
- Epistaxis.
- Suspected airway trauma.

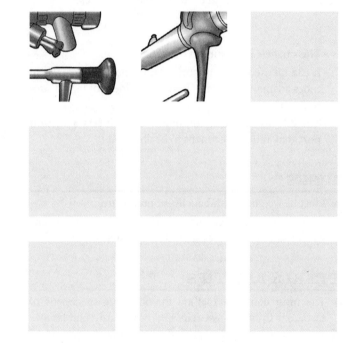

CONTRAINDICATIONS

Relative

- Severe bleeding problems.
- Severe airway stenosis.
- Severe hypoxia.
- Severe bronchospasm.

EQUIPMENT

- Rigid or flexible bronchoscope (Figures 56–1 and 56–2).
- Many different size flexible bronchoscopes allow visualization in a wide range of children.

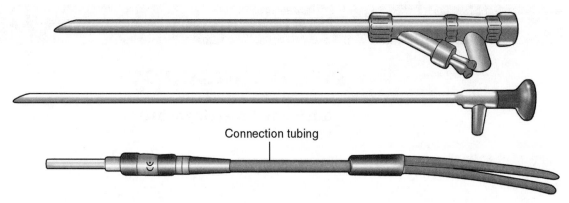

Connection tubing

Figure 56–1. *Rigid bronchoscope.*

• The smallest is 2.2 mm in diameter.
• It can be used in premature infants and in endotracheal tubes as small as 2.5 mm; however, it does not have a suction port.
• The 2.8 mm is most commonly used; it has a suction port that allows specimens to be obtained.

RISKS

■ Must be weighed with benefits of procedure.
■ Information obtained through less invasive, less expensive, or safer procedures should be explored.

PEARLS AND TIPS

■ The most common method for obtaining specimens of secretions from the lower airway is bronchoalveolar lavage.
■ The specimen can be sent to the laboratory for infectious evaluation (eg, bacterial, fungal, viral cultures) and to pathology for additional evaluation.
■ Lipid-laden macrophages are a common pathologic evaluation and help diagnose aspiration.
■ Other specimens can be obtained with various instruments passed through the suction port (eg, biopsies and brushing).

PATIENT PREPARATION

■ Explain to the family what symptoms are being evaluated and describe the procedure.

PROCEDURE

Rigid Bronchoscopy

■ Most often done with sedation or anesthesia.
■ Uses a stiff tube to visualize airways to about the level of the carina.

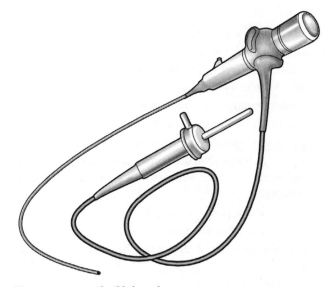

Figure 56–2. *Flexible bronchoscope.*

- Airway has traction placed on it, allowing for improved visualization of posterior airway structures.
- Major advantage is the ability to pass a variety of instruments through the tube, allowing for surgical intervention including removal of a foreign body.

Flexible Bronchoscopy

- Most often done with sedation or anesthesia.
- Can be performed at the bedside in intensive care unit.
- Introduce bronchoscope through the nasal passages or through an artificial airway, allowing the airways to be visualized without traction on airway.
- This method can also be used in patients with tracheostomy.
- The entire airway can be visualized, starting at the nasal passages and extending down to multiple generations of right and left bronchi.

COMPLICATIONS

- Hypoxia.
- Hypercapnia.
- Laryngospasm.
- Bronchospasm.
- Arrhythmias.
- Bradycardia.
- Hypotension.
- Fever.
- Pneumothorax.
- Pneumomediastinum.
- Hemoptysis.
- Laryngeal and nasal trauma.
- Epistaxis.
- Mucosal or subglottic edema.

—————[■■■]—————

- Overall, complications are very rare.

REFERENCES

Perez CR. Update on pediatric flexible bronchoscopy. *Pediatr Clin North Am.* 1994;41:385–400.

Wood RE. Spelunking in the pediatric airways: explorations with the flexible fiberoptic bronchoscope. *Pediatr Clin North Am.* 1984;31:785–799.

Wood RE. The emerging role of flexible bronchoscopy in pediatrics. *Clin Chest Med.* 2001;22:311–317.

CHAPTER 57

Internal Jugular and Subclavian Catheterization

Kelly Michelson, MD

INDICATIONS

- Emergency resuscitation requiring administration of large amounts of fluids.
- Need for central venous pressure monitoring.
- Placement of a pulmonary artery catheter.
- Need for frequent blood draws.
- Infusion of hyperalimentation.
- Infusion of agents that can extravasate and cause soft tissue necrosis.
  - Concentrated solutions (ie, KCl, dextrose concentrations > 12.5%, chemotherapeutic agents, hyperosmolar saline).
  - Vasoactive drugs (ie, dopamine and norepinephrine).
- Need for hemodialysis.
- Central access needed in a patient for which femoral vein catheterization is not possible due to poor landmarks or known thrombus.

RISKS

- Infection.
- Bleeding.
- Arrhythmias; can occur if the catheter or guidewire comes in contact with the heart.
- Cardiac tamponade.

PEARLS AND TIPS

- Internal jugular and subclavian catheters have certain advantages over femoral venous catheters, including the following:
  - A pulmonary artery catheter is placed more easily from the internal jugular vein because there is an almost a straight course to the superior vena cava and right atrium of the heart.
  - Placement of a subclavian catheter uses a "blind" approach with good external landmarks; therefore, the operator may have more success in patients in shock or cardiopulmonary arrest where arterial pulsations are difficult to palpate.

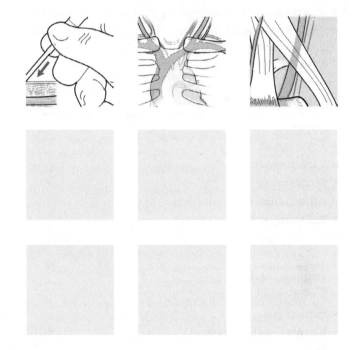

- Internal jugular and subclavian catheters are central lines placed percutaneously; they provide an alternative to femoral venous catheterization (see Chapter 10) when central venous access is needed.

- Catheters are minimally affected by ambulation and may be preferable in very mobile patients.
- Site of insertion is considered relatively "clean," compared with the femoral location.

■ Keep in mind that in a patient receiving anticoagulation therapy, bleeding can be controlled more easily using internal jugular puncture.

■ However, there is a slightly higher incidence of failure using the internal jugular approach compared with the subclavian approach.

■ Securing the catheter can be difficult in a child with a small neck.

■ To avoid aspiration during intubation or conscious sedation, the procedure should be delayed 6 hours after the ingestion of solid food and 4 hours after the ingestion of clear liquids, unless central access is needed emergently.

PATIENT PREPARATION

■ Inform parents of the indications and risks of the procedure.

■ Inform parents about how long the catheter is likely to remain in place.

■ Inform parents in advance that their child may be sedated or intubated for the procedure and what risks each incurs.

PROCEDURE

■ Internal jugular and subclavian catheters are placed using the Seldinger technique (Figure 57–1) based on identifying external landmarks (Figure 57–2).

■ Please see Chapter 10, Femoral Venous Catheterization, for a detailed description of this technique.

COMPLICATIONS

■ Bleeding; avoid placing a subclavian catheter in a patient with coagulopathy because it is not possible to apply direct pressure to the subclavian vein or artery.

■ Local hematomas.

■ Air embolus.

■ Catheter embolus.

■ Creating an arteriovenous fistula.

■ Creating a pneumothorax or hemothorax.
- Obtain a chest radiography immediately after the procedure to rapidly identify such complications.

FOLLOW-UP

■ The catheter should be removed as soon as it is not needed.
- Remove the sutures and pull the catheter out slowly and carefully.

■ Because of the risks and potential complications, only anesthesiologists, intensivists, some cardiologists, and surgeons perform this procedure.

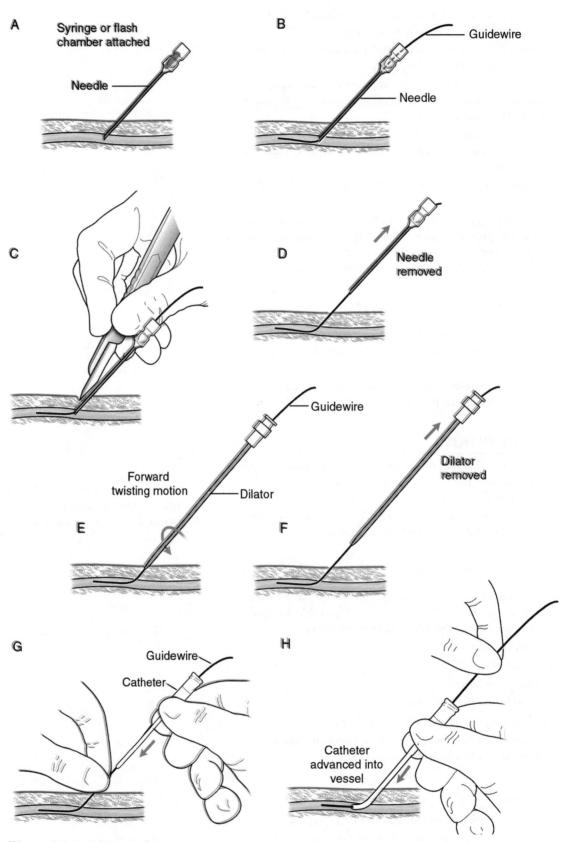

Figure 57–1. *Seldinger technique.*

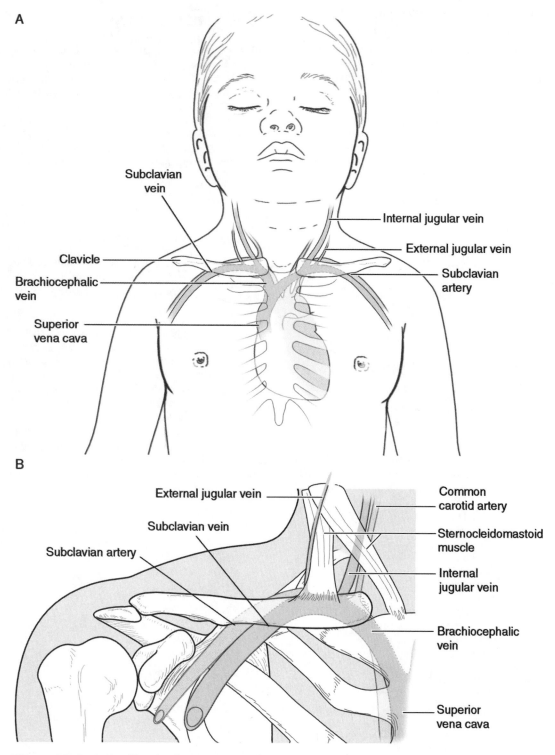

Figure 57–2. *A: Vessel location for percutaneous placement of central venous catheters. B: Landmarks used to guide central venous catheter placement.*

- If possible, pull the catheter out on the patient's exhalation to avoid creating an air embolus.
- Apply pressure at the insertion site until the bleeding stops.

REFERENCES

Advanced Trauma Life Support Program for Doctors: ATLS. 6th ed. Chicago: American College of Surgeons; 1997.

Domino KB, Bowdle TA, Posner KL, Spitellie PH, Lee LA, Cheney FW. Injuries and liability related to central vascular catheters: a closed claims analysis. *Anesthesiology.* 2004;100: 1411–1418.

Hazinski MF et al, eds. *PALS Provider Manual.* Dallas, TX: American Heart Association; 2002.

Journeycake JM, Buchanan GR. Thrombotic complications of central venous catheters in children. *Curr Opin Hematol.* 2003;10:369–374.

Merrer J, De Jonghe B, Golliot F et al. Complications of femoral and subclavian venous catheterization in critically ill patients: a randomized controlled trial. *JAMA.* 2001;286:700–707.

Mickiewicz M, Dronen SC, Younger JG. Central venous catheterization and central venous pressure monitoring. In: Roberts JR, Hedges JR, eds. *Clinical Procedures in Emergency Medicine.* 4th ed. Philadelphia: WB Saunders Company; 2004.

O'Grady NP, Alexander M, Dellinger EP et al. Guidelines for the prevention of intravascular catheter-related infections. The Hospital Infection Control Practices Advisory Committee, Centers for Disease Control and Prevention, U.S. *Pediatrics.* 2002;110(5):e51.

Roberts JR, Hedges JR, Chanmugam AS. *Clinical Procedures in Emergency Medicine.* 4th ed. Philadelphia: WB Saunders; 2004.

Rosen P. *Emergency Medicine Concepts and Clinical Practice.* 5th ed. St. Louis: MD Consult LLC; 2002.

CHAPTER 58

Venous Cutdown

Marybeth Browne, MD, Anthony Chin, MD, and Marleta Reynolds, MD

INDICATIONS

- In general, the cutdown procedure is used for the operative placement of an intermediate or long-term central catheter or in an emergency setting when percutaneous access is unachievable.

CONTRAINDICATIONS

Absolute

- Infection on the skin over the area of the intended cutdown.
- Percutaneous access that can be safely achieved.

Relative

- Bleeding disorder.
- Coagulopathy.
- Irritation of skin over area of the intended cutdown.

EQUIPMENT

- Antiseptic solution.
- Sedative or analgesic.
- Surgical protective wear (sterile gloves, mask, hat, sterile gown).
- Tourniquet.
- 4–6 sterile towels.
- 10-mL syringe, 20–25-gauge needle, 0.5% lidocaine.
- 2 scalpels (#10 and #11 blades).
- 4 × 4 gauze sponges.
- 1 curved hemostat.
- 1 forceps.
- Single-toothed spring retractors (optional).
- Sutures, 4-0 silk ties (1 package), 4-0 nylon suture with cutting needle (1 package).
- Needle holder.
- 2 cutdown catheters (depends on size of child and vein; can use between a #14 and #22 gauge).

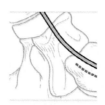
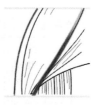

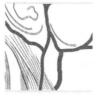

{ ■ ■ ■ }

- In the emergent setting, a venous cutdown procedure is potentially lifesaving; however, it is considered a last resort procedure and should only be performed by a clinician familiar with the technique.
- With the development of modern vascular devices, a traditional vascular cutdown is less commonly used.

■ Sterile dressing.

■ Topical antibiotic ointment.

RISKS

■ Bleeding.

■ Infection.

■ Thrombosis.

■ Arterial or nerve injury.

■ Air embolus, catheter migration or erosion, and arrhythmias (more often seen with central venous access cutdowns).

PATIENT PREPARATION

■ Apply eutectic mixture of local anesthetic (EMLA) over intended incision site 30 minutes prior to procedure, and administer morphine or diazepam for sedation.

■ Prepare a large area of skin over the intended dissection site with antiseptic solution and drape the area with sterile towels.

ANATOMY REVIEW

Greater Saphenous Vein

■ This vein is the preferred site in emergency situations due to its anatomic reliability and ease of access.

■ Runs slightly anterior to the anterior malleolus (Figure 58–1).

■ The knee should be abducted and the ankle turned laterally to achieve adequate exposure of the medial ankle and calf for the procedure.

■ A small transverse skin incision should be made slightly anterior and cephalad to the medial malleolus perpendicular to the vein.

■ With fine dissection, the greater saphenous vein is found in the subcutaneous tissue.

Cephalic and Basilic Veins

■ Both veins can be used for both central and peripheral access.

■ The median basilic vein runs transversely across the medial border of the antecubital fossa (Figure 58–2).

■ The cephalic vein runs more vertically toward the lateral aspect of the fossa (Figure 58–2).

■ With the aid of a tourniquet, a central incision can be used to expose both the cephalic and basilic veins, which are found in the subcutaneous tissue of the antecubital fossa.

■ The cephalic vein can also be accessed in the deltopectoral groove.

■ The most common sites for possible venous cutdown include greater saphenous, cephalic, basilic, and jugular (in neonates) veins.

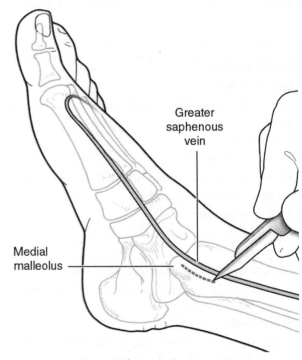

Greater saphenous vein

Medial malleolus

Figure 58–1. *Greater saphenous vein.*

Saphenofemoral Vein

■ The greater saphenous vein drains into the femoral vein at the infrainguinal area; and the saphenofemoral vein lies just medial to the femoral artery (Figure 58–3).

■ Flex and abduct the hip to place the leg in frog-like position for exposure of the inguinal region.

■ A transverse skin incision is made just below the inguinal ligament, medial to the femoral pulse.

■ With fine dissection, the greater saphenous vein is identified in the subcutaneous fat, superficial to the femoral fascia.

External Jugular Vein

■ This vein begins behind the angle of the mandible near the union of the posterior auricular vein and the posterior retromandibular vein (Figure 58–4).

■ It obliquely crosses the sternocleidomastoid muscle and drains into the subclavian vein just above the clavicle.

■ To provide adequate access to the external jugular vein, the neck must be fully extended and the head slightly turned away from the intended site of dissection.

■ A transverse incision should be made at the midpoint between the mandible and the clavicular head over the anterior border of the sternocleidomastoid muscle.

■ A long catheter may be difficult to advance in the external jugular because of the angulation at its junction with the subclavian vein.

Common Facial Vein

■ This vein is joined by the anterior retromandibular vein and drains directly into the internal jugular vein (Figure 58–4).

■ For adequate exposure, the neck must be fully extended and the head slightly turned away from the intended site of dissection.

■ A transverse incision is made halfway between the inferior tip of the ear and the sternal notch, along the anterior border of the sternocleidomastoid muscle.

■ With delicate dissection, the common facial vein is found just inferior to the superficial cervical fascia.

Internal Jugular Vein

■ This vein runs posterior to the sternocleidomastoid muscle and joins the subclavian vein posterior to the clavicular head.

■ Although sacrifice of a unilateral internal jugular vein may be without morbidity, it should be the last vein of choice, especially in a premature infant.

■ The positioning and incision site should be similar to the common facial vein cutdown.

■ The internal jugular vein can be found by following the common facial vein to where it drains into the internal jugular.

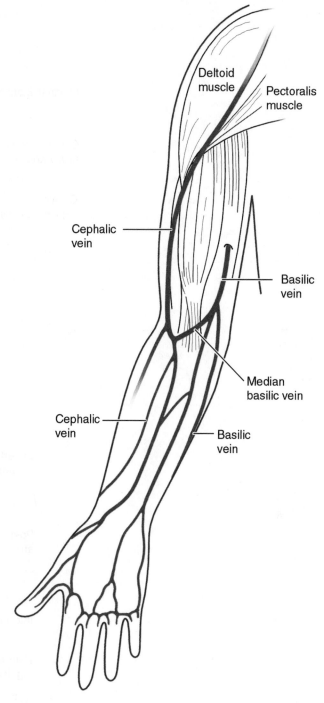

Figure 58–2. *Cephalic and basilic veins.*

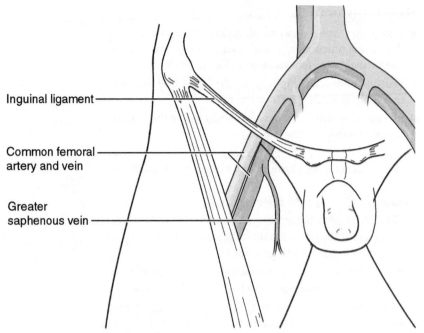

Figure 58–3. *Saphenofemoral vein.*

Inguinal ligament

Common femoral
artery and vein

Greater
saphenous vein

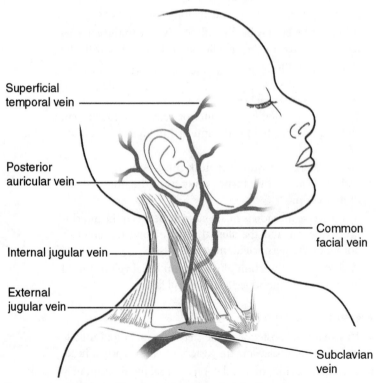

Figure 58–4. *External jugular and common facial veins.*

Superficial
temporal vein

Posterior
auricular vein

Internal jugular vein

External
jugular vein

Common
facial vein

Subclavian
vein

PROCEDURE

- After proper sterilization and draping of the area, infiltrate the skin over the intended incision site with 0.5% lidocaine. (Maximum dose of lidocaine is 5 mg/kg.)
- Make a full thickness 2.5-cm skin incision using the #10 scalpel over the infiltrate area.
- Be careful not to cut too deep to avoid accidentally injuring the vein.
- Using a curved hemostat, bluntly dissect the subcutaneous tissue until the intended vein is identified (Figures 58–5A and 58-5B).
- Free the vein from any accompanying structure, being aware of the local nerves and arteries.
- Elevate and dissect the vein for a distance of about 1 cm.
- Pass a tie around the most distal end and ligate the vein. Leave the suture in place for traction (Figure 58–5C).
- Pass a second tie around the vein and place it cephalad to your intended venotomy (Figure 58–5C).
- Make a small transverse venotomy using the #11 scalpel, and gently dilate the venotomy with the tips of the curved hemostats (Figure 58–5D).
- Introduce the access catheter through the venotomy, and secure it in place by tying the proximal suture around the vein and cannula.
- Insert the cannula a sufficient distance to prevent inadvertent dislodging (Figure 58–5E).
- Attach the intravenous tubing to the catheter being watchful for air embolization.
- Close the incision with interrupted sutures (Figure 58–5F).
- Suture the catheter to the skin.
- Apply topical antibiotic ointment and a sterile dressing.

COMPLICATIONS

- Cellulitis.
- Hematoma.
- Phlebitis.
- Venous thrombosis.
- Nerve injury.
- Arterial injury.
- Air embolus.
- Catheter migration or malposition.
- Arrhythmias.

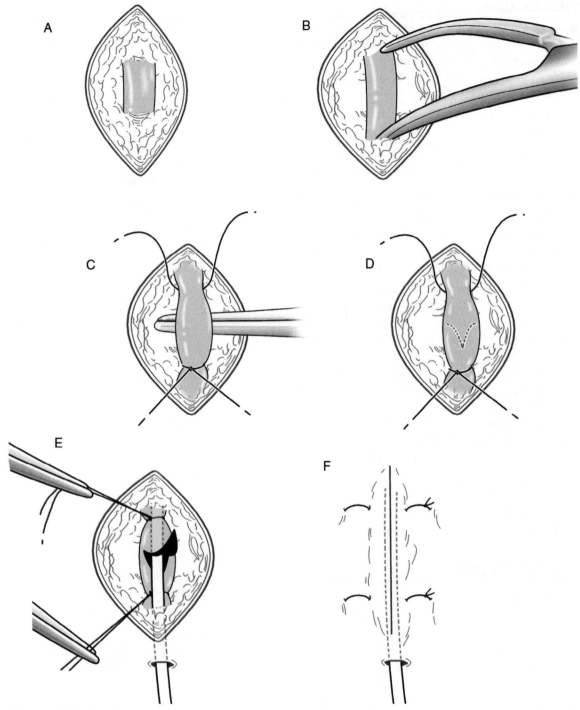

Figure 58–5. *Procedure of venous cutdown.*

REFERENCES

Gauderer MW. Vascular access techniques and devices in the pediatric patient. *Surg Clin North Am.* 1992;72:1267–1284.

Iverson KV, Criss EA. Pediatric venous cutdowns: utility in emergency situations. *Pediatr Emerg Care.* 1986;2:231–234.

Chung DH, Ziegler MM. Vascular access procedures. Chapter 8.

Shock. Chapter 3. Advanced trauma life support student course manual. 6th edition. Chicago: American College of Surgeons; 1997:121–124.

CHAPTER 59

Cardiac Catheterization

David Wax, MD and Stephen Pophal, MD

INDICATIONS

Diagnostic Catheterization

- To obtain information about the physiology and anatomy of the circulatory system, frequently in the setting of structural congenital heart disease.
- To assess patients with the following:
  - Pulmonary atresia and tetralogy of Fallot who have complex collateral pulmonary blood supply.
  - Pulmonary atresia with intact ventricular septum to evaluate coronary anatomy.
  - Single ventricle prior to their second and third stage repairs.

Therapeutic Catheterization

- To treat heart disease, usually taking the place of a more invasive surgical procedure.
- To open stenotic valves or vessels.
  - Stenotic valves (in order of frequency, pulmonary, aortic, mitral, and tricuspid).
  - Stenotic blood vessels (eg, pulmonary artery, coarctation of the aorta).
- To close such abnormalities as patent ductus arteriosus, atrial septal defect, and collateral blood vessels.

CONTRAINDICATIONS

- The trend is toward reserving diagnostic catheterization for cases in which noninvasive imaging is insufficient to provide the information necessary for management decisions.
- Examples of congenital heart disease where routine diagnostic catheterization is no longer performed prior to surgical repair include the following:
  - Uncomplicated ventricular septal defect.
  - Atrioventricular canal.
  - Transposition of the great arteries.
  - Tetralogy of Fallot.
  - Most types of single ventricle prior to their initial palliation.

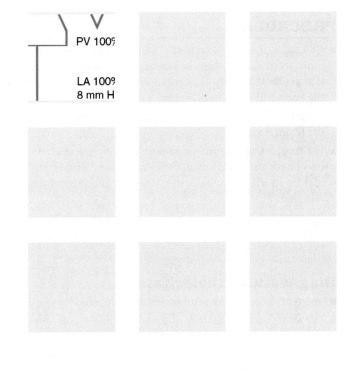

- Cardiac catheterization can be roughly divided into diagnostic and therapeutic procedures although there is often overlap between the two.

■ Some persons with the above conditions may be candidates for palliative therapeutic catheterizations (eg, balloon atrial septostomy for patients with transposition of the great arteries).

PATIENT PREPARATION

■ Estimate the length of the procedure to prepare the patients and family.
  • Accurate predictions are easier for simple diagnostic cases.
  • Endomyocardial biopsy may take about 20 minutes.
  • A multi-part therapeutic procedure may take half a day.

PROCEDURE

■ Cardiac catheterization is the invasive evaluation, and more recently, treatment of heart disease, using catheters that are threaded into the various chambers and vessels of the heart and circulatory system.

■ Vascular access for most pediatric catheterizations is via the femoral vessels.

■ For complex procedures or anatomy, multiple access sites may be required and include bilateral femoral vessels, jugular or subclavian veins; rarely, transhepatic puncture is required.

■ Patients who have femoral access are generally required to remain supine with legs straight from 4 to 6 hours after the procedure to prevent rebleeding.

Diagnostic Catheterization

■ Procedure does not require significant analgesia.

■ However, anxiety and lack of understanding usually preclude young patients from cooperating sufficiently, so most procedures are performed with patients under deep sedation.

■ Sometimes patient may perceive ectopic beats associated with catheter manipulation.

■ Radiopaque contrast is instilled into area of interest while a fluoroscopic cine recording is made to obtain anatomic information.

■ Instillation of contrast may be associated with a warm feeling and the need to urinate; both sensations pass quickly.

■ Saturation and pressure measurements in the different chambers of the heart and circulatory system can be used to calculate quantitative information.

Therapeutic Catheterization

■ General anesthesia is reserved for the longest procedures, those likely to be associated with persistent discomfort, patients who are deeply cyanotic, or those likely to have unguarded airways with deep sedation.

- The use of general anesthesia remains largely a preference of the individual physician. NPO orders are routine for the sedation to be used.
- Therapeutic angioplasty, especially of the arteries, can be painful although narcotic analgesia is usually sufficient to control discomfort.

INTERPRETATION

- Hemodynamic information commonly obtained includes measurement of pressure and oxygen saturation in the various chambers of the heart (Figure 59–1).
- Using the oxygen consumption (usually taken from tables), oxygen saturation and hemoglobin, the systemic and pulmonary blood flow can be calculated via the Fick equation.

$$Qs = \frac{VO_2}{C_{AO} - C_{MV}}$$

- where VO_2 = oxygen consumption, C_{AO} = arterial oxygen content, C_{MV} = mixed venous oxygen content. For pulmonary blood flow (Qp), pulmonary venous and pulmonary arterial oxygen content is substituted. Qp = Qs in a patient with no intracardiac shunts. Normal cardiac index is 3.1 ± 0.4 L/min/m^2.
- Cardiac index is usually reported as the ratio of pulmonary to systemic blood flow in patients with a left to right shunt.
- A pulmonary blood flow > 1.5 times the systemic blood flow represents a significant shunt.
- Pressure and blood flow data are combined to calculate systemic vascular resistance (SVR) and pulmonary vascular resistance (PVR). For SVR, mean aortic pressure, mean right atrial pressure, and Qs are substituted.

$$PVR = \frac{\text{Mean PA pressure} - \text{Mean LA pressure}}{Qp}$$

- This may be used to distinguish pulmonary hypertension caused by high blood flow in left to right shunt lesions from pulmonary hypertension secondary to pulmonary vascular disease.
- Resistance ≤ 3 units/m^2 is normal.
- Interpretations of the angiograms are presented as a radiologic report.

COMPLICATIONS

- Factors that increase the risk of complications include the following:
  - Younger and smaller patients.
  - Therapeutic as opposed to diagnostic procedure.
  - Clinical condition of the patient at the time of the procedure.

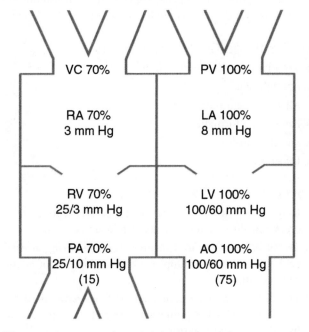

Figure 59–1. *Hemodynamic information.*

- Arrhythmias account for most of the major complications.
- Decreased pulse at the site of arterial access accounts for most of the minor complications.
  - Transient loss of pedal pulse is relatively common after arterial access.
  - Occurs in up to 10% of patients under 5 kg.
  - May require systemic heparinization or thrombolytic therapy if it does not spontaneously resolve.

Diagnostic Catheterization

- Vascular or cardiac perforation.
- Arrhythmia.
- Allergic reaction to contrast.
- Hematoma formation.
- Vessel occlusion.
- Infection.

Therapeutic Catheterization

- Most interventions require larger sheaths leading to a greater likelihood of vascular complications.
- This is especially true with procedures requiring arterial access like aortic valvuloplasty and angioplasty of aortic coarctation.
- The difficult catheter course and stiff wires required for interventions in the pulmonary arterial tree can lead to hypotension and cyanosis.
- Occlusion devices may embolize with the seriousness of this complication related to the size and location of the device.

FOLLOW-UP

- Most patients are discharged the day of the procedure after the prescribed period of bed rest.
- They can ambulate that night and return to school or most jobs the next day or after 1 additional day of rest.

- Parents of young children, patients having complex procedures, and patients with procedures starting later in the day are instructed that an overnight hospital stay is possible and should plan accordingly.
- Patients with large and multiple catheters (generally after interventional procedures) may have discomfort and bruising at the access site for weeks that keep them from feeling comfortable with vigorous physical activity. This discomfort is almost always self-limited and is rarely treated with anything stronger than nonsteroidal anti-inflammatory drugs.
- Patients who have increasing rather than decreasing discomfort over time or those with any sign of infection at the access site are seen for follow-up.

REFERENCES

Allen HD, Beekman RH III, Garson A Jr et al. Pediatric therapeutic cardiac catheterization: a statement for healthcare professionals from the Council on Cardiovascular Disease in the Young, American Heart Association. *Circulation.* 1998; 97:609–625.

Bonhoeffer P, Boudjemline Y, Saliba Z et al. Percutaneous replacement of pulmonary valve in a right-ventricle to pulmonary-artery prosthetic conduit with valve dysfunction. *Lancet.* 2000;356:1403–1405.

Cambier PA, Kirby WC, Wortham DC, Moore JW. Percutaneous closure of the small (less than 2.5 mm) patent ductus arteriosus using coil embolization. *Am J Cardiol.* 1992;69:815–816.

Kan JS, White RI Jr, Mitchell SE, Gardner TJ. Percutaneous balloon valvuloplasty: a new method for treating congenital pulmonary-valve stenosis. *N Engl J Med.* 1982;307:540–542.

King TD, Thompson SL, Steiner C, Mills NL. Secundum atrial septal defect. Nonoperative closure during cardiac catheterization. *JAMA.* 1976;235:2506–2509.

Vitiello R, McCrindle BW, Nykanen D, Freedom RM, Benson LN. Complications associated with pediatric cardiac catheterization. *J Am Coll Cardiol.* 1998;32:1433–1440.

CHAPTER 60

Echocardiography

Frederique Bailliard, MD and Luciana T. Young, MD

INDICATIONS

Cardiovascular Disease in the Newborn

- To monitor normally occurring physiologic changes during the transitional circulation of the newborn.
- Helps define structural anomaly, if present.
- Helps determine hemodynamics and ventricular function.
- To assess the presence and degree of pulmonary artery hypertension in premature infants with respiratory failure related to lung disease.
- Doppler echocardiography can show ductal patency as well as amount and direction of shunting.
- Cyanosis in newborns without evidence of severe lung disease but whose chest radiograph, ECG, and extremity blood pressures are abnormal.
- Arrhythmias, nonimmune hydrops, and sepsis.
- Chromosomal abnormalities and certain extracardiac anomalies.

Murmurs in Infants and Children

- Innocent heart murmurs do not warrant echocardiography.
  - Still's murmur.
  - Flow murmur of the pulmonary artery.
  - Peripheral pulmonic stenosis.
  - Supraclavicular murmur.
  - Systolic flow murmur.
- Maintain low threshold for obtaining echocardiogram in children with a murmur and abnormal results on accompanying studies (eg, ECG, chest radiograph).
- Diastolic murmur or gallop.

Acquired Heart Disease

- Examples include Kawasaki disease, rheumatic fever, myocarditis, and endocarditis.
- Provides important information regarding the following:
  - Chamber sizes.

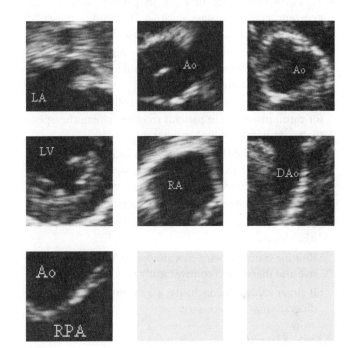

- Guidelines for the clinical application of echocardiography have been formulated by the American College of Cardiology and the American Heart Association in collaboration with the American Society of Echocardiography.

• Valve and ventricular function.

• Pericardial involvement.

• Presence of intracardiac masses.

■ Can also be used for serial evaluation throughout the disease process and to determine whether therapy is effective.

Systemic Disease

■ To evaluate patients with connective tissue diseases, such as Marfan syndrome and Ehlers-Danlos syndrome, which are associated with valve prolapse, aortic root dilation, and dissection.

■ To assess ventricular function in patients with certain neuromuscular disorders, such as Duchenne's muscular dystrophy, that can affect the heart muscle.

■ To assess left ventricular hypertrophy and dysfunction in children with chronic renal disease and long-standing systemic hypertension.

■ To obtain baseline and serial echocardiograms to assess for cardiomyopathy in patients receiving chemotherapeutic agents, which can be cardiotoxic.

■ Useful in additional disease processes including HIV, serial assessment for rejection in cardiac transplant patients, and screening of patients with a family history of cardiomyopathy.

■ Newly diagnosed thromboembolic disease.

• Searches for sources of thrombus and potential intracardiac shunts.

• Routine transthoracic echocardiogram is often inconclusive and therefore, a contrast study may be necessary.

• If either study is inconclusive, a transesophageal echocardiogram may be necessary.

Arrhythmia

■ Determines whether there is associated structural heart disease (eg, Ebstein's anomaly, mitral valve prolapse, and cardiac tumors).

■ Evaluates cardiac function (ie, myocarditis, cardiomyopathy).

■ If tachycardia has been present for an extended period of time, an echocardiogram may help determine whether an intracardiac thrombus is present and if ventricular function is preserved.

Chest Pain/Syncope

■ Chest pain is not an absolute indication for echocardiography, since < 5% of chest pain is cardiac in origin.

■ Abnormal ECG or chest radiography in those rare patients with cardiac disease.

■ Chest pain associated with exercise, a family history of hypertrophic cardiomyopathy or long QT syndrome.

■ Syncope in children is most frequently vasovagal or neurogenic and does not require an echocardiogram.

■ However, when syncope occurs during exercise, an echocardiogram can rule out an anomalous coronary artery or left ventricular outflow obstruction.

CONTRAINDICATIONS

■ Do not perform transesophageal echocardiogram in patients with the following:

• Esophageal obstruction or bleeding.

• Unrepaired tracheoesophageal fistula.

• Inadequate control of the airway.

■ Relative contraindications to TEE include the following:

• Esophageal varices or diverticuli.

• Previous esophageal surgery.

• Coagulopathy.

• History of a cervical spine injury.

• Small patient size (< 3 kg).

RISKS

■ Transesophageal echocardiography may pose a risk because of its invasive nature.

• Hypoxia due to tracheal compression.

• Hypotension.

• Nonsustained ventricular tachycardia.

• Supraventricular tachycardia.

• Esophageal tear.

■ Risks associated with sedation should also be considered.

PEARLS AND TIPS

■ Be specific regarding the purpose of the echocardiogram; this helps the sonographer perform the examination.

■ A "normal" echocardiogram does not necessarily mean a normal heart.

• Someone with a family history of hypertrophic cardiomyopathy may have a normal study as a child, but hypertrophy may develop later in life.

• Likewise, the presence of an anomalous coronary artery may not be detected if the coronary anatomy is not specifically examined.

• Therefore, clinical correlation of the echocardiographic findings with history, physical examination, and other testing is always essential.

■ When a discrepancy exists between the clinical picture and the echocardiographic findings, the patient should be reevaluated and additional testing (ie, computed tomoangiography, MRI, cardiac catheterization) should be considered.

■ An echocardiogram can cost up to 3–5 times more than a cardiology consultation with an ECG. Therefore, it may be more cost-effective to consult with a cardiologist to determine whether an echocardiogram is indicated.

- When an echocardiogram is obtained without cardiology consultation, it is important to know how to interpret the results.
  - A patent foramen ovale is considered a normal finding in infants and trivial tricuspid and pulmonary regurgitation are almost always present.
  - However, the presence of aortic insufficiency is almost always considered an abnormal finding.

PATIENT PREPARATION

- Conscious sedation is often necessary in infants and young children to obtain accurate information.
- Electrodes are placed to document the ECG throughout the study.
- Water-soluble gel is applied to the chest and acts as a medium for ultrasound waves to travel through.

PATIENT POSITIONING

- The patient needs to lie still in the supine position for the echocardiogram.
- Infants can be calmed with a pacifier or bottle.
- A videotaped cartoon or movie may be used to hold the attention of older children.

ANATOMY REVIEW

- Five standard views are obtained on all patients.
  - **Subcostal view (Figure 60–1):** Situs, abdominal aorta, inferior vena cava and superior vena cava return to right atrium, atrial septum (best view), right and left ventricular outflow tracts, ventricular septum.
  - **Parasternal long and short axis views (Figures 60–2, 60–3, and 60–4):** Mitral and aortic valves, great vessel relationship, pulmonary valve and main pulmonary artery, ventricular septum, tricuspid valve, coronary arteries, m-mode assessment of ventricular function (fractional shortening).
  - **Apical view (Figure 60–5):** Mitral and tricuspid valve inflow, ventricular size, ventricular septum, great vessel relationship, ejection fraction for assessment of ventricular function.
  - **Suprasternal arch and coronal views (Figures 60–6 and 60–7):** Aortic sidedness, ascending and descending aorta, superior vena cava, patent ductus arteriosus, pulmonary venous return, branch pulmonary arteries.

PROCEDURE

- Because of its complex nature, an echocardiogram should not be ordered without cardiology consultation.

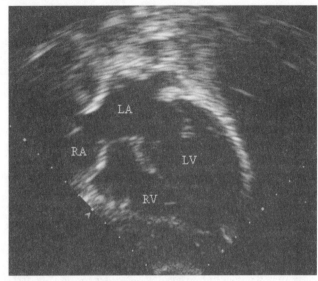

Figure 60–1. *Subcostal 4-chamber view in a normal patient. Intracardiac connections may be determined by scanning from posterior to anterior in this plane. This view (in combination with the subcostal short axis view) is also useful for assessing the atrial septum. LA, left atrium; RA, right atrium; RV, right ventricle; LV, left ventricle.*

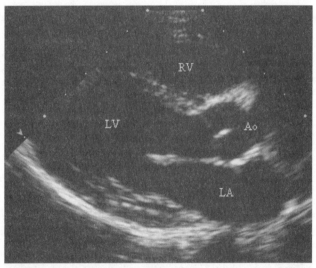

Figure 60–2. *Parasternal long axis view in a normal patient is helpful for visualizing the RV, LA, LV, and mitral and aortic valves. Imaging of the tricuspid and pulmonary valves is achieved by additional scanning from right to left in this plane. RV, right ventricle; LV, left ventricle; LA, left atrium; Ao, aorta.*

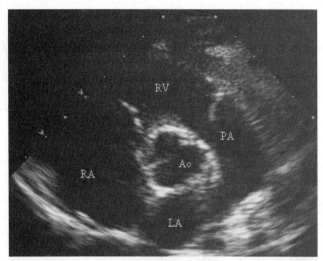

Figure 60–3. *Parasternal short axis view in a normal patient. The aortic valve is seen in cross section at the base of the heart. With clockwise rotation of the transducer, the coronary arteries may also be examined. This view also provides information regarding the tricuspid valve, RV outflow tract, and pulmonary valve. RA, right atrium; RV, right ventricle; LA, left atrium; PA, main pulmonary artery; Ao, aorta.*

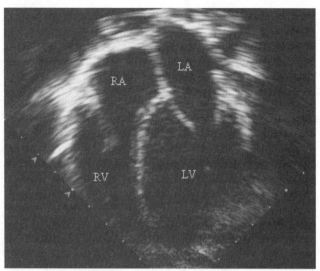

Figure 60–5. *Apical view in a normal patient. All 4 cardiac chambers, the tricuspid and mitral valves, and the atrial and ventricular septae are demonstrated. Additional information regarding the coronary sinus and outflow tracts may be obtained by tilting the transducer from posterior to anterior in this plane. This view is also used to obtain the ejection fraction for assessment of LV function. RA, right atrium; RV, right ventricle; LA, left atrium; LV, left ventricle.*

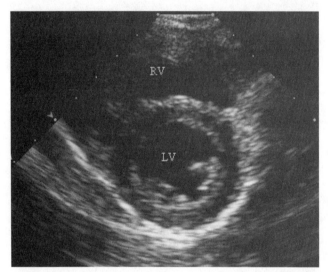

Figure 60–4. *Parasternal short axis view at the level of the mitral valve in a normal patient. The left ventricle is seen in cross section. This view is used for m-mode assessment of LV function. RV, right ventricle; LV, left ventricle.*

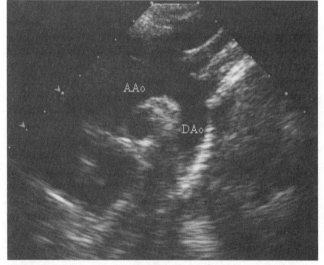

Figure 60–6. *Suprasternal long axis view of the aortic arch in a normal patient. This view provides visualization of the entire aortic arch and origins of the head and neck vessels. AAo, ascending aorta; DAo, descending aorta.*

- Transesophageal echocardiography.
  - Used as an adjunct to transthoracic echocardiography in older patients or for those in whom obesity, lung disease, or chest wall deformities preclude reliable imaging.
  - Useful in searching for sources of intracardiac thrombus or shunting in patients who have had a stroke.
  - Useful for detecting vegetations in endocarditis.
  - Useful for evaluating patients who have undergone previous valve replacement.
  - Commonly used to provide guidance during transcatheter interventions and for intraoperative assessment of surgical repair and function in patients with congenital heart disease.
  - To perform, pass a probe similar in size to an endoscope into the esophagus to obtain high-resolution images of the heart.
  - Oral analgesic sprays are often used to decrease discomfort associated with probe insertion.
  - Requires sedation and the ability to provide rapid airway protection if necessary.
  - Typically performed in a specialized unit with close monitoring such as the endoscopy suite, operating room, or intensive care unit.

INTERPRETATION AND MONITORING

- Monitor pulse oximetry and ECG continuously if sedation is used.
- Assess blood pressure, heart rate, and respiratory effort frequently.
- Z-scores are used to determine whether a measurement falls within 2 standard deviations of the expected normal value.
- Assess ventricular function by measuring the ejection fraction, which is obtained from the apical view.
- The normal ejection fraction range is $67 \pm 8\%$.

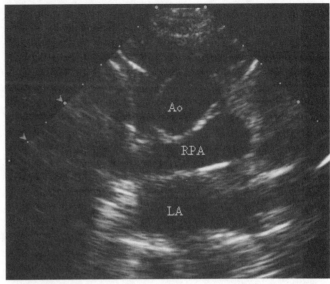

Figure 60–7. *Suprasternal coronal view in a normal patient. The transverse aorta is seen in cross section. This view is used to determined arch sidedness. It also provides good visualization of the RPA and LA. Ao, aorta; RPA, right pulmonary artery; LA, left atrium.*

REFERENCES

ACC/AHA/ASE 2003 Guideline update for the clinical application of echocardiography. www.acc.org/clinical/guidelines/echo/index.pdg.

Baddour LM, Wilson WR, Bayer AS et al; Committee on Rheumatic Fever, Endocarditis and Kawasaki Disease; Council on Cardiovascular Disease in the Young; Council on Clinical Cardiology, Stroke and Cardiovascular Surgery and Anesthesia; American Heart Association; Infectious Disease Society of America. Infective endocarditis: diagnosis, antimicrobial therapy and management of complications: a statement for healthcare professionals from the Committee on Rheumatic Fever, Endocarditis and Kawasaki Disease, Council on Cardiovascular Disease in the Young, and the Council on Clinical Cardiology, Stroke and Cardiovascular Surgery and Anesthesia, American Heart Association: endorsed by the Infectious Disease Society of America. *Circulation.* 2005;111: e394–434.

Danford DA, Martin AB, Fletcher SE, et al. Echocardiographic yield in children when innocent murmur seems likely but doubts linger. *Pediatr Cardiol.* 2002;23:410–414.

Garson A, Bricker JT, Fisher DJ, Neish SR. *The Science of Pediatric Cardiology.* 2nd ed. Williams and Wilkins; 1998.

McMorrow Tuohy AM, Tani LY, Cetta F et al. How many echocardiograms are necessary for follow-up evaluation of patients with Kawasaki disease? *Am J Cardiol.* 2001;88:328–330.

Meyer RA, Hagler D, Huhta J, Smallhorn J, Snider R, Williams R. Guidelines for physician training in pediatric echocardiography. Recommendations of the Society of Pediatric Echocardiography Committee on Physician Training. *Am J Cardiol.* 1987;60:164–165.

Minich LL, Tani LY, Pagotto LT et al. Doppler echocardiography distinguishes between physiologic and "pathologic" mitral regurgitation in patients with rheumatic fever. *Clin Cardiol.* 1997;20:924–926.

Newburger JW, Takahashi M, Gerber M et al; Committee on Rheumatic Fever, Endocarditis and Kawasaki Disease; Council on Cardiovascular Disease in the Young; American Heart Association; American Academy of Pediatrics. Diagnosis, treatment and long-term management of Kawasaki disease: a statement for health professionals from the Committee on Rheumatic Fever, Endocarditis and Kawasaki Disease, Council on Cardiovascular Disease in the Young, American Heart Association. *Circulation.* 2004:110:2747–2771.

Oh JK, Seward JB, Tajik AJ. *The Echo Manual.* Philadelphia: Lippincott Williams and Wilkins; 1999.

Park MK. *Pediatric Cardiology for Practitioners.* St. Louis: Mosby; 1996.

Scott JS, Ettedgui JA, Neches WH. Cost-effective use of echocardiography in children with Kawasaki disease. *Pediatrics.* 1999;104:54–60.

Snider RA, Serwer GA, Ritter SB. *Echocardiography in Pediatric Heart Disease.* St Louis: Mosby; 1997.

Yi MS, Kimball TR, Tsevat J et al. Evaluation of heart murmurs in children: cost-effectiveness and practical implications. *J Pediatr.* 2002;141:504–511.

*Thanks to Kaliope Berdusis, MBA, RDCS, FASE, for her help in preparing the echocardiographic images in this chapter.

CHAPTER 61

Intracardiac Electrophysiology Studies

Barbara J. Deal, MD

INDICATIONS

- Evaluation of tachycardia mechanism, in preparation for catheter ablation procedure.
- Evaluation of wide QRS tachycardia, where ECG interpretation does not clarify mechanism of tachycardia.
- Evaluation of sudden cardiac arrest.
- Evaluation of unexplained syncope.
- Risk stratification for risk of cardiac arrest in patients with repaired congenital heart disease.
- Evaluation of conduction system, or risk of tachycardia, particularly prior to surgery for congenital heart disease.

CONTRAINDICATIONS

- Lack of vascular access.

EQUIPMENT

- Cardiac catheterization laboratory; nursing and technical support staff.
- Biplane fluoroscopy.
- Electrode catheters, usually multiple, with recording equipment.
- Sedation and intravenous access as necessary.
- Cardiac defibrillator.
- Resuscitation medications.

RISKS

- Vascular injury, peripheral or coronary.
- Bleeding.
- Infection.
- Pneumothorax.
- Cardiac perforation.
- Thromboembolism.
- Initiation of hemodynamically unstable arrhythmia, or conversion of one mechanism of tachycardia into another tachycardia.

- Arrhythmias may require direct current cardioversion or defibrillation.
- Radiation exposure.
- Risk of death: < 0.5%.

PEARLS AND TIPS

- Invasive electrophysiology studies are performed prior to virtually all ablation procedures.
- Patients with unexplained cardiac arrest, particularly with congenital heart disease, may undergo electrophysiologic studies to identify cause and direct therapy.
- In the setting of structural heart disease, electrophysiologic studies may help identify patients at increased risk of sudden cardiac arrest, such as patients with repaired tetralogy of Fallot.
- Patients with cardiac ion channelopathies, such as long QT syndrome, do not generally undergo invasive electrophysiology studies.

PATIENT PREPARATION

- Patient should not have any oral intake for at least 4 hours before the study.
- Sedation is administered; general anesthesia is often preferred for lengthy procedures or for younger patients.
- Intravenous access is necessary, usually femoral venous, often bilaterally and multiple, in addition to internal jugular or subclavian venous access.

PATIENT POSITIONING

- Supine, with protection of airway.
- Arms are positioned at sides for long procedures, to avoid potential brachial plexus injury.
- Adequate padding to avoid pressure injury is needed for extremities and head.
- Shielding of gonads from radiation is necessary.

ANATOMY REVIEW

- Catheters are positioned in atria, at atrioventricular nodal region, and in right ventricular apex for basic procedures.
- Additional catheters are positioned in coronary sinus, coursing posteriorly to mitral valve, to record left atrial activation.
- Left ventricular or esophageal recordings may be added.

PROCEDURE

- Using sterile preparation with Seldinger percutaneous entry technique into veins or an artery, electrode catheters are advanced to the heart through vascular sheaths, and positioned using fluoroscopy.

- Catheters are connected to recording equipment and filter box to allow electrogram display and recording; real-time and review mode of tracings available.
- Catheter positioning is optimized based on size of electrograms recorded, pacing capture thresholds, and anatomic positioning.
- For diagnostic purposes, pacing may initiate *reentrant* cardiac arrhythmias, allowing interpretation of mechanism of tachycardia.
- Mapping may be performed to precisely localize critical part of tachycardia circuit, or origin of *automatic* arrhythmia; performed in preparation for ablation procedures.
- For therapeutic purposes, pacing may be performed from catheter, using narrow pulse width (2 msec), and pacing output (2–8 mA).
- Pacing is generally performed at rates 10–20% faster than the underlying rhythm, for brief intervals of 2–4 beats, up to 30 seconds or longer as needed.
- Following completion of procedure, catheters and sheaths are removed, and hemostasis is obtained with pressure.
- Monitoring of peripheral pulse needed after arterial access.

INTERPRETATION AND MONITORING

- Interpretation of tachycardia mechanisms, conduction system, and risk stratification for cardiac arrest are performed.

COMPLICATIONS

- Occur in 1–2% of procedures.
- Vascular complications are more frequent in smaller patients.
- Most intracardiac electrophysiology studies are performed in children > 12 kg, to minimize vascular complications.
- Cardiac perforation may occur, particularly during transseptal procedures for access to the left atrium.
- Sedation complications.

FOLLOW-UP

- Relative to arrhythmia diagnosis.

REFERENCES

Tracy CM, Akhtar M, DiMarco JP et al. American College of Cardiology/American Heart Association clinical competence statement on invasive electrophysiology studies, catheter ablation, and cardioversion. *Circulation.* 2000;102:2309–2320.

Zipes DP, DiMarco JP, Gillette PC et al. Guidelines for clinical intracardiac electrophysiological and catheter ablation procedures. *J Am Coll Cardiol.* 1995;26:555–573.

CHAPTER 62

Catheter Ablation

Barbara J. Deal, MD

INDICATIONS

- Treatment of supraventricular tachycardia (SVT).
  - Life-threatening arrhythmia unresponsive to medications.
  - Younger children with arrhythmia refractory to antiarrhythmic medications.
  - Older children with recurrent SVT.
  - Older children with SVT associated with preexcitation.
- Treatment of ventricular tachycardia.
  - Younger children with life-threatening ventricular tachycardia refractory to medications.
  - Older children with recurrent ventricular tachycardia refractory to medications.
  - Older children with recurrent ventricular tachycardia who are unable to tolerate medications due to side effects, or who choose to have procedure.

CONTRAINDICATIONS

Absolute

- Lack of vascular access.

Relative

- Infants with arrhythmia controlled by medications.
- Patients with multiorgan system disease.
- Patients with hemodynamic instability unable to tolerate procedure or anesthesia.

EQUIPMENT

- Cardiac catheterization laboratory.
- Biplane fluoroscopy.
- Monitoring for continuous heart rate, blood pressure, oxygen saturation.
- Respiratory monitoring and support.
- Vascular access.
- Anesthesia.

- Resuscitation equipment, including medications and cardiac defibrillator.
- Electrode catheters, ablation catheters, energy delivery generator.

RISKS

- Hemodynamically unstable arrhythmias.
- Bleeding.
- Infection.
- Vascular injury, including coronary artery damage.
- Pneumothorax.
- Cardiac perforation.
- Thromboembolism.
- Stroke.
- Radiation exposure.
- Cardiac valve injury.
- Conduction system injury, including complete heart block; may necessitate implantation of permanent pacemaker.
- Risk of injuring the normal conduction system is highest for right septal ablation sites.
- Cardiac arrest.

—[■■■]—

- Risks are higher for small children (< 12–15 kg); lesion growth occurs in the immature heart.

PEARLS AND TIPS

- Not all arrhythmias are amenable to catheter ablation.
- Highest success rates are for SVT due to accessory connections or for atrioventricular nodal reentry tachycardia.
- Automatic atrial tachycardias, especially due to a single automatic focus, are amenable to ablation, with slightly lower success rates than above.
- Ablation of ventricular tachycardias: Lower success rate than SVT.
- Primary electrical disorders, such as long QT syndrome, are not amenable to catheter ablation.
- Availability of noncontact mapping systems and "global positioning" systems reduces fluoroscopy time.
- Neonatal SVT often improves substantially during first 18 months of life and frequently recurs later, such as ages 5–8 and 10–13 years.
- Delaying intervention until child is older and larger may be indicated.

PATIENT PREPARATION

- Patient should not have any oral intake for at least 4 hours before the study.
- Antiarrhythmic medications are generally withdrawn for at least 5 half-lives prior to ablation.
- Sedation is administered; general anesthesia is often preferred for lengthy procedures or for younger patients.

■ Intravenous access is necessary, usually femoral venous, often bilaterally and multiple, in addition to internal jugular or subclavian venous access.

PATIENT POSITIONING

■ Supine, with protection of airway.

■ Arms are positioned at sides for long procedures, to avoid potential brachial plexus injury.

■ Adequate padding to avoid pressure injury is needed for extremities and head.

■ Shielding of gonads from radiation is necessary.

ANATOMY REVIEW

■ **Accessory connections** are located along atrioventricular valve annuli.
  • Tricuspid or mitral valve ring.
  • Most common location is at left lateral mitral annulus.

■ **Atrioventricular nodal reentry tachycardia:** Ablation performed between tricuspid valve and coronary sinus os region below compact atrioventricular node region.

■ **Automatic atrial foci**
  • More commonly located in right atrium, near atrial appendage or along crista terminalis.
  • Left atrial foci, particularly near entrance of pulmonary veins, are also present.

■ **Atrial reentry tachycardia**
  • Usually in setting of repaired congenital heart disease (atrial septal defects, Senning or Mustard repair of transposition of the great arteries, Ebstein anomaly of tricuspid valve, Fontan-type repairs for single ventricle).
  • Atrial circuits often near inferior right atrium/tricuspid valve isthmus but may have multiple circuits related to surgical incisions.

■ **Ventricular tachycardia** is often in right ventricular outflow tract or near surgical incision/patch of repaired congenital heart disease.

PROCEDURE

■ Following intracardiac electrophysiology study, including mapping of tachycardia circuit or focus, ablation catheter is introduced into heart either transvenously or retrogradely via aorta.

■ Ablation catheter is positioned at optimal site, based on tachycardia mapping and electrogram appearance.

■ Energy is delivered via catheter; by damaging tissue, the electrical activity producing or participating in tachycardia is eliminated.

■ Present energy sources include the following:
  • Radiofrequency energy (thermal).
  • Cryoablation.

■ Newer sources, such as microwave, are under development.

■ To assess efficacy of lesion delivery, test with pacing, baseline and with catecholamine infusion; repeat testing after waiting period.

■ Anticoagulation is used during mapping of left atrium and ventricle.

■ At conclusion of procedure, catheters and sheaths are removed, and hemostasis is obtained.

MONITORING

■ Due to risk of cardiac perforation or vascular injury, careful monitoring of vital signs and rhythm is needed, with prompt echocardiogram to assess for pericardial effusion as needed.

COMPLICATIONS

■ Occur in 1–8% of procedures.

■ Major complications occur in less than 2% of cases.

CAVEATS

■ **Acute success rates** vary depending on type of arrhythmia and ablation site.
  • 98% for left lateral accessory connections.
  • 90% for right-sided accessory connections.
  • 60–80% for atrial reentry tachycardia.
  • For VT, acute success rates of 60–90%.

■ **Recurrence risks** also vary depending on arrhythmia mechanism and location.
  • Lowest for left lateral accessory connections (5–10%).
  • Highest for atrial reentry tachycardia (30–80%), followed by right-sided accessory connections (10–25%).

■ Most recurrences occur in first several months after procedure, although late recurrences years later are also seen.

FOLLOW-UP

■ Immediate.
  • Monitor peripheral pulses.
  • Chest pain or respiratory distress may indicate coronary artery injury, pericardial effusion, embolic phenomenon, or pneumothorax.
  • Obtain electrocardiogram and monitor rhythm.

■ Late follow-up for long-term complications: Studies are ongoing to assess late complications, such as scarring.

REFERENCES

Dubin AM, Van Hare GF. Radiofrequency catheter ablation: indications and complications. *Pediatr Cardiol.* 2000;21:551–556.

Friedman RA, Walsh EP, Silka MJ et al. NASPE Expert Consensus Conference: Radiofrequency catheter ablation in children with and without congenital heart disease. *Pacing Clin Electrophysiol.* 2002;25:1000–1017.

Van Hare GF, Javitz H, Carmelli D et al. Prospective assessment after pediatric cardiac ablation: demographics, medical profiles, and initial outcomes. *J Cardiovasc Electrophysiol.* 2004; 15:759–770.

Van Hare GF, Javitz H, Carmelli D et al. Prospective assessment after pediatric cardiac ablation: recurrence at 1 year after initially successful ablation of supraventricular tachycardia. *Heart Rhythm.* 2004;1:188–196.

CHAPTER 63

Tilt-Table Testing

Barbara J. Deal, MD

INDICATIONS

- Evaluation of syncope of uncertain origin.
- Evaluation of symptoms suggestive of autonomic dysfunction, such as
  - Presyncope.
  - Atypical seizures.
  - Orthostatic symptoms.
- Distinguish between psychosomatic and neurally mediated symptoms.

CONTRAINDICATIONS

- Complete heart block or profound bradycardia at rest.
- Significant left or right ventricular outflow obstructive lesions.
- Generally not performed in patients with structural heart disease and syncope, unless all other testing, including invasive electrophysiology testing, is unrevealing.

EQUIPMENT

- Tilt table: Motor-driven table, capable of 70-degree upright positioning.
- Monitoring for continuous heart rate and blood pressure recording.
- Intravenous access.
- Resuscitation equipment, including medications and cardiac defibrillator.

RISKS

- Prolonged asystole.
- Hypotension.
- Seizures.
- Cardiac arrest (very rare).

PEARLS AND TIPS

- Most episodes of vasovagal or neurally mediated syncope can be elucidated by careful history of the events surrounding clinical episodes.
- Tilt-table testing does not provide additional useful information for most straightforward cases of vasovagal syncope.
- Tilt-table testing is helpful in the following settings:
  - Recurrent syncope of uncertain etiology.
  - Syncope without prodromal symptoms.
  - Patients with normal electroencephalogram and a diagnosis of a seizure disorder.
  - Symptoms occurring while standing.
- Patients with syncope should have an ECG performed to exclude possibility of long QT syndrome.

PATIENT PREPARATION

- Patient should not have any oral intake for at least 4 hours before the study.

PATIENT POSITIONING

- Initially supine.
- Patient is secured to table with straps and given a footrest for support.

ANATOMY REVIEW

- During standing, with decreased filling of ventricular chambers, C-reactive fibers in myocardium are stimulated and initiate afferent response to brain.
- In response, neural reflex is initiated with drop in blood pressure or heart rate, or both.
- Patients with neurally mediated syncope have profound decrease in blood pressure or heart rate or both, resulting in the following:
  - Dizziness.
  - Nausea.
  - Headache.
  - Abdominal discomfort.
  - Syncope (often).
- With profound hypotension or asystole, patient may experience seizure due to cerebral hypoperfusion.

PROCEDURE

- Obtain intravenous access.

- Monitor heart rate and blood pressure in baseline state while patient is supine.
- Slowly raise table to 60–80-degree angle.
  - Patient remains in this position for 15–60 minutes, depending on protocol.
  - Test is terminated promptly if significant symptoms develop.
- Return the patient to the supine position at end of baseline testing or when significant symptoms develop.
- Test may be repeated with pharmacologic challenge, usually isoproterenol infusion of 1–3 mcg/min.

INTERPRETATION AND MONITORING

- Positive tilt-table responses to upright positioning trigger symptoms similar to clinical complaints.
- The following responses describe positive responses:
  - Vasodepressor response: Drop in systolic blood pressure.
  - Cardio-inhibitory response: Significant bradycardia.
  - Mixed response: Both drop in blood pressure and heart rate.
  - Postural tachycardia response: Increase in heart rate > 30 bpm during first 10 minutes of upright position.
  - Psychogenic: Cerebral vasoconstriction, without change in heart rate or blood pressure.

COMPLICATIONS

- Occur rarely.
- Asystole and seizures occur during profound response to upright positioning.

CAVEAT

- Reproducibility (60–90%), specificity (90%), and false-positivity (10%) are limiting factors.

FOLLOW-UP

- Relative to management of symptoms.

REFERENCES

Grubb BP. Neurocardiogenic syncope and related disorders of orthostatic intolerance. *Circulation.* 2005;111:2997–3006.

Massin MM. Neurocardiogenic syncope in children. Current concepts in diagnosis and management. *Pediatr Drugs.* 2003; 5:327–334.

McLeod KA. Dysautonomia and neurocardiogenic syncope. *Curr Opin Cardiol.* 2001;16:92–96.

CHAPTER 64

Colonoscopy

Boris Sudel, MD and B U.K. Li, MD

INDICATIONS

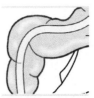

- Chronic diarrhea.
- Lower gastrointestinal bleeding.
- Abdominal pain.
- Evaluation of radiographic abnormalities.
  - Ulcerations.
  - Filling defects.
  - Strictures.
- Initial diagnosis and follow-up evaluation of inflammatory bowel disease.
- Removal of foreign bodies.
- Dilatation of colonic strictures.
- Diagnosis and removal of polyps.
- Histopathologic evaluation of pinhead-sized biopsy specimens.

CONTRAINDICATIONS

Absolute

- Cardiorespiratory collapse.
- Hemodynamically unstable patient.
- Unstable airway.
- Intestinal perforation.
- Peritonitis.
- Cervical spine trauma.
- Toxic, fulminant colitis.

Relative

- Coagulopathy (prothrombin time > 18 sec).
- Thrombocytopenia (platelet count < 100,000/μL).
- Intestinal tract surgery within previous month.
- Food intake within previous 6 hours.
- Bowel obstruction.

EQUIPMENT

- Fiberoptic or video endoscopes.
- Biopsy forceps.
- Snares.
- Nets and baskets.
- Heater probes.
- Electrocautery probes and snares.
- Balloon-dilation devices.

RISKS

- Anesthesia complications.
- Bleeding.
- Perforation.

PEARLS AND TIPS

- Biopsies are required because characteristics of many disorders may only be detectable under the microscope.

PATIENT PREPARATION

- Obtain medical history and physical examination for clearance from pulmonary, cardiovascular, and hematologic standpoints.
- Obtain laboratory tests, if needed.
  - Hemoglobin levels.
  - Platelet count.
  - Prothrombin time.
  - Partial thromboplastin time.
- Primary care providers can prepare patients and families by explaining that the colonoscopy provides detailed diagnostic information and rarely causes complications (1/2000 chance of significant bleeding or perforation).
- Have parents sign a consent form.
- Bowel preparation.
  - Clear liquids for 24 hours prior to procedure (infants: 12 hours); avoid red-colored fluids.
  - Sodium phosphate, magnesium citrate, MiraLax (for 4 days), polyethylene glycol (PEG) lavage solution, enemas (saline or phosphate) if needed.
  - No oral intake after midnight before procedure.
- Antibiotics for endocarditis prophylaxis in at-risk patients.
- Antibiotics for immunosuppressed patients or those with central lines (controversial).

PATIENT POSITIONING

- Left lateral decubitus.
- Supine.

ANATOMY REVIEW

- The colon is divided into 5 sections:
  - Sigmoid.
  - Descending.
  - Transverse.
  - Ascending.
  - Cecum.
- The rectum as well as the sigmoid and descending colon are the areas where juvenile polyps and ulcerative colitis are commonly seen.
- The junction between the descending and transverse colons is usually marked by the bluish blush of the spleen.
- The transverse colon can be recognized by the triangular-shaped folds.
- The junction between the transverse and ascending (or right colon) is usually marked by the bluish blush of the liver.
- The cecum can be verified by finding the small appendiceal opening, the ileocecal valve, or seeing light transilluminate the right lower quadrant.
- The cecum and terminal ileum are often involved in Crohn disease.

PROCEDURE

- Administer oxygen by nasal cannula.
- Start intravenous sedation or gas anesthesia via an endotracheal catheter.
  - Heavier sedation is required for colonoscopy than for upper endoscopy.
  - Sedation options include midazolam plus fentanyl for conscious sedation, but it is rarely sufficient for full colonoscopy; propofol; and general anesthesia.
- Vital signs are monitored continuously.
- Place child in a left lateral position.
- Introduce the colonoscope tip into the rectum and advance in sequence:
  - Sigmoid colon.
  - Descending colon.
  - Transverse colon.
  - Ascending colon.
  - Cecum (Figure 64–1).
- In suspected inflammatory bowel disease, cannulation of the terminal ileum is important but is challenging because the ileocecal valve cannot be directly visualized.
- Multiple biopsies are taken from the terminal ileum, ascending colon, transverse colon, descending colon, and rectum as the colonoscope is removed.

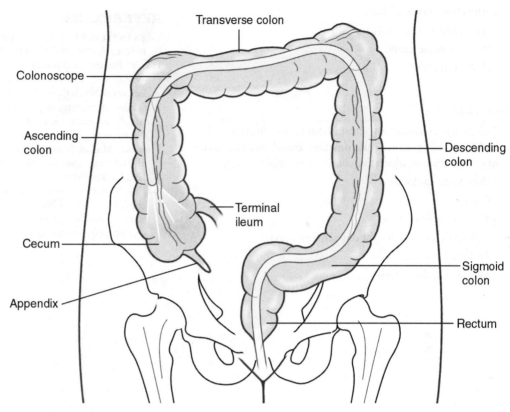

Figure 64–1. *Anatomy of colon with colonoscope in place.*

INTERPRETATION AND MONITORING

- Pulse oximetry.
- Cardiac monitor.
- Blood pressure monitor.
- Macroscopic picture interpretation.
- Histopathology.
- Special tests: Cultures.

COMPLICATIONS

- Overall in < 2% of cases.
- Anesthesia related.
  - Hypoxia.
  - Aspiration.
  - Postoperative nausea and vomiting.
  - Allergy to medications or latex, or both.
  - Hypotension.
  - Respiratory and cardiac arrest.
  - Malignant hyperthermia.
- Intramural duodenal hematoma.
- Bleeding.

---[■■■]---

- Colonoscopy is challenging because of the tendency of the scope to become looped.

- Perforation, mucosal tears.
- Fatal massive air embolism.
- Infection, bacteremia.
- Splenic laceration.

FOLLOW-UP

- Follow-up colonoscopy examinations are indicated in children with chronic inflammatory bowel disease, such as Crohn disease, ulcerative colitis, or multiple polyps.
- When to call a doctor:
  - Fever.
  - Nausea and vomiting.
  - Melanotic stool or bright red hematochezia.
  - Abdominal pain.
  - Abdominal distention.

REFERENCES

Faigel DO et al. Preparation of patients for GI endoscopy. *Gastrointest Endosc.* 2003;57:446–450.

Fox V. Patient preparation and general considerations. In: Walker WA et al. *Pediatric Gastrointestinal Diseases.* 4th ed. Lewiston, NY: B.C. Decker; 2004.

Principles of training in gastrointestinal endoscopy. From the ASGE. American Society for Gastrointestinal Endoscopy. *Gastrointest Endosc.* 1999;49:845–853.

Thomson M et al. Ileoscopy and enteroscopy. In: Walker WA et al. *Pediatric Gastrointestinal Diseases.* 4th ed. Lewiston, NY: B.C. Decker; 2004.

Waring JP et al; American Society for Gastrointestinal Endoscopy, Standards of Practice Committee. Guidelines for conscious sedation and monitoring during gastrointestinal endoscopy. *Gastrointest Endosc.* 2003;58:317–322.

CHAPTER 65

Esophagogastroduodenoscopy

Boris Sudel, MD and B U.K. Li, MD

INDICATIONS

- Vomiting.
- Hematemesis.
- Melena.
- Chronic diarrhea.
- Failure to thrive.
- Abdominal pain.
- Dysphagia, odynophagia.
- Foreign body.
- Caustic ingestion.
- Histopathologic, biochemical, and microbial evaluations of pinhead-sized biopsy specimens and sampled fluids (eg, pancreatic).

CONTRAINDICATIONS

Absolute

- Cardiorespiratory collapse.
- Unstable airway.
- Intestinal perforation.
- Peritonitis.
- Cervical spine trauma.

Relative

- Coagulopathy (prothrombin time > 18 sec).
- Thrombocytopenia (platelet count < 100,000/μL).
- Intestinal tract surgery within previous 1 month.
- Food intake within previous 6 hours.
- Bowel obstruction.

EQUIPMENT

- Fiberoptic or video endoscopes.
- Biopsy forceps.
- Snares.
- Nets and baskets.

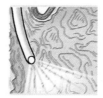

- Sclerotherapy needles.
- Banding devices.
- Heater probes.
- Electrocautery probes.
- Balloon-dilation devices.
- Guidewires and wire-guided bougie dilators.

RISKS

- Anesthesia complications.
- Bleeding.
- Perforation.

PEARLS AND TIPS

- Biopsies are required because characteristics of many disorders may only be detectable under the microscope.
- Retroflection with a good view of the cardia may demonstrate source of bleeding or prolapse gastropathy.

PATIENT PREPARATION

- Obtain medical history and physical examination for clearance from pulmonary, cardiovascular, and hematologic standpoints.
- Obtain laboratory tests, if needed.
  - Hemoglobin levels.
  - Platelet count.
  - Prothrombin time.
  - Partial thromboplastin time.
- Primary care providers can prepare patients and families by explaining that the procedure provides detailed diagnostic information and rarely causes complications (1/2000 chance of significant bleeding or perforation).
- Have parents sign a consent form.
- No oral intake for 6 hours before the procedure.
- Antibiotics for endocarditis prophylaxis in at-risk cardiac patients.

PATIENT POSITIONING

- Left lateral decubitus.
- Supine.

ANATOMY REVIEW

- The esophagus is divided into proximal, middle (8–10 cm above the gastroesophageal junction), and distal regions.
- Peptic injuries are usually located in the distal portion.

- Eosinophilic (allergic) injuries are usually located in both the middle and distal regions.
- The stomach is composed of the cardia (underside of the gastroesophageal junction), fundus or dome of the stomach, body or main portion with rugal folds, and antrum the distal portion without rugae containing the pylorus (Figure 65–1).
- Peptic gastritis and *Helicobacter pylori* infection are usually located in the antrum.
- The duodenum consists of the bulb, the smooth portion immediately after the pylorus and the second portion with circular valvulae conniventes and the ampulla of Vater.
- Peptic injuries are found in the bulb.
- Celiac disease is found in the second portion and beyond.

PROCEDURE

- Administer oxygen by nasal cannula.
- Start intravenous sedation or gas anesthesia via an endotracheal catheter.
  - Sedation options include midazolam plus fentanyl or meperidine for conscious sedation, propofol, or general anesthesia.
- Topical anesthesia is sprayed into the oropharynx.
- Vital signs are monitored continuously.
- Place the child in a left lateral position.
- The endoscope tip is set in a slightly curved arc and introduced in the midline plane through the mouth past the upper esophageal sphincter.
- The esophagus is examined for peptic and allergic injuries.
- Next, the gastric body, antrum, and pylorus are examined for peptic and *H pylori*–associated gastritis.
- After that, the duodenal bulb is examined for peptic erosions, and the second portion is assessed for celiac and Crohn disease.
- Finally, the stomach fundus is examined by 180-degree retroflexion of the endoscope.
- Multiple biopsies are taken from the duodenum, gastric antrum and body, and distal and middle esophagus as the endoscope is removed.

MONITORING

- Pulse oximetry.
- Cardiac monitor.
- Blood pressure monitor.
- Macroscopic picture interpretation.
- Histopathology.
- Special tests include the following:
  - Cultures.

- Disaccharidase enzyme levels.
- CLO test.
- *H pylori* culture.
- Pancreatic enzymes (following CCK/secretin stimulation).

COMPLICATIONS

- Anesthesia related.
  - Hypoxia.
  - Aspiration.
  - Postoperative nausea and vomiting.
  - Allergy to medications, latex.
  - Hypotension.
  - Respiratory and cardiac arrest.
  - Malignant hyperthermia.
- Intramural duodenal hematoma.
- Bleeding.
- Perforation, mucosal tears.
- Fatal massive air embolism.

FOLLOW-UP

- Follow-up esophagogastroduodenoscopies are indicated in children with peptic ulcers, allergic esophagitis, and Crohn disease.
- When to call a doctor:
  - Fever.
  - Nausea and vomiting.
  - Melanotic stool or bright red hematemesis.
  - Abdominal pain.
  - Abdominal distention.
  - Chest pain.

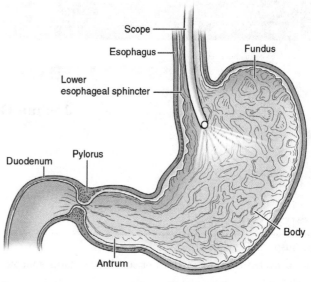

Figure 65–1. *Anatomy of the esophagus and stomach with esophagogastroduodenoscope in place.*

- Overall, complications are less than 1%.

REFERENCES

Fox V. Patient preparation and general considerations. In: Walker WA et al. *Pediatric Gastrointestinal Diseases.* 4th ed. Lewiston, NY: B.C. Decker; 2004.

Schaeppi M et al. Upper gastrointestinal endoscopy. In: Walker WA et al. *Pediatric Gastrointestinal Diseases.* 4th ed. Lewiston, NY: B.C. Decker; 2004.

Waring JP, Baron TH, Hirota WK et al; American Society for Gastrointestinal Endoscopy, Standards of Practice Committee. Guidelines for conscious sedation and monitoring during gastrointestinal endoscopy. *Gastrointest Endosc.* 2003;58: 317–322.

Principles of training in gastrointestinal endoscopy. From the ASGE. American Society for Gastrointestinal Endoscopy. *Gastrointest Endosc.* 1999;49:845–853.

Faigel DO, Eisen GM, Baron TH et al. Preparation of patients for GI endoscopy. *Gastrointest Endosc.* 2003;57:446–450.

[CHAPTER 66]

Electroencephalography

Joshua Goldstein, MD

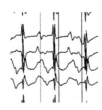
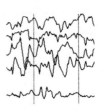
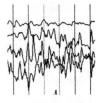

INDICATIONS

- Suspected epilepsy.
- Suspected ongoing seizures or subclinical status epilepticus.
- Epilepsy characterization.
- Unexplained encephalopathy or coma.
- Monitoring medication-induced coma.
- Paralyzed patients with possible seizures.
- Medication titration.

RISKS

- Scalp abrasion after prolonged monitoring is a minor risk.

PEARLS AND TIPS

- Automatic spike and seizure detection paradigms are not sensitive or specific enough to base clinical decisions on at this time.
- Cardiac and respiratory artifacts are often misinterpreted as epileptiform.
- Patients with focal (localization related) epilepsy may have normal or near normal interictal electroencephalograms (EEGs).
- In neonates, there is a paucity of clear epileptiform abnormalities even in patients with frequent seizures, thus prolonged monitoring should be strongly considered in place of routine studies.
- EEG must be considered in clinical context.
- An abnormal EEG is not always suggestive of epilepsy and may reflect a nonepileptic encephalopathy.

PATIENT PREPARATION

- The EEG is not painful or dangerous, although the placement of the electrodes may require the child's restraint for a few minutes.

- Patient's hair should be washed and free of oils and chemical agents prior to the study; any braids in hair need to be removed.
- Metal EEG electrodes are placed over the scalp in standardized positions and fixed with a variety of specialty adhesives.
  - The glue can leave a small red welt on the scalp, which will resolve in a few days.
  - Alcohol can be helpful in removing stuck adhesive.
- Impedance is checked to determine appropriate electrical connectivity.
- The electrode wires are attached to the head box, which is then attached to the monitoring unit (usually a computer with screen for EEG display).

PROCEDURE

- The study is performed by placing electrodes each approximately the size of a pea on the scalp and affixing them with some type of adhesive (usually paste or glue).
- Most commonly, 21 electrodes are affixed.
- The electrodes are connected to the EEG machine by thin wires usually pulled together into a "ponytail."
- The patient may be asked to perform certain "maneuvers" that may bring out EEG abnormalities.
  - Intermittently closing his or her eyes.
  - Watching flashing strobe lights.
  - Hyperventilating for 2–3 minutes.
- Sleep is often important to capture as well, and parents may be asked to keep their child awake on the night before the study.
- A routine outpatient EEG usually is performed for approximately 45–60 minutes but longer studies may be required.
- After the EEG is complete, the electrodes can be easily removed after the EEG machine is turned off.

INTERPRETATION

- A normal EEG result rarely rules out the possibility of seizures just as an abnormal EEG may not diagnose epilepsy or risk of recurrent seizures.
- EEG must be used in the context of a neurologic evaluation and only rarely can replace it entirely.
- Appropriate filters should be placed on the recording to minimize electrical and mechanical interference.
- A montage (display paradigm for the electrodes) is selected for appropriate review.
- The study should be read and intermittently reviewed by a trained electroencephalographer.

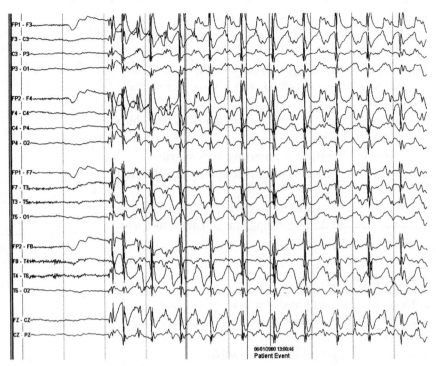

Figure 66–1. *Generalized seizure (absence seizure).*

- Background architecture can be compared with age norms and may be correlated with degree or cause of encephalopathy.

- Focal findings (focal slowing, attenuation, interictal epileptiform discharges) suggest a focal structural abnormality but are not always etiologically specific.

- Interictal epileptiform discharges (spikes, spike waves, and generalized discharges) suggest the predisposition toward seizures but are not always diagnostic.

- Generalized discharges suggest generalized epilepsy.

- Focal discharges (spikes and spike waves) suggest focal epilepsy (Figures 66–1 and 66–2).

- Background continuity can be useful in following medication as well as physiologically induced comas (Figure 66–3).

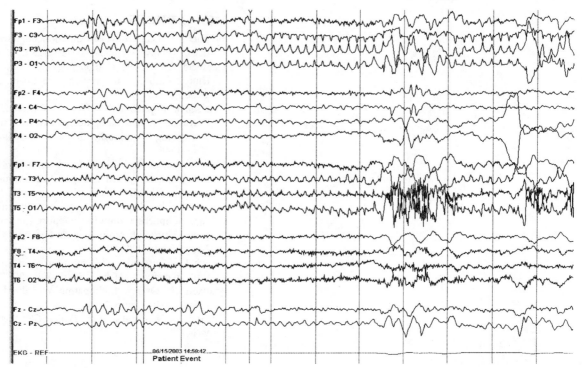

Figure 66–2. *Focal seizure.*

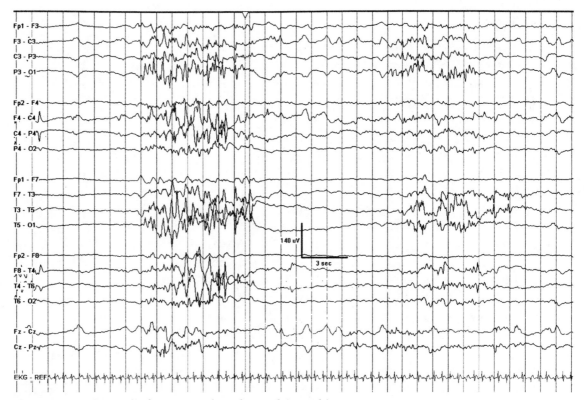

Figure 66–3. *Suppression burst pattern (note shortened time scale).*

REFERENCES

Brenner RP. EEG in convulsive and nonconvulsive status epilepticus. *J Clin Neurophysiol.* 2004;21:319–331.

Camfield P, Camfield C. Epileptic syndromes in childhood: clinical features, outcomes, and treatment. *Epilepsia.* 2002; 43 Suppl 3:27–32.

Claassen J, Mayer SA, Kowalski RG, Emerson RG, Hirsch LJ. Detection of electrographic seizures with continuous EEG monitoring in critically ill patients. *Neurology.* 2004;62: 1743–1748.

Flink R et al; Commission of European Affairs of the International League Against Epilepsy: Subcommission on European Guidelines. Guidelines for the use of EEG methodology in the diagnosis of epilepsy. International League Against Epilepsy: commission report. Commission on European Affairs: Subcommission on European Guidelines. *Acta Neurol Scand.* 2002;106:1–7.

Hirsch LJ. Continuous EEG monitoring in the intensive care unit: an overview. *J Clin Neurophysiol.* 2004;21:332–340.

Mattson RH. Overview: idiopathic generalized epilepsies. *Epilepsia.* 2003;44 Suppl 2:2–6.

Zupanc ML. Neonatal seizures. *Pediatr Clin North Am.* 2004;51: 961–978.

CHAPTER 67

Percutaneous Kidney Biopsy

Jerome C. Lane, MD

INDICATIONS

- Persistent or recurrent gross hematuria of glomerular origin (ie, not related to urinary infection or bladder abnormalities).
- Persistent, nonorthostatic proteinuria.
- Nephrotic syndrome.
  - Younger than 18 months or older than 8 years.
  - As a result of systemic disease (eg, systemic lupus erythematosus or other collagen vascular disease, vasculitis).
  - As a result of glomerulonephritis (low C3, hypertension, hematuria, or decreased renal function).
  - Corticosteroid-resistant nephrotic syndrome.
- Acute nephritis.
  - As a result of systemic disease (systemic lupus erythematosus, vasculitis).
  - Normal C3.
  - Low C3 for > 8 weeks (unlikely to be postinfectious nephritis).
  - With nephrotic syndrome.
  - With deteriorating kidney function.
- When the cause of acute kidney insufficiency is not apparent, consider obtaining a biopsy in selected cases:
  - Nephrotic syndrome.
  - Glomerulonephritis.
  - Vasculitis.
  - Systemic lupus erythematosus or other systemic disease.
- Obtain biopsy in selected cases of chronic kidney insufficiency to establish diagnosis, prognosis, and risk of recurrence.
- Follow up on prior biopsy in chronic kidney disease to establish disease progression, severity, and prognosis.
- Kidney transplant with rise in creatinine.

CONTRAINDICATIONS

Absolute

- Solitary, ectopic, or horseshoe kidney.
- Bleeding diathesis.
- Uncontrolled hypertension.
- Abnormal kidney vascular supply or arteriovenous malformation.
- Kidney tumor.
- Large kidney cysts.
- Kidney abscess.
- Pyelonephritis.
- Patient who is unwilling or unable to cooperate (insufficient sedation when indicated).

Relative

- Severe obesity.
- Hydronephrosis.
- Small kidney (as seen in end-stage kidney disease, for example).

EQUIPMENT

- Ultrasound.
- Biopsy needle (in general, automated, spring-loaded system preferred).
- Biopsy tray (sterile drapes, scalpel, syringes and needles for injecting local anesthetic, gauze).
- Specimen container with saline, on ice.

PATIENT PREPARATION

- Before the procedure obtain following tests:
  - Complete blood count.
  - Prothrombin time.
  - Partial thromboplastin time.
- Patient should have nothing by mouth as indicated by sedation protocol.
- No nonsteroidal anti-inflammatory drugs for 1–2 weeks prior to procedure.
- Obtain informed consent prior to procedure.
- Review indications, procedure, and risks with patient and family.

PATIENT POSITIONING

- Prone with roll under abdomen (native biopsy).
- Supine (transplant).

ANATOMY REVIEW

- Lower pole of left kidney is preferred but either kidney may be biopsied.

- In many cases of kidney disease, laboratory evaluation of the blood and urine fails to yield a specific diagnosis.
- Occasionally, a clinical syndrome or constellation of laboratory findings might narrow the differential diagnosis; examples include the following:
  - Post-streptococcal glomerulonephritis (acute onset, transient hypocomplementemia, recent streptococcal infection).
  - Systemic lupus erythematosus (positive antinuclear antibody and anti-ds-DNA antibodies, hypocomplementemia, joint pains, and rashes).
  - Minimal change nephrotic syndrome (nephrosis in a school-age child without azotemia, hypocomplementemia, or other complications).
- In these instances, a kidney biopsy might not be required.
- However, in most cases, a tissue specimen is required to establish a specific etiology.

- Consider open biopsy in cases in which relative contraindications are present.

■ For kidney transplant, the lower pole is generally biopsied but depends on placement of kidney and location of adjacent structures (bladder, bowel, blood vessels).

PROCEDURE

■ Administer conscious sedation or general anesthesia.
■ Localize lower pole of kidney by ultrasound and mark on skin.
■ Note the depth of kidney on ultrasound.
■ Prepare and drape site with sterile technique.
■ Infiltrate site with local anesthetic down to capsule of kidney.
■ Make small cutaneous incision.
■ Perform biopsy with needle of choice.
■ Biopsy can be performed safely using skin markings or using "real-time" ultrasound as biopsy needle is advanced toward the kidney.
■ Obtain 2–3 cores of tissue.
■ Ultrasonography may be performed after biopsy to look for large hematoma or other complications.
■ Apply sterile bandage; pressure dressing preferred by some clinicians.

INTERPRETATION AND MONITORING

■ Tissue specimens are generally processed using light microscopy, immunofluorescence, and electron microscopy.
■ Light microscopy.
  • Specimens processed using a number of specialized stains, such as H&E, PAS, Mason's trichrome, and Jones' stains.
  • Particularly useful in identifying inflammatory cells, fibrosis, sclerosis, vascular, and endocapillary changes.
  • Jones' stain, in particular, is useful in visualizing changes in the basement membrane.
■ Immunofluorescence is an essential tool in diagnosing immune-mediated renal diseases, such as systemic lupus erythematosus, IgA nephropathy, and others.
■ Electron microscopy.
  • Particularly useful in examining basement membrane changes and detecting the presence of immune deposits.
  • Also helpful in demonstrating the reticular inclusions characteristic of systemic lupus erythematosus and HIV nephropathy.
■ Traditionally: Supine bedrest and **overnight monitoring** in hospital for 24 hours; hemoglobin checked 6–8 hours after procedure and following morning.
■ More recently, studies suggest safety and efficacy of **same day procedure** and discharge after 4–6 hours of supine bedrest in uncomplicated cases as defined by the following:

■ Kidney biopsy is usually performed as a percutaneous procedure under ultrasound guidance.
■ In high-risk circumstances, an open biopsy is preferred, in which a surgeon exposes and visualizes the kidney directly before performing the biopsy.
■ For a kidney transplant patient, kidney biopsy is usually an outpatient procedure, in which the patient is discharged home after a 4–6 hour period of observation.

• No gross hematuria.

• Normal anatomy (2 kidneys).

• Stable vital signs.

• Fully alert.

• Tolerating oral fluids.

• Minimal pain.

• No history of bleeding diathesis or vascular disease.

• Normal pre-biopsy laboratory test results.

• No azotemia.

• Reliable family who can be easily contacted, understand and agree to instructions, and live within reasonable distance to medical care.

■ Post-biopsy complete blood count might not be performed in this setting.

COMPLICATIONS

■ Minor complications (~15%).

■ Major complications (~5%).

■ Gross hematuria (5–25%).

■ Severe bleeding requiring transfusion (1–2%).

■ Perirenal hematomas can be detected in up to 85% of cases on computed tomography and are usually asymptomatic.

■ Symptomatic hematomas (resulting in decrease of hemoglobin or requiring transfusion, for example) occur in < 2% of cases.

■ Arteriovenous fistula (AVF) is usually asymptomatic and resolves spontaneously; symptomatic AVF occurs in < 0.5% of cases.

■ Injury of other viscera (rare).

■ Injury of renal vessels (rare).

■ Infection (rare).

■ Death: < 0.1%.

■ Pain is generally mild; occasionally, it is severe in up to 3% of patients.

■ Unable to obtain adequate tissue during biopsy (1–2%).

FOLLOW-UP

■ As indicated by results of biopsy.

■ Instruct parents to call immediately should any of the following occur:

• Severe or persistent pain.

• Bleeding at biopsy site.

• Gross hematuria after the first day of biopsy.

• Signs of infection at biopsy site.

■ Sports, strenuous exertion, and heavy lifting are prohibited for 2 weeks following the procedure, after which the patient can return to usual activities.

REFERENCES

al Rasheed SA, al Mugeiren MM, Abdurrahman MB, Elidrissy AT. The outcome of percutaneous renal biopsy in children: an analysis of 120 consecutive cases. *Pediatr Nephrol.* 1990;4: 600–603.

Bohlin AB, Edstrom S, Almgren B, Jaremko G, Jorulf H. Renal biopsy in children: indications, technique and efficacy in 119 consecutive cases. *Pediatr Nephrol.* 1995;9:201–203.

Feneberg R, Schaefer F, Zieger B, Waldherr R, Mehls O, Scharer K. Percutaneous renal biopsy in children: a 27-year experience. *Nephron.* 1998;79:438–446.

Fogo A. Renal pathology. In: Avner ED, Harmon WE, Niaudet P, eds. *Pediatric Nephrology.* 5th ed. Baltimore: Lippincott Williams and Wilkins; 2004:475–500.

Hergesell O, Felten H, Andrassy K, Kuhn K, Ritz E. Safety of ultrasound-guided percutaneous renal biopsy-retrospective analysis of 1090 consecutive cases. *Nephrol Dial Transplant.* 1998;13:975–977.

Simckes AM, Blowey DL, Gyves KM, Alon US. Success and safety of same-day kidney biopsy in children and adolescents. *Pediatr Nephrol.* 2000;14:946–952.

CHAPTER 68

Renal Replacement Therapy

Jerome C. Lane, MD

PERITONEAL DIALYSIS

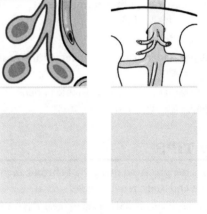

INDICATIONS

- End-stage renal disease.
- Acute kidney failure accompanied by 1 or more of the following:
  - Oliguria or anuria.
  - Uremia (azotemia accompanied by platelet dysfunction and bleeding, change in mental status, or other uremic symptoms).
  - Electrolyte or metabolic disturbance unresponsive to medical management (eg, hyperkalemia, hyponatremia or hypernatremia, acidosis, hypocalcemia, hyperphosphatemia).
  - Inability to provide adequate nutrition or other intravenous therapy due to fluid restriction.
- Inborn error of metabolism: urea cycle disorders, propionic acidemia, maple syrup urine disease (hemodialysis and CRRT more effective and are preferred).
- Dialyzable toxin (hemodialysis and CRRT more effective and are preferred).

CONTRAINDICATIONS

Absolute

- Lack of adequate peritoneal membrane or cavity.
  - Omphalocele.
  - Diaphragmatic hernia.
  - Gastroschisis.

Relative

- Recent abdominal surgery.
- Prior extensive abdominal surgery that might have resulted in adhesions or peritoneal scarring.
- Ventriculo-peritoneal shunt.
- Unsuitable social situation for home dialysis.

EQUIPMENT

- Peritoneal dialysate solutions.
  - Lactate-buffered, electrolyte-balanced dextrose solution most often used.
  - Available as 1.5%, 2.5%, and 4.25% dextrose.
  - Bicarbonate-buffered solutions are available.
  - Icodextrin (glucose polymer) solution available; useful for patients with poor fluid removal.
- Solution warmer (blood transfusion warmer for continuous ambulatory peritoneal dialysis [CAPD] or warming tray on cycler).
- Automated cycler for intermittent peritoneal dialysis (IPD) or continuous cycling peritoneal dialysis (CCPD) or manual exchange set for CAPD.
- Peritoneal dialysis catheter.
  - Surgically placed permanent catheter preferred in most situations.
  - Temporary percutaneous catheter in unstable patients or per center preference for acute kidney failure.

PEARLS AND TIPS

- Peritoneal dialysis is the preferred method of chronic dialysis in children with end-stage renal disease.
- Children receiving peritoneal dialysis have less daytime disruption of school and social activities.
- Because peritoneal dialysis is performed every day, a more liberal fluid and dietary regimen is possible.
- Peritoneal dialysis might be the only option available to small infants who cannot tolerate the large fluid shifts and large extracorporeal circuit volume of hemodialysis, and to those patients who do not have adequate vascular access for hemodialysis.
- However, hemodialysis might be the only option for RRT for those children who have had extensive abdominal surgery, who have a social situation that precludes home dialysis, or in whom peritoneal dialysis has already failed due to repeated bouts of peritonitis or other complications.
- Hemodialysis and CRRT remain the treatments of choice for inborn errors of metabolism and toxic ingestions because peritoneal dialysis does not provide efficient and rapid clearance of metabolites and toxins.

PATIENT PREPARATION

- Educate and train family to use home dialysis in patients with end-stage renal disease.
- Counsel patients with end-stage disease extensively about long-term dialysis options (hemodialysis vs. peritoneal dialysis) and advantages, disadvantages, and risks of each option.

- Renal replacement therapy (RRT) refers to any procedure whereby solute or water, or both, are removed from the body, generally during acute or chronic kidney insufficiency.
- RRT can be divided into intermittent or continuous therapies.
  - Intermittent therapies include hemodialysis and peritoneal dialysis and are indicated for maintenance dialysis in end-stage renal disease or for acute dialysis in stable patients with acute or chronic kidney failure.
  - Continuous renal replacement therapies (CRRT) consist of several types of procedures; the most well known to non-nephrologists is continuous venovenous hemofiltration (CVVH).
  - CRRT is indicated for critically ill, unstable patients and situations in which meticulous continuous control of fluid and electrolytes is indicated.
  - In general, CRRT is performed in the intensive care setting, whereas intermittent RRT can be performed in the inpatient setting, outpatient dialysis unit, or even home.

- Before starting peritoneal dialysis, a peritoneal dialysis catheter must be placed.
  - After insertion, a healing period of several weeks or longer may be needed.
  - Catheter can be used immediately for urgent dialysis, but there is a risk of increased rates of leakage and peritonitis.
  - Surgical placement of the catheter is preferred.
  - However, the catheter can be placed percutaneously at the bedside in unstable patients.

PATIENT POSITIONING

- Generally supine or on side.

ANATOMY REVIEW

- The peritoneum consists of connective tissue covered by mesothelium.
- The visceral peritoneum covers the intraperitoneal organs and receives its arterial blood supply from celiac, superior mesenteric, and inferior mesenteric arteries (Figure 68–1).
- The parietal peritoneum lines the inner abdominal and pelvic walls and the diaphragm and receives its arterial blood supply from adjacent structures.
- Venous drainage of the peritoneum occurs via the portal vein.

PROCEDURE

- Dialysate fluid is instilled into the peritoneal cavity via a peritoneal dialysis catheter manually or by automated cycler.
- Dialysate fluid is drained into a drainage bag and the peritoneal cavity is refilled with fresh fluid at regular intervals.
- Dialysis prescription is individualized for each patient regarding:
  - Modality (eg, CAPD, CCPD, IPD).
  - Type and concentration of dialysis solution.
  - Volume of fluid (fill volume).
  - Length of time in abdomen (dwell time).
  - Number of cycles.
  - Total treatment time.
  - Additives to dialysis solution (potassium, heparin, antibiotics, amino acids).
- The peritoneal dialysis solution generally contains a prescribed concentration of dextrose (1.5, 2.5, or 4.25%)and a fixed amount of electrolytes and buffer (sodium chloride, lactate, magnesium, and calcium).
- The concentration of dextrose provides an osmotic gradient for movement of water from the blood vessels lining

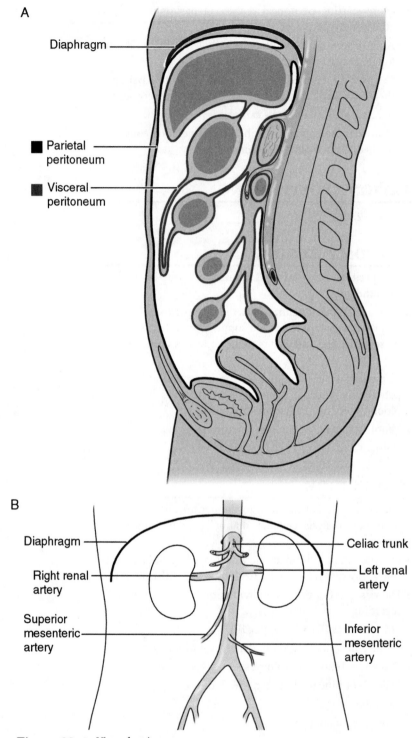

Figure 68–1. *Visceral peritoneum.*

the peritoneal cavity into the dialysate solution, which then is drained.

■ Adjustment of dextrose concentration, dialysate volume, number of cycles, and length of time the solution remains in the peritoneal cavity affect the removal of solute and water.

INTERPRETATION AND MONITORING

- For acute kidney failure, the following should be monitored carefully:
  - Fluids and electrolytes.
  - Strict intake and output.
  - Daily weight.
  - Blood pressure and vital signs.
- For long-term peritoneal dialysis, the following may be monitored at home:
  - Total fluid drainage.
  - Daily weight.

COMPLICATIONS

- Peritonitis.
- Bleeding.
- Perforation of bladder or other viscera by dialysis catheter.
- Pain.
- Dialysate leakage.
- Catheter obstruction.
- Electrolyte imbalance.
- Respiratory compromise due to increased intraperitoneal pressure or hydrothorax.
- Hypotension.
- Hypoalbuminemia from loss of protein into dialysate.
- Hyperglycemia, especially with higher dextrose concentrations.
- Inguinal or umbilical hernia.

FOLLOW-UP

- For acute kidney failure, as indicated following discontinuation of dialysis.
- For end-stage renal disease, regular follow-up (about once a month) by an experienced nephrologist and peritoneal dialysis nurse is required to manage dialysis prescription, complications, and other aspects of end-stage kidney disease.

HEMODIALYSIS

INDICATIONS

- End-stage renal disease.
- Acute kidney failure accompanied by 1 or more of the following:
  - Oliguria or anuria.
  - Hypervolemia.
  - Uremia (azotemia accompanied by platelet dysfunction and bleeding, change in mental status, or other uremic symptoms).
  - Electrolyte or metabolic disturbance unresponsive to medical management (eg, hyperkalemia, hyponatremia or hypernatremia, acidosis, hypocalcemia, hyperphosphatemia, tumor lysis syndrome).
  - Inability to provide adequate nutrition or other intravenous therapy due to fluid restriction.
- Electrolyte or metabolic disturbance unresponsive to medical management in the absence of kidney failure, as in inborn errors of metabolism (urea cycle disorders, propionic acidemia, maple syrup urine disease) or tumor lysis syndrome.
- Dialyzable toxin.

CONTRAINDICATIONS

Absolute

- Lack of vascular access.

Relative

- Hemodynamic instability.

EQUIPMENT

- Hemodialysis machine.
- Hemodialyzer cartridge and tubing.
- Dialysate solution.
- Blood prime for small children and infants to prevent hypotension during initiation of extracorporeal circuit.
- Heparin.
- Water treatment system (to remove pathogens, sediment, and hazardous substances from water).
- Vascular access via arteriovenous fistula (AVF), arteriovenous graft (AVG), or hemodialysis catheter.

PEARLS AND TIPS

- Hemodialysis might be the only option for those children who have had extensive abdominal surgery, who have a social situation that precludes home dialysis, or in whom peritoneal dialysis has already failed due to repeated bouts of peritonitis or other complications.
- Hemodialysis and CRRT remain the treatments of choice for inborn errors of metabolism and toxic ingestions.
- Hemodialysis usually is performed 3 times per week, for 3–4 hours per session.

PATIENT PREPARATION

- Counsel patients with end-stage disease extensively about long-term dialysis options (hemodialysis vs. peritoneal dialysis) and advantages, disadvantages, and risks of each option.
- Before starting hemodialysis, some form of vascular access is required.

■ For the patient with impending or current end-stage renal failure, surgical placement of an AVF is preferred due to its superior survival and decreased risk of thrombosis and infection compared with other access.

■ In the patient whose veins or anatomy prevents construction of an AVF, the placement of an intervening prosthetic graft (AVG) can be performed.

■ An AVF usually requires at least 4–6 weeks to heal before usage; an AVG can be used sooner but preferably requires a similar healing period.

■ Therefore, patients requiring urgent dialysis require a central venous, double-lumen hemodialysis catheter.

■ A dialysis catheter also might be necessary in small children or in those lacking adequate vessels for construction of an AVF or AVG.

■ In general, the preferred site for a venous hemodialysis catheter is the internal jugular vein, although sometimes the femoral vein and, least preferred, the subclavian vein is used for acute situations.

■ Long-term hemodialysis catheters are generally cuffed and inserted via a subcutaneous tunnel to provide more secure anchoring.

PATIENT POSITIONING

■ Generally supine or on side.

ANATOMY REVIEW

■ AVFs are constructed by joining an artery to a vein.

■ As the AVF heals and matures, the vein dilates, allowing eventual cannulation by large bore needles and accommodating the large blood flow rates needed for hemodialysis.

■ Common sites for AVF construction include the wrist (radiocephalic or Brescia-Cimino fistula) and the brachial artery to cephalic vein.

■ In addition to the above sites, the AVG can also be constructed in the thigh.

■ The internal jugular vein is preferred for long-term hemodialysis catheters, with placement of the catheter tip in the right atrium.

■ For urgent dialysis, the femoral vein also can be used.

■ The subclavian vein is least commonly used due to risk of venous stenosis.

PROCEDURE

■ Dialysis prescription is individualized for each patient regarding:
  • Modification of dialysate.
  • Type of hemodialyzer membrane and size of circuit tubing.
  • Need for blood prime.
  • Blood flow rate.
  • Duration of each dialysis session.
  • Number of dialysis sessions per week.
  • Dose of heparin.
  • Amount of fluid removed.

■ Hemodialysis is an extracorporeal therapy, in which blood is removed from the patient, circulated through a cartridge (hemodialyzer) containing a semipermeable membrane, and then returned to the patient.

■ A dialysate solution is circulated through the cartridge on the opposite side of the membrane from the patient's blood.

■ The dialysate solution contains a fixed amount of electrolytes and buffer (sodium chloride, bicarbonate, magnesium, calcium, and dextrose or glucose), which can be adjusted for special circumstances.

■ Fluid is removed from the patient by the application of hydrostatic pressure across the dialysis membrane, resulting in the transit of water from the blood across the membrane to the dialysate compartment.

■ Solute is removed from the blood by diffusion of substances such as urea and potassium down their concentration gradients across the membrane from the blood to the dialysate solution.

■ Fluid removal (ultrafiltration) is highly accurately controlled by adjusting the amount of transmembrane hydrostatic pressure.

■ The efficiency of solute removal is determined primarily by the blood and dialysate flow rates, the duration of the dialysis treatment, the frequency of dialysis treatments, and the characteristics of the dialysis membrane (eg, surface area, porosity).

■ The patient is weighed before and after to confirm the amount of fluid removed.

■ Heparin is used to prevent clotting of the circuit during hemodialysis.
  • Hemodialysis can be performed with low-dose ("tight") heparin or no heparin, with an increased risk of circuit clotting, in surgical patients or patients with acute bleeding.
  • Methods of anticoagulation other than heparin have been described but are not commonly used.

INTERPRETATION AND MONITORING

■ For acute kidney failure, the following should be monitored carefully:
  • Fluids and electrolytes.
  • Strict intake and output.
  • Daily weight.
  • Blood pressure and vital signs.

■ Circuit pressures are monitored throughout the circuit for signs of clotting or access thrombosis or obstruction.

■ Air detection monitors and air traps are placed throughout the circuit to detect and prevent air embolism.

COMPLICATIONS

■ Disequilibrium syndrome (too rapid removal of urea, resulting in cerebral edema, change in mental status, seizures).
■ Anaphylaxis (primarily due to reaction to dialysis membrane or preservatives used to process membrane).
■ Catheter complications.
  • Obstruction.
  • Infection.
  • Pneumothorax.
  • Hemothorax.
  • Arterial or venous perforation.
  • Air embolism.
  • Cardiac perforation.
  • Cardiac tamponade.
  • Hemopericardium.
■ Nausea, vomiting, abdominal pain, muscle cramps (usually due to fluid removal).
■ Heparin.
  • Bleeding.
  • Thrombocytopenia.
■ Hypovolemia.
■ Hypotension.
■ Electrolyte imbalance.
■ Air embolism.
■ Infection of dialysis catheter.
■ Temperature instability.
■ Blood-borne pathogens if blood prime used (HIV, hepatitis).

FOLLOW-UP

■ For acute kidney failure, as indicated following discontinuation of dialysis.
■ For end-stage kidney disease, regular follow-up by an experienced nephrologist and hemodialysis nurse is required to manage dialysis prescription, complications, and other aspects of end-stage renal disease.
■ The patient usually returns to the hemodialysis unit 3 times per week for dialysis.

CONTINUOUS RENAL REPLACEMENT THERAPY

INDICATIONS

■ Acute kidney failure in the critically ill patient in the intensive care unit, accompanied by 1 or more of the following:

• Oliguria or anuria.
• Hypervolemia.
• Uremia (azotemia accompanied by platelet dysfunction and bleeding, change in mental status, or other uremic symptoms).
• Electrolyte or metabolic disturbance unresponsive to medical management (eg, hyperkalemia, hyponatremia or hypernatremia, acidosis, hypocalcemia, hyperphosphatemia, tumor lysis syndrome).
• Inability to provide adequate nutrition or other intravenous therapy due to fluid restriction.
■ Electrolyte or metabolic disturbance unresponsive to medical management in the absence of kidney failure, as in inborn errors of metabolism (urea cycle disorders, propionic acidemia, maple syrup urine disease) or tumor lysis syndrome.
■ Dialyzable toxin.

CONTRAINDICATIONS

Absolute

■ Lack of vascular access.

Relative

■ Severe hemodynamic instability unresponsive to pressor support.
■ Active bleeding (heparin anticoagulation only).
■ Uncorrected hypocalcemia (citrate anticoagulation only).

EQUIPMENT

■ CRRT machine.
■ Hemofilter cartridge and circuit tubing.
■ Blood warmer.
■ Vascular access via central venous catheter.
■ Solutions as indicated by modality (replacement solution, dialysate solution).
■ Anticoagulation.
  • Heparin.
  • Sodium citrate (ACD-A).
  • Calcium chloride infusion via separate central line during citrate anticoagulation.
  • Bedside activated clotting time monitor for heparin anticoagulation.
■ Packed red cells to prime the circuit in small children to prevent hypotension during initiation of extracorporeal circuit.
■ Hemodialysis dialysis catheter.

PEARLS AND TIPS

■ CRRT is the preferred method of RRT for unstable patients in the intensive care setting.

- CRRT also is useful for inborn errors of metabolism and toxic ingestions.
- The continuous nature of the procedure might prevent the rebound of toxins or metabolites that can otherwise occur with intermittent hemodialysis.
- Experimental uses of CRRT include sepsis, multiorgan dysfunction, and liver failure.

PATIENT PREPARATION

- Placement of dialysis access (AVF, AVG, or catheter).

PATIENT POSITIONING

- Generally supine or on side.

ANATOMY REVIEW

- A double-lumen, central venous hemodialysis catheter is placed in the internal jugular, femoral, or subclavian vein.
- The subclavian vein is least commonly used due to risk of venous stenosis.
- In small children and infants, if a double-lumen venous catheter is too large to be placed, 2 separate single lumen venous catheters may be used.

PROCEDURE

- In infants and small children, the circuit first is filled ("primed") with blood to prevent hypotension.
- CRRT prescription is individualized for each patient regarding:
  - Modality (SCUF, CVVH, CVVHD, or CVVHDF).
  - Modification of dialysate or replacement solutions.
  - Type of hemofilter membrane and size of circuit tubing.
  - Need for blood prime.
  - Blood, dialysate, and replacement flow rates.
  - Type and flow rates of anticoagulation (heparin or citrate).
  - Amount of fluid removed (ultrafiltration rate).
- CRRT is an extracorporeal therapy, in which blood is removed from the patient, circulated through a cartridge (hemofilter) containing a semipermeable membrane, and then returned to the patient.
- Clearance of solute is achieved by **convective** or **diffusive** means.
- **Convective clearance** is performed by the addition of an isotonic replacement solution to the blood side of the membrane.
- The replacement solution allows large volumes of fluid to be removed without causing hypovolemia.

- Various modalities of CRRT combine different combinations of diffusive and convective clearance.
- Slow continuous ultrafiltration (SCUF) uses no dialysate or replacement solution and relies on hydrostatic pressure alone to achieve slow, gentle fluid removal with little solute clearance.
- CVVH uses only replacement solution and no dialysate, achieving clearance by convective means alone.
- Continuous venovenous hemodialysis (CVVHD) uses only dialysate and no replacement solution, achieving clearance by diffusive means alone.
- Finally, continuous venovenous hemodiafiltration (CVVHDF) uses both dialysis and replacement solutions to achieve both diffusive and convective clearance.
- Although each method has its own theoretical advantages, the clearances achieved by CVVH, CVVHD, and CVVHDF are roughly equivalent and, in practice, the choice of modality usually depends on the personal preference of the prescriber.

- The movement of water across a semipermeable membrane under hydrostatic pressure, with resultant "drag" of solute by water across the membrane, results in convective clearance of solute.
- **Diffusive clearance** is performed by circulating dialysis solution on the side of the membrane opposite to the blood and in countercurrent direction to the flow of blood.
- Similar to hemodialysis, solute diffuses down its concentration gradient into the dialysis solution.
- As in hemodialysis, anticoagulation must be used to prevent clotting of the circuit during CRRT.
- Heparin was the primary means of anticoagulation until recently.
- Given the continuous nature of CRRT, the use of constant heparin infusion results in systemic patient anticoagulation and a significantly increased risk of bleeding.
- The use of regional anticoagulation through citrate infusion into the circuit is achieving widespread use.
- Citrate is infused directly into the CRRT circuit.
- The citrate binds calcium and prevents clotting.
- The calcium level of the circuit is monitored and the citrate infusion is adjusted to keep the filter calcium level within a target range to prevent clotting.
- A calcium infusion is administered to the patient, and calcium levels are monitored to prevent systemic hypocalcemia.
- Citrate anticoagulation does not result in systemic anticoagulation and reduces the risk of bleeding.
- Citrate, however, can cause hypernatremia, alkalosis, and hypocalcemia and requires careful monitoring and practitioners experienced with this technique.

INTERPRETATION AND MONITORING

- Monitor the following carefully:
  - Fluids and electrolytes.
  - Strict intake and output.
  - Daily weight.
  - Blood pressure and vital signs.
- Activated clotting time is monitored for adjustment of heparin anticoagulation.
- Filter and patient ionized calcium is monitored for adjustment of citrate and calcium infusion rates during citrate anticoagulation.
- Rate of fluid removal is monitored and adjusted according to patient's volume status as determined by physical examination, weight, vital signs, central venous pressure, and electrolytes.
- Circuit pressures are monitored throughout the circuit for signs of clotting or access thrombosis or obstruction.

- Air detection monitors and air traps are placed throughout the circuit to detect and prevent air embolism.

COMPLICATIONS

- Heparin.
  - Bleeding.
  - Thrombocytopenia.
- Citrate.
  - Hypocalcemia.
  - Hypernatremia.
  - Alkalosis.
  - Citrate toxicity.
- Disequilibrium syndrome (too rapid removal of urea, resulting in cerebral edema, change in mental status, seizures).
- Anaphylaxis (primarily due to reaction to hemofilter membrane or preservatives used to process membrane).
- Hypovolemia.
- Hypotension.
- Electrolyte imbalance.
- Air embolism.
- Catheter complications.
  - Obstruction.
  - Infection.
  - Pneumothorax.
  - Hemothorax.
  - Arterial or venous perforation.
  - Air embolism.
  - Cardiac perforation.
  - Cardiac tamponade.
  - Hemopericardium.
- Temperature instability.
- Blood-borne pathogens if blood prime used (HIV, hepatitis).

FOLLOW-UP

- For acute kidney failure, as indicated following discontinuation of CRRT.
- If kidney function does not recover once patient stabilizes (ie, end-stage renal disease), extensive counseling needs to be provided regarding long-term dialysis options (hemodialysis vs. peritoneal dialysis) and advantages, disadvantages, and risks of each option.
- For end-stage renal failure, regular follow-up by an experienced nephrologist and dialysis nurse is required to manage dialysis prescription, complications, and other aspects of end-stage renal disease.

REFERENCES

Benfield MR, Bunchman TE. Management of acute renal failure. In: Avner ED, Harmon WE, Niaudet P, editors. *Pediatric Nephrology.* 5th ed. Baltimore: Lippincott Williams and Wilkins; 2004:1253–1266.

Blowey DL, Alon US. Dialysis principles for primary healthcare providers. *Clin Pediatr.* 2005;44:19–27.

Goldstein SL, Jabs K. Hemodialysis. In: Avner ED, Harmon WE, Niaudet P, editors. *Pediatric Nephrology.* 5th ed. Baltimore: Lippincott Williams and Wilkins; 2004:1395–1410.

Warady BA, Morgenstern BZ, Alexander SR. Peritoneal dialysis. In: Avner ED, Harmon WE, Niaudet P, editors. *Pediatric Nephrology.* 5th ed. Baltimore: Lippincott Williams and Wilkins; 2004:1375–1394.

Warady BA, Schaefer FS, Fine RN, Alexander SR, editors. *Pediatric Dialysis.* Boston: Kluwer Academic Publishers; 2004.

CHAPTER 69

Bone Marrow Aspiration and Biopsy

Robert I. Liem, MD

INDICATIONS

- Pancytopenia.
- Unexplained anemia, leukopenia, or thrombocytopenia (aspiration only).
- Acute or chronic leukemia (aspiration only).
- Myelodysplasia.
- Myeloproliferative disease.
- Non-Hodgkin or Hodgkin lymphoma.
- Childhood solid tumors (including sarcoma, Wilms tumor, neuroblastoma, germ cell tumor).
- Bone marrow failure (including acquired aplastic anemia, Fanconi anemia, Diamond-Blackfan syndrome).
- Fever of unknown origin.
- Storage disease.
- Monitoring during chemotherapy or following stem cell transplantation (aspiration only).

CONTRAINDICATIONS

Relative

- Congenital factor deficiency or acquired coagulation defect.
- Anticoagulation with warfarin or heparin.
- Severe thrombocytopenia.
- Infection or prior radiation at sample site.

EQUIPMENT

Site Preparation

- 10% povidone-iodine.
- Alcohol preparation pads or swabs.
- Sterile gloves, gown, and drape.
- Spinal and subcutaneous needles, 20 to 26 gauge.
- 1% lidocaine hydrochloride, injection.
- 8.4% sodium bicarbonate, injection, USP.

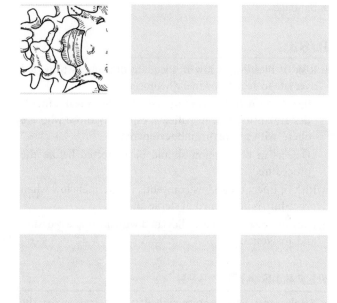

- Bone marrow examination provides critical information in the diagnosis of various hematologic and oncologic conditions in children.
- Bone marrow aspiration also permits immunophenotyping, cytogenetic analysis, and other molecular studies.

Marrow Aspiration and Biopsy

- Sodium heparin, injection, 1000 USP units/mL, preservative free.
- Bone marrow aspiration needles (15 and 18 gauge, adjustable lengths).
- Bone marrow biopsy needles (11 and 13 gauge, 4 or 2 inches in length).
- Sterile syringes, 10 to 20 mL.
- Container with fixative for trephine biopsy specimen.
- Vacutainers; one for sodium heparin and one for ethylenediaminetetraacetic acid (EDTA).
- Gauze sponges.
- Bandages.

RISKS

- Risk of bleeding is low if adequate pressure is provided over site to achieve primary hemostasis.
  - Platelet transfusion is indicated when technical difficulties are anticipated in patients, especially those who are obese, with severe thrombocytopenia.
  - Defects in coagulation should be corrected before the procedure.
- Risk of infection and osteomyelitis is extremely low when procedure is performed in sterile fashion.
- Pain and discomfort are alleviated with adequate sedation and analgesics.

PEARLS AND TIPS

- Adolescents may require only local anesthesia for the procedure.
- Conscious sedation or general anesthesia is generally necessary in young children, particularly if repeated procedures are required.
- Adding local anesthesia in young patients also decreases postprocedural discomfort at the site.
- Lidocaine used for local anesthesia should be buffered with sodium bicarbonate (sodium bicarbonate mixed with lidocaine in a 1:4 ratio) to reduce burning during injection.
- Obtaining spicules (bone marrow particles rich in hematopoietic elements) on the first pull of the aspiration may be easier using a larger syringe (30 or 60 mL).
- Aspirating more than 0.25 mL of marrow initially dilutes the sample with sinusoidal blood and interferes with morphologic studies.
- If an aspirate is "dry" and an adequate specimen cannot be obtained, a touch imprint of the biopsy core may be helpful for cytologic examination.
- A dry tap usually indicates myelofibrosis or a marrow cavity packed with malignant cells.

■ All equipment, tubes, and syringes should be ready and available before preparing the patient.

- Lidocaine should be drawn.
- Syringes that will be used to collect any additional marrow after the first pull should be heparinized to prevent clotting.
- A laboratory assistant should be ready to help in the immediate preparation of bone marrow smears and handling of the core biopsy.

PATIENT PREPARATION

■ Obtain a thorough medical history and perform physical examination.

- Examine peripheral blood smear.
- Obtain laboratory tests and radiographs as needed.

■ Primary care providers may prepare patients and families by emphasizing the diagnostic usefulness of the procedure and reviewing such risks as pain, bleeding, and infection.

■ Assure patients and families that pain may be minimal with use of analgesics and sedation.

■ Obtain written informed consent.

■ Minimize anxiety in adolescents and young adults who receive only local anesthesia; be honest about the pain and discomfort associated with aspiration and biopsy.

■ Inform patients who are not receiving general anesthesia that an unpleasant, lightening-like sensation down their lower extremities may be felt at the time of suction during aspiration.

PATIENT POSITIONING

■ The posterior superior iliac crest is the optimal location for bone marrow aspiration and biopsy in most children (Figure 69–1).

■ Alternative sites include the anterior iliac crest in obese patients and the tibia in infants younger than 3 months.

■ The sternum, which is used in some adults, should be avoided in children.

■ If the posterior iliac crest is used, the patient is placed in the right or left decubitus position, with the hips flexed and the knees drawn up.

■ If the anterior iliac crest is used, the patient is placed in the supine position with the hips and knees flexed.

■ Occasionally, thin patients who do not receive general anesthesia may be placed in the prone position.

ANATOMY REVIEW

■ The posterior superior iliac crest can usually be identified by a dimple in the skin located at the lateral edge of Michaelis' rhomboid.

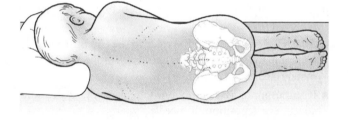

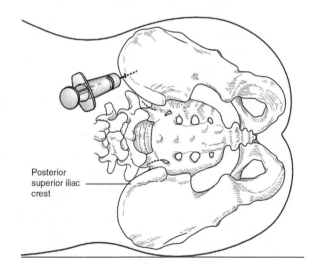

Posterior superior iliac crest

Figure 69–1. *Posterior superior iliac crest is optimal location.*

- Michaelis' rhomboid is a diamond-shaped area over the posterior aspect of the pelvis formed by the posterior superior iliac spines, the gluteal muscles, and the groove at the distal end of the vertebral column.
- This area can be located in most patients by palpation with the thumb, even if anatomic landmarks are not visible.

PROCEDURE

Bone Marrow Aspiration

- Clean the site with povidone-iodine followed by alcohol swab.
- Place sterile drape.
- Inject buffered lidocaine intradermally with a subcutaneous needle to produce a small wheal.
- Use a larger bore needle to push through the skin and subcutaneous tissue and inject 2–3 mL (maximum 3 mg/kg/dose) more lidocaine along the periosteum.
- Hold the bone aspirate needle horizontally using the index finger near the tip of the needle for control.
- Advance the needle through the skin, subcutaneous tissue, and the surface of the cortical bone with steady pressure and a twisting motion.
- An abrupt decrease in resistance occurs when the needle penetrates the cortex and enters the spongy marrow cavity.
- Advance the needle 1 cm more before the stylet is removed.
- Attach a 10-mL or 20-mL syringe to the end of the needle and pull the plunger back quickly to aspirate approximately 0.25 mL of bone marrow.
- If an aspirate is not obtained, replace the stylet and advance or reposition the needle.
- This first pull contains the marrow particles or spicules that should be used for preparing initial smears.
- A heparinized, larger syringe (30 mL) may be used to obtain additional marrow for cytogenetic analysis, flow cytometry, and other studies.

Bone Marrow Biopsy

- The trephine biopsy is the preferred method to evaluate cellularity and detect bone marrow metastasis in lymphoma and many childhood solid tumors.
- Biopsy specimen is obtained through the same incision site.
- Hold the biopsy needle in the same manner as the aspiration needle but angle it to sample a different area from the aspiration.
- Advance the needle with steady pressure to the periosteum and twist into the surface of the cortical bone.
- Remove the obturator and push the needle through the cortex using a rotating, twisting motion until decreased resistance is met.

- Advance the needle another 1–2 cm.
- Reinsert the obturator until resistance is met to gauge the length of the specimen.
- Rotate the needle 360 degrees vigorously several times while moving it back and forth vertically and horizontally to break the biopsy core off the surrounding bone.
- Carefully remove the needle and insert a separate blunt obturator into the distal end of the needle to force the core out through the hub onto a glass slide.
- Touch preparations of the core biopsy should be performed.
- Specimen should be at least 1.5 to 2 cm in length for optimal processing.
- If the specimen is inadequate or consists mostly of cartilage or cortical bone rather than core marrow, which appears dark red with a fine, white trabecular network, attempt additional biopsies.
- The specimen should be placed in an appropriate fixative.
- Apply direct pressure to the site for at least 5 minutes once the procedure is completed and the needle removed.
- Place a pressure dressing.

INTERPRETATION AND MONITORING

- Prepare the initial aspirate at the bedside immediately.
- Various techniques for spreading the film have been described, including the traditional wedge technique, particle crush method, and cover slip preparation.
- Slides are then dried, fixed in methanol and stained by the Wright-Giemsa technique.
- Systematic analysis of the aspirate slides includes assessment of the adequacy of spicules, cellularity, megakaryocyte count as well as maturation and morphologic features of other cell lineages.
- The biopsy specimen, once fixed, is decalcified.
- Further processing includes hematoxylin and eosin (H&E), reticulin, and immunohistochemical staining when necessary.
- Comprehensive analysis of the biopsy specimen should include evaluation of the specimen's adequacy, cellularity, and bone structure and detection of focal lesions or metastatic disease.

COMPLICATIONS

- Bleeding at any site, with or without development of a hematoma, is rare if adequate pressure is applied.
- Bleeding risk has been reported to be increased in adults with osteoporosis or extensive bony involvement by disease, such as multiple myeloma.
- Retroperitoneal hemorrhage, osteomyelitis, and needle breakage have also been rarely described.
- Infection (rare).

FOLLOW-UP

- Multiple evaluations are often required to monitor efficacy and recovery following chemotherapy or stem cell transplantation.

- Patients should lie on their backs for an additional 15–20 minutes for procedures performed on the posterior iliac crest.

- Patients should be reminded that a dull ache may be felt for several days following the procedure.

- Routine post-procedural monitoring should be performed when heavy sedation or general anesthesia is administered.

REFERENCES

Aboul-Nasr R, Estey EH, Kantarjian HM et al. Comparison of touch imprints with aspirate smears for evaluating bone marrow specimens. *Am J Clin Pathol.* 1999;111:753–758.

Bain BJ. Bone marrow aspiration. *J Clin Pathol.* 2001;54:657–663.

Bain BJ. Bone marrow biopsy morbidity and mortality. *Br J Haematol.* 2003;121:949–951.

Bain BJ. Bone marrow trephine biopsy. *J Clin Pathol.* 2001;54:737–742.

Barone MA, Rowe PC. Pediatric procedures. In: McMillan JA, DeAngelis CD, Feigin RD, Warshaw JB, editors. *Oski's Pediatrics: Pediatrics and Practice.* Philadelphia: Lippincott Williams & Wilkins; 1999:2273.

Penchansky L. Bone marrow biopsy in the metastatic work-up of solid tumors in children. *Cancer.* 1984;54:1447–1448.

Riley RS, Hogan TF, Pavot DR et al. A pathologist's perspective on bone marrow aspiration and biopsy: I. Performing a bone marrow examination. *J Clin Lab Anal.* 2004;18:70–90.

[CHAPTER 70]

Exchange Transfusion of the Newborn

Robin H. Steinhorn, MD

INDICATIONS

- Prevent neurotoxicity induced by hyperbilirubinemia.
- Jaundice and intermediate to advanced stages of acute bilirubin encephalopathy are present even if the serum bilirubin level does not exactly fit the guidelines.
  - Early phase: Severely jaundiced infants become lethargic, hypotonic, and feed poorly.
  - Intermediate phase: Moderate stupor; irritability; and hypertonia, manifested by backward arching of the neck (retrocollis) and trunk (opisthotonos); fever; and high-pitched cry that may alternate with drowsiness.
- Treat coagulopathy due to disseminated intravascular coagulation and life-threatening metabolic disorders.
- Correct polycythemia using a partial exchange transfusion, meaning that < 1 blood volume is removed and then replaced with normal saline.
- Treat severe anemia associated with heart failure with partial exchange transfusion, using packed red blood cells as the replacement solution.
- Recommended after intensive phototherapy fails.

RISKS

- Quantifying the risks of morbidity and mortality accurately is difficult because exchange transfusions are now rarely performed.
- Death has been reported in approximately 0.3% of all procedures; although in otherwise well term and near-term infants (> 35 weeks' gestation), the risk is probably much lower.
- Significant morbidity occurs in as many as 5% of cases.
  - Infection.
  - Complications of vascular catheters (vasospasm, thrombosis).
  - Apnea and bradycardia.
  - Necrotizing enterocolitis.

- The risks associated with the use of blood products must always be considered.
- Hypoxic-ischemic encephalopathy and AIDS have been reported in otherwise healthy infants receiving exchange transfusions.

PEARLS AND TIPS

- In general, phototherapy is initiated at lower TSB levels in an attempt to avoid exchange transfusion.
- Additional risk factors for neurotoxicity, such as prematurity, sepsis, and acidosis, should be carefully considered when deciding whether to proceed with an exchange transfusion.
- Intravenous gamma-globulin has been shown to reduce the need for exchange transfusions in Rh and ABO hemolytic disease.
- Therefore, in isoimmune hemolytic disease, administration of intravenous gamma-globulin (0.5–1 g/kg over 2 hours) is recommended.
  - If the TSB is rising despite intensive phototherapy.
  - If the TSB level is within 2–3 mg/dL of the exchange level.
- The fluid volume required to administer the dose of gamma-globulin is considerable and needs to be factored into its use for critically ill newborns.

PATIENT PREPARATION

- The possible need for exchange transfusion should be discussed with the family at the onset of severe hyperbilirubinemia, particularly if hemolysis is present.
- Generally, this discussion takes place while initiating intensive phototherapy, contacting the blood bank, and instituting other measures to avoid the need for exchange, such as administering gamma-globulin.
- The infant should be transferred to a neonatal intensive care unit capable of full monitoring and resuscitation, and a neonatologist should assist with counseling the family.
- Feedings are stopped prior to the procedure.
- Rh-negative mothers who are known to be antibody-positive are monitored closely during pregnancy, and counseling about the possible need for exchange transfusion can occur prior to birth.

PROCEDURE

- Place 1 or 2 large bore catheters, and an additional intravenous catheter is needed to maintain access for delivery of intravenous fluids and emergency medications.
- Perform procedure using single umbilical venous catheter ("push-pull") or isovolumetrically using both an umbilical venous and arterial catheter.

- While there are multiple causes of hyperbilirubinemia, severe disease is most commonly the result of isoimmune hemolytic disease of the newborn secondary to Rh, ABO, or other antigen incompatibility.
- Perhaps the most difficult aspect of this procedure is determining when the level of hyperbilirubinemia warrants its use.
  - A clinical practice guideline was recently published by the American Academy of Pediatrics Subcommittee on Hyperbilirubinemia.
  - Recommended total serum bilirubin (TSB) levels for exchange transfusion are provided in this document and are based largely on keeping TSB levels below those at which kernicterus has been reported.
- Exchange transfusion is performed infrequently due to improved prenatal prevention and management of hemolytic disease of the newborn.

- Exchange transfusions should be performed only by trained personnel in neonatal intensive care units with full monitoring and resuscitation capabilities.
- Blood used is usually modified whole blood (red cells and plasma) that is type O negative, cytomegalovirus negative, irradiated, cross-matched against the mother, and compatible with the infant.
- Enough blood for 2 of the infant's blood volumes (1 blood volume in a term infant is 80 mL/kg) as well as enough volume to prime the tubing and blood warmer is needed.
- As cross-matching to both the mother and infant may require additional time, blood should be ordered *before* the infant meets criteria for the procedure.

- The second method maintains more stable blood volumes and may be better tolerated in a critically ill newborn but requires additional personnel.

- After catheter placement, draw blood from the infant in small aliquots and replace using banked blood over a 1- to 2-hour period.

- Monitor glucose, ionized calcium, and platelet counts during and after the procedure.

- Most infants will require additional calcium during the procedure.

- The platelet count typically drops to ~50% of the preexchange value; some critically ill infants will require platelet transfusions after the procedure.

- The procedure removes variable amounts of medications, including antibiotics and anticonvulsants; redosing is often necessary.

- Approximately 85% of the infant's blood volume is replaced during a double-volume exchange transfusion.

- However, the serum bilirubin usually drops to about 50% of the preexchange value due to equilibration with extravascular bilirubin and/or ongoing hemolysis.

FOLLOW-UP

- Resume phototherapy immediately after the procedure, and a rebound of the bilirubin should be anticipated within 2–4 hours of completing the exchange transfusion.

REFERENCES

American Academy of Pediatrics. Subcommittee on Hyperbilirubinemia. Management of hyperbilirubinemia in the newborn infant 35 or more weeks of gestation. *Pediatrics.* 2004; 114:297–316.

Gottstein R, Cooke RW. Systematic review of intravenous immunoglobulin in haemolytic disease of the newborn. *Arch Dis Child Fetal Neonatal Ed.* 2003;88:F6–10.

Harris MC, Bernbaum JC, Polin JR, Zimmerman R, Polin RA. Developmental follow-up of breastfed term and near-term infants with marked hyperbilirubinemia. *Pediatrics.* 2001; 107:1075–1080.

Jackson JC. Adverse events associated with exchange transfusion in healthy and ill newborns. *Pediatrics.* 1997;99:E7.

Keenan WJ, Novak KK, Sutherland JM, Bryla DA, Fetterly KL. Morbidity and mortality associated with exchange transfusion. *Pediatrics.* 1985;75(2 Pt 2):417–421.

Ramesethu J. Exchange transfusions. In: MacDonald MG, Ramesethu J, editors. *Procedures in Neonatology.* 3rd ed. Philadelphia: Lippincott Williams & Wilkins; 2002:348–356.

[CHAPTER 71]

Extracorporeal Membrane Oxygenation

Robin H. Steinhorn, MD

INDICATIONS

- Meconium aspiration syndrome.
- Congenital diaphragmatic hernia.
- Idiopathic pulmonary hypertension.
- Severe, reversible respiratory failure.
- Cardiac disease.

CONTRAINDICATIONS

- Preterm infants (< 34 weeks).
- Small infants(< 2 kg) because of the increased risk of hemorrhage during heparinization.
- Significant intracranial hemorrhage.
- Lethal anomalies (eg, trisomy 18).

EQUIPMENT

- Extracorporeal membrane oxygenation (ECMO) bypass circuit (Figure 71–1), which includes the following:
  - Large vascular catheters.
  - Servo-regulated pump.
  - Silicone membrane artificial lung.
  - Heat exchanger.

PEARLS AND TIPS

- The UK Collaborative ECMO Trial Group demonstrated that ECMO decreased mortality (32% vs. 59%) and reduced severe disability at 1 year of age (33% vs. 62%).
- There are no universally accepted criteria for referral and initiation of ECMO; rather each center develops its own criteria based on experience.
- Infants are cannulated for ECMO when their mortality is predicted to be 80% or greater.
- Most centers factor in the severity of hypoxemia, the level of respiratory support, and severity of cardiac failure into the decision-making process.

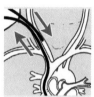

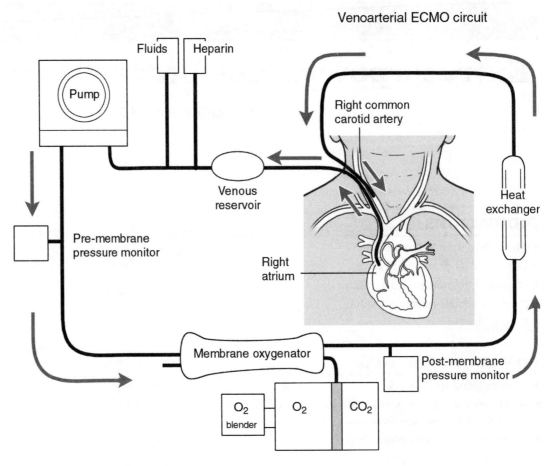

Figure 71–1. *ECMO bypass circuit.*

- An important consideration is reversibility of lung disease.
- Infants who have received prolonged mechanical ventilation and exposure to high oxygen concentrations (more than 10–14 days) may be excluded from consideration due to concerns about irreversible lung injury.
- Therefore, discussion with an ECMO center should occur relatively early in the disease process.

PATIENT PREPARATION

- ECMO is only provided at highly specialized centers, and most infants cannulated for ECMO must be transported from the hospital of birth to the ECMO center.
- Therefore, the additional time and difficulty associated with the transport should be taken into account when considering a referral for ECMO.
- Most often, the need for ECMO cannot be anticipated prior to birth, and families require a great deal of support to understand and cope with the unexpected severe illness of their infant.

- However, prenatal diagnosis of congenital diaphragmatic hernia is often possible.
  - Discussion of ECMO criteria and outcomes will ideally occur prior to birth.
  - Delivery plans can be made with the possible need for ECMO in mind.

PROCEDURE

- Support is most often provided using a venoarterial (VA) technique, meaning that catheters are inserted into the right atrium and right common carotid artery.
- VA ECMO bypasses both the heart and lungs, providing both pulmonary and cardiac support.
- Some infants can be supported with venovenous (VV) ECMO, in which blood is removed and returned to the right atrium through a double-lumen catheter.
- VV ECMO does not provide cardiac support but can effectively remove CO_2 and deliver additional oxygen.
- Because contact of blood with the ECMO circuit activates the clotting cascade, patients must receive systemic heparin.
- ECMO is continued until the lungs and heart recover.
- Care is provided by a specialized interdisciplinary team.
  - Surgeons.
  - Medical specialists.
  - Bedside intensive care nurse.
  - ECMO specialist trained specifically in ECMO circuit management.
- The usual duration of ECMO treatment is 5 days, although infants with congenital diaphragmatic hernias usually require support for longer periods.
- It is possible to maintain ECMO support for several weeks, although the risk of complications rises.

COMPLICATIONS

- Hemorrhage.
- Intracranial hemorrhage occurs in about 5% of patients.
  - Most devastating hemorrhagic complication.
  - Most common cause of death.

- Nonhemorrhagic infarction of the central nervous system.
- Renal failure.
- Infection.
- Mechanical failure of circuit components.

CAVEATS

- Infants with severe respiratory failure are at increased risk for neurodevelopmental abnormalities and should be referred to a comprehensive neurodevelopmental follow-up program after hospital discharge.
- Up to 15% of infants will display a major handicap, most commonly mental retardation.
- However, in infants without intracranial hemorrhage, need for ECMO does not appear to increase the risk of handicap.
- Delayed-onset sensorineural hearing loss occurs in up to 20% of ECMO-treated infants; therefore, these infants should be screened regularly for the first 3 years of life.
- Survival rates differ depending on underlying disease; they are lowest for congenital diaphragmatic hernia (53%).

REFERENCES

Bahrami KR, Van Meurs KP. ECMO for neonatal respiratory failure. *Semin Perinatol.* 2005;29:15–23.

Dalton HJ, Rycus PT, Conrad SA. Update on extracorporeal life support 2004. *Semin Perinatol.* 2005;29:24–33.

Extracorporeal Life Support Organization. Neonatal ECMO Registry: Extracorporeal Life Support Organization (ELSO); July 2004.

Farrow KN, Fliman P, Steinhorn RH. The diseases treated with ECMO: focus on PPHN. *Semin Perinatol.* 2005;29:8–14.

UK Collaborative ECMO Trial Group. UK collaborative randomised trial of neonatal extracorporeal membrane oxygenation. *Lancet.* 1996;348:75–82.

Appropriate Equipment for a General Pediatrics Office

Sharon M. Unti, MD

AIRWAY MANAGEMENT

- Masks for bag ventilation (in premature, infant, pediatric, adult sizes)
- Oxygen source with flow meter
- Self-inflating bag with reservoir (500 mL and 1000 mL)
- Oxygen masks (simple, Venturi type, and nonrebreather in premature, infant, child, adult sizes)
- Suction, wall, or portable/Yankauer suction catheters (8F, 10F, 14F)
- Cardiac arrest board
- Emergency drug dosing card or Broselow Pediatric Emergency Tape
- Adhesive tape to secure airway
- Nasal airways (infant to adult sizes)
- Nasogastric tubes (8F, 10F, 14F)
- Oral airways (infant to adult sizes)

FLUID AND MEDICATION ADMINISTRATION

- Butterfly needles (23 gauge)
- IV catheters: Short over-the-needle (18 gauge, 20 gauge, 22 gauge, 24 gauge) several of each size
- IV boards, tape, alcohol swabs, tourniquet
- D5 ½ normal saline
- Isotonic fluids (normal saline or lactated Ringer's solution)
- Syringes
- Sphygmomanometer (manual plus, if desired, mechanical) and blood pressure cuffs (in premature, infant, child, adult sizes)
- Pediatric drip chambers and tubing

MEDICATION LIST

- Albuterol, 0.5% nebulization solution, 20 mL
- Ceftriaxone, 5 g

- Dextrose 25% or 50%, 200 mL
- Epinephrine, 1:1000, 10 amp of 1 mg/mL (also effective when nebulized for croup in place of racemic epinephrine)
- Lidocaine, 1%, 50-mL vial
- Lorazepam or diazepam
- Naloxone, 1 mg/mL, 2-mL vial
- Activated charcoal, 125 g
- Atropine (0.1 mg/mL), 1-mL vials (at least 5 vials)
- Corticosteroids (methylprednisolone or dexamethasone)
- Epinephrine, 1:10,000, 10 mL
- Phenytoin, fosphenytoin, or phenobarbital
- Sodium bicarbonate, 4.2%, 5 50-mL vials or premeasured syringes

MISCELLANEOUS

- Portable monitor/defibrillator with pediatric paddles and skin electrode contacts (peel and stick)
- Splints
- Pulse oximeter with reusable (older children) and non-reusable (small children) sensors
- Device to check serum glucose
- Strips to check urine for glucose, blood, and so on
- Ophthalmoscope
- Otoscope
- Infant scale
- Standing scale
- View box

Index

Note: Page numbers followed by *f* indicate figures, and those followed by *t* indicate tables.